MINDFULNESS AND YOGA
IN SCHOOLS

Catherine P. Cook-Cottone, PhD, is a certified school psychologist, licensed psychologist, registered yoga teacher (200 RYT-E and 500 RYT), and associate professor at SUNY at Buffalo. She is an associate editor of the journal *Eating Disorders: Journal of Treatment and Prevention*. She is also the founder and president of Yogis in Service, Inc., a not-for-profit organization that creates access to yoga. The mother of two teenage girls, Dr. Cook-Cottone is married to Jerry Cottone, PhD, a fellow psychologist and yogi. *Mindfulness and Yoga in Schools* brings together Dr. Cook-Cottone's experience working with children and youth in schools and neighborhood settings. Dr. Cook-Cottone graduated from the Utica College of Syracuse University in 1989, receiving a BS degree in preprofessional psychology. She attended the State University of New York at Oswego for her MS degree in school psychology. In 1997, she received her PhD degree from the University at Buffalo, SUNY, in counseling psychology with a specialization in school psychology. She became a licensed psychologist in New York State the following year. Before entering academia, Dr. Cook-Cottone worked as a group worker and residential counselor for children in need, including adolescents classified as Persons in Need of Supervision and Juvenile Delinquents. She also worked in a neighborhood center for underserved, urban youth. As a school psychologist, she worked in both rural and urban settings, eventually transitioning to academia.

Dr. Cook-Cottone is an associate professor at the University at Buffalo, SUNY, in the Department of Counseling, School, and Educational Psychology within the Graduate School of Education. Her research specializes in embodied self-regulation (i.e., yoga, mindfulness, and self-care) and psychosocial disorders. She has written four books and over 50 peer-reviewed articles and book chapters. Her most recent book is titled *Mindfulness and Yoga for Self-Regulation: A Primer for Mental Health Professionals*. Presenting nationally and internationally, Dr. Cook-Cottone uses her model of embodied self-regulation to structure discussions on empirical work and practical applications. She teaches courses on mindful therapy, yoga for health and healing, self-care and service, and counseling with children and adolescents. She also maintains a private practice specializing in the treatment of anxiety-based disorders, eating disorders (including other disorders of self-care), and development of emotion regulation skills.

Dr. Cook-Cottone has a passion for yoga and for serving others. She has been a yoga researcher since 2002 when she began implementing her eating disorder prevention program, *Girls Growing in Wellness and Balance: Yoga and Life Skills to Empower*. She became a certified and registered yoga instructor in 2010. In 2013, she began the work that evolved into Yogis in Service, Inc. This work began as informal yoga classes for an urban summer camp and evolved into what is now an official not-for-profit with a community yoga studio on the east side of Buffalo. Specifically, Yogis in Service, Inc. offers yoga to those who would not otherwise have access in settings such as after-school programs, hospitals, rehabilitation centers, and universities. Dr. Cook-Cottone is honored to work with a collective of compassionate yoga teachers and students that are as excited as she is to share their love of yoga and yoga's effective tools for self-regulation.

MINDFULNESS AND YOGA IN SCHOOLS
A Guide for Teachers and Practitioners

Catherine P. Cook-Cottone, PhD

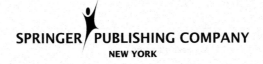

SPRINGER PUBLISHING COMPANY
NEW YORK

Copyright © 2017 Springer Publishing Company, LLC

Springer Publishing Company, LLC
11 West 42nd Street
New York, NY 10036
www.springerpub.com

Acquisitions Editor: Debra Riegert
Compositor: diacriTech

ISBN: 978-0-8261-3172-0
e-book ISBN: 978-0-8261-3173-7

17 18 19 20 / 5 4 3 2 1

The author and the publisher of this Work have made every effort to use sources believed to be reliable to provide information that is accurate and compatible with the standards generally accepted at the time of publication. The author and publisher shall not be liable for any special, consequential, or exemplary damages resulting, in whole or in part, from the readers' use of, or reliance on, the information contained in this book. The publisher has no responsibility for the persistence or accuracy of URLs for external or third-party Internet websites referred to in this publication and does not guarantee that any content on such websites is, or will remain, accurate or appropriate.

Library of Congress Cataloging-in-Publication Data
Names: Cook-Cottone, Catherine P., author.
Title: Mindfulness and yoga in schools: a guide for teachers and
   practitioners / Catherine Cook-Cottone, PhD.
Description: New York, NY: Springer Publishing Company, LLC, [2017] |
   Includes bibliographical references and index.
Identifiers: LCCN 2016054626 | ISBN 9780826131720
Subjects: LCSH: Hatha yoga for children—United States. | Classroom
   management—Psychological aspects—United States. | Self-control in children.
Classification: LCC RJ133.7 .C66 2017 | DDC 613.7/046083—dc23 LC record available at
https://lccn.loc.gov/2016054626

Special discounts on bulk quantities of our books are available to corporations, professional associations, pharmaceutical companies, health care organizations, and other qualifying groups. If you are interested in a custom book, including chapters from more than one of our titles, we can provide that service as well.

For details, please contact:
Special Sales Department, Springer Publishing Company, LLC
11 West 42nd Street, 15th Floor, New York, NY 10036-8002
Phone: 877-687-7476 or 212-431-4370; Fax: 212-941-7842
E-mail: sales@springerpub.com

Printed in the United States of America by Gasch Printing.

This book was written in honor of my mother, Elizabeth Glenn Cook,
who taught me what it means to truly love reading
and for whom it has been said,
"Mrs. Cook's English classroom was always Zen."

It is dedicated to the loves of my life:
Jerry Cottone, Chloe Jordan Cottone, and Maya Elizabeth Cottone.

CONTENTS

FOREWORD

Welcome to this important and comprehensive exploration of mindfulness and yoga for schools. It's a pleasure for us to say a few words about the exceptional work of Catherine Cook-Cottone on this book, and we are glad that you've found it. You'll find within a combination of thoughtful and well-developed analyses of the field, and practical, timely, and immediately useful information for teaching yoga and mindfulness in schools and setting up sustainable and effective programs.

As a certified school psychologist, licensed psychologist, and yoga researcher, as well as a certified yoga teacher, Dr. Cook-Cottone has a unique set of experiences that contribute to the critical eye she brings to the topic in *Mindfulness and Yoga in Schools*. Specifically, she has explored yoga and mindfulness in schools from a variety of perspectives that situate the conversation firmly within the intersecting topics of education, psychology, neuropsychology, and embodiment.

At a time when today's youth are facing increased stress levels, mental health challenges, mood disorders, health issues related to nutrition and exercise, and many other challenges to their well-being, yoga and mindfulness are practices that can positively impact our young people. Schools, where children spend most of their time, are increasingly focused on producing reportable academic results such as high test scores, contributing to a culture of stress and anxiety among students and staff alike. In this type of environment, a young person's natural inclination to explore, experiment, grow, and learn is often diminished. Yoga and mindfulness can help to restore and maintain this innate curiosity and support the creation of a positive learning environment.

The research on yoga and mindfulness in schools, and in the lives of children, continues to grow. Dr. Cook-Cottone's work is timely and necessary. *Mindfulness and Yoga in Schools* provides insight into how these practices support children to become effective learners. This book invites the reader to consider not just the tools of yoga and meditation, but also the way that these practices bridge the experiences of young people. It asks us to consider the vast scope of growing up by contextualizing learning as something that integrates the experiences of the body, the emotions, the thoughts, as well as the external reality that frames learning, for example, the culture, the community, and the school. Her framework, which postures "the self as effective learner" who practices the integration of "self-regulation and care" and "intentional reflective engagement," is profound and provides a framework for discussing yoga and mindfulness that is broad enough to move the field forward in invaluable ways.

This book is grounded in research and provides the insight that only an experienced practitioner, researcher, and teacher can provide. The delivery of the empirically supported methods and theory demonstrates Dr. Cook-Cottone's significant experience in the field. An extensive literature review supports the information about implementing programs in schools. From an opening chapter that discusses learning and explores how yoga influences learning, the book moves through chapters that examine the individual experience of learners and the efficacy of the practices to increase student engagement and to reduce stress. The carefully crafted figures, tables, and images are helpful to any reader looking to implement programs in schools. The reader will move from chapters that frame the work of yoga as an intervention model for developing self-regulation into sections that take a close look at programs and interventions offered in schools, paying close attention to the philosophical influences of these protocols.

Dr. Cook-Cottone also integrates the essential element of success for anyone stepping into a school to offer this important work: She provides a tool for teacher reflection and self-care. The work of taking yoga into schools demands that a teacher be mindful, aware of research, and fully educated about the practice, but it also requires that we bring joy, compassion, and an acceptance of the process to each encounter. *Mindfulness and Yoga in Schools* concludes with a carefully structured and user-friendly tool for self-care; an essential, and often overlooked, part of offering successful yoga in schools programs.

While reading through this book will give you a lot to consider, the best way to truly understand these practices, and the many benefits they can offer our children (and us!), is to explore them yourself. We encourage you to read slowly, and take time to experiment with and experience both the practices described in the text and the wide variety of mindfulness and yoga offerings available. Notice if connecting to your own body changes your experience—emotionally and intellectually—and imagine how the practices could affect children's health, well-being, and learning.

While implementing yoga and mindfulness programming in schools is important and has tremendous potential to support our children, often the greatest gift we can give a child is a mindful adult! When we can slow down, stay grounded in the present moment, curious about our own experiences and the experiences of our kids as well as the world around us, dedicated to kindness and to inquiry rather than judgment, then we can truly share these practices by creating an immersive experience of mindfulness for our students. Rather than just teaching practices, we are creating a space for them in which mindfulness is a core part of how the community engages with each other and with the world. Ideally, we offer our students both the gift of our own mindful attention, and the tools to use these practices out in the world when things get challenging. This takes a commitment to our own practice, and our own path of self-reflection and inquiry. Catherine Cook-Cottone's book is a wonderful resource on this journey.

Jennifer Cohen Harper
Founder, Little Flower Yoga
Board President, Yoga Service Council
Editor, *Best Practices for Yoga in Schools*

Traci Childress
Cofounder, Children's Community School
Executive Director, Saint Mary's Nursery School
Editor, *Best Practices for Yoga in Schools*

PREFACE

It is that openness and awareness of sorts that I try to cultivate...
to be aware of the poignancy of life at that moment.

I would like to feel that I had, in some way,
given them the gift of themselves.

—Martha Graham (1991, 1998)

Mindfulness and embodiment can give students the gift of themselves. It is in the present moment, completely embodied and engaged, and full of intention that our lives happen and futures are made. It is in the present moment that real learning occurs. No matter how sophisticated, research based, and wonderful your curriculum is, if your students are not present, they will not learn. Yes, presence and embodiment are crucial factors in educating our children and youth. Unfortunately, it is getting increasingly difficult for us and our students to be in the present moment and embodied. We chronically leave ourselves. We check out. For adults, it shows up as a not-quite-noticing that we have been *spacing out* for the last few minutes (i.e., dissociating), or it is a few drinks, a Netflix binge, Facebook distraction, compulsive shopping, overeating, or a whole host of other distractions. For students, it's not much different. Maybe it is a never-ending group text message, Twitter drama, binge-watching shows, or, unfortunately, drinking, using, self-harm, and worse. Why are we doing this? Why is it so hard for us to just be present?

We have good reason. Technological advances are happening faster than we can effectively adapt to them. Media has become increasingly sensationalized, grabbing our attention at every turn. We have real stress. The United States has been at war since many of our students were born. We are climbing out of recession, yet many are still feeling financial hardship. There are regular terror attacks and mass shootings, leaving few places seemingly safe (e.g., movie theaters, clubs, schools, universities, large gatherings, and malls). Even if your neighborhood or city has been spared violence, you see violent images roll across your newsfeed and repeated on headline news almost daily. These images of violence can come unexpectedly and be extremely graphic. Innocently scrolling through your newsfeed, you see a puppy, children laughing, and then, without warning, a shooting being streamed live. Being humans, with brains designed to keep us safe, we focus on the threats and negative news. It is our nature. It feels like we can't help it and many of us are not even aware that we have a choice. More, school systems have their own set of challenges as we try to keep students safe, include families, and teach the curriculum of the day. We are stressed and the students are stressed. In all of this stress, it is easy to lose yourself.

Still, we ask our students over and over to pay attention, do their work, and try. We teach the math, reading, science, art, social studies, and music. Yet we don't always teach them how to cope with the stress they are feeling as they walk into school, handle the frustration they experience when they do try, or pay attention in the first place. Often, we take ownership of their self-regulation through sophisticated behavior plans with rewards and consequences. Of course, behavior plans and class-wide systems are helpful. However, with no eye on our students' ultimate ability to be the masters of their own attention, impulse control, and sustained effort, we leave them without a set of tools to negotiate the stress inherent not only in third, eighth, and 12th grades, but also in life and all of its challenges. Our schools are the perfect environment for teaching our students how to be mindfully aware, manage frustration, engage with persistent effort and attention, embody intentional action, and be kind and caring to each other. We know that it takes embodied learning, in real time, to internalize these skills and construct knowledge. School is where this can be done.

I know all of this can feel too big and overwhelming. As a teacher you might ask yourself, "How can I fix this? How can I make a difference with so many students in need?" I find inspiration in *The Starfish Story*. It was a favorite of my mom's, an English teacher. She taught literature for decades in a rural upstate New York high school. No matter how big the challenge, my mom focused on one student at a time, one book at a time, one journal entry at a time, and one moment at a time. They called her classroom Zen-like. When I began writing this book, I asked my dad if I could have mom's notes so I could use her favorite quotes to begin each chapter. In the files, I kept coming across copy after copy of *The Starfish Story*. It goes like this.

> Once, there was a young man walking down a deserted beach at dawn. The tide was out, the beach wide. In the distance, he saw an old man. Was he dancing? What was he doing? As he approached the old man, he saw that he was picking up beached starfish and throwing them back into the ocean. The young man gazed in wonder as he watched the old man throw starfish after starfish into the ocean waves. Bewildered, the young man asked the star thrower, "Why are you doing this?" The old man explained that the starfish would die if they were left in the morning sun. The young man looked down the expanse of the beach, "But there must be thousands of starfish. How can you possibly make any difference at all?" Smiling, the old man looked down at the starfish in his hand and threw it safely into the ocean. He said, "It makes a difference to this one."

> —Eiseley (1969)

This story emphasizes the importance of present moment awareness and embodied, intentional action. It speaks as much to our role as teachers as it does to a student doing math. It is in *this moment* and *this action* that we can make a difference. Stop, refocus, breathe, and see how you can support *this student* learning right here and right now. For the student, it is not in the 30 math problems ahead, the thought "How will I ever finish?," or the fear "Can I even get into college if math is this hard?" It is *this math problem*, right here, right now. Stop, refocus, breathe, and let's look at this problem,

"You've got this." In this way, we can all learn to be starfish throwers for whom problems, and moments, seldom feel too big.

Schools are adopting mindfulness and yogic techniques at increasing rates. In 2002, my research team began the first ever yoga-based eating disorder prevention program in schools. For over 14 years, we have studied the outcomes among hundreds of students. When I first began this work, the field of yoga in schools did not really exist. Mindfulness programs were making their way to schools. Still, the initiatives were small and happening in large cities next to the few universities looking at mindfulness. Now, a simple Google News search of "mindfulness and yoga in the schools" yields tens of thousands of stories. The Kripalu Yoga in Schools Symposium is heading into its fourth year. The former first lady, Michelle Obama, is known for her yoga practice and fitness. Under her tenure, I was part of a team that taught yoga at the White House Easter Egg Roll as part of the administration's commitment to health and fitness for children and youth. For years, Ohio Congressional Representative Tim Ryan passionately and consistently argued for mindfulness and yoga in the schools as a pathway to well-being (see http://www.mindful.org/ohio-congressman-tim-ryan-talks-about-a-mindful-nation-video/).

Accordingly, there is a demand for teacher, school psychology, school counseling, school social work, and school administration training programs to integrate mindfulness and yoga content into their curricula. To support training and continuing education, this text explicates mindfulness and yoga as tools for cultivating embodied self-regulation within healthy, active, engaged learners. The learner is the student (primary object of focus), as well as teachers, counselors, psychologists, and parents. Embracing the mindful and yogic perspective, mindfulness and yoga are considered this way—we are all on the path and we can instruct most effectively from our own experience in mindfulness and embodied practice. To help you get a sense of the bigger picture, this text offers a conceptual framework within the first three chapters, which is then distilled into 12 embodied practices that are woven through the more practical, application-based chapters that follow. The methodology is presented in a clear, easy-to-follow format that integrates theory, empirical evidence, and hands-on, school-based practices.

The only comprehensive text integrating the files of mindfulness, yoga, and schools, *Mindfulness and Yoga in Schools: A Guide for Teachers and Practitioners* is structured in four parts, each comprised of one to five chapters. Part I sets the stage for mindfulness and yoga interventions in schools. First, a review of the conceptual model for embodied self-regulation is presented (Chapter 1). Also, this section addresses the risks and outcomes associated with a lack of self-regulation and engagement among students (Chapter 2). Chapter 2 also includes the three-tiered model of intervention used in education and a framework for implementing mindfulness and yogic practices within the three-tier approach. Chapter 3 introduces 12 embodied practices that promote self-regulation and student engagement.

Parts II and III explicate the philosophical underpinnings of mindfulness and yoga, detail the formal and informal practices in an on-the-cushion/mat and off-the cushion/mat format, and critically review the mindfulness and yoga protocols that have been implemented and studied in schools. Specifically, Part II focuses on mindfulness interventions and Part III focuses on yoga interventions. These sections interweave the mindful and yogic principles presented in Chapter 3. They are presented in parallel formats for ease of reading and accessibility. You will find tips for implementing a program in your classroom and school, overviews of school-based programs, and reviews of the research. There are photographs, scripts, figures, and tables to help you implement your own program or strengthen the program you have.

Part IV addresses mindful self-care for students and teachers. The mindful self-care scale is presented as a framework for presenting actionable self-care goals for students and teachers. Both the longer form and the shorter form are offered with a scoring system and research on each of the aspects of self-care. This chapter provides a centered focus on the self and closure for the text.

I love this work because, in its essence, it brings us to the best versions of ourselves, fully present, aware, and embodied. Mindfulness and yoga practices help us be on-purpose, intentional in our teaching and in our lives. That said, this book is for you. It is designed not only to help you be the best version of you in the classroom, but also to help you be the best version of you in your life. In this way, you will be able to teach without even using words. You will be exactly what and where you are asking your students to be—right here—in this moment, learning, and in the beautiful creation of your life.

> There is a vitality, a life force, an energy, a quickening
> that is translated through you into action,
> and because there is only one of you in all time,
> this expression is unique.
> And if you block it,
> it will never exist through
> any other medium and will be lost.

—Martha Graham
(Martha Graham in De Mille, 1979)

REFERENCES

De Mille, A. (1979). *Dance to the piper: A promenade home: A two-part autobiography*. New York, NY: Da Capo Press.

Eiseley, L. (1969). *The unexpected universe: The starfish thrower*. New York, NY: Harcourt.

Graham, M. (1991). *Blood memory*. New York, NY: Doubleday.

Graham, M. (1998). I am a dancer. In A. Carter (Ed.), *Routledge dance studies reader* (pp. 66–71). New York, NY: Routledge.

ACKNOWLEDGMENTS

Be who God meant you to be and you will set the world on fire.

—St. Catherine of Siena[1]

When contemplating how the writing of a book is possible, I think of the pinecone sitting—without growth—on the shelf at work. It has been a few years since I first found that old pinecone at the lake and brought it to work. Day after day it sits, not growing at all. That pinecone reminds me that *seeds without soil, water, and love don't grow*. It is the support all around us that creates the context in which dreams can thrive, even bear fruit. From a seed of an idea to the fruit of a book, I have so many to thank.

There are numerous people who played an integral role in the creation of this book. First, thank you to Jerry Cottone, Chloe Cottone, and Maya Cottone, who agreed (in a tight vote) that they would let me write another book. Thank you! More specifically, thank you for all of the grocery shopping, dinner cooking, and comedic and dramatic relief you gave me so that I could write. I love you guys.

I would like to thank Nancy Hale, who shared my vision and worked with me to create the proposal. Once the idea and the contract were in place, I had a host of helpers. A big thank you to Janel Anthony, a rehabilitation counselor (then a student), who helped me collect and organize hundreds of articles on mindfulness and yoga. She did all of this with a smile and the thoughtfulness that comes with multicolored tabs and gigantic binders. Thank you also to Heather Cahill, Jillian Cherry, and Rebeccah Sivecz for your hard work searching for mindfulness and yoga programs in schools. As always, thank you to Christopher Hollister, associate librarian at the University at Buffalo, State University of New York, and seeker of quote origins and citations extraordinaire.

Critical to my research trajectory and forthcoming work, Lindsay Travers, elementary school teacher, Melissa LaVigne, social worker, and Erga Lemish, doctoral student, helped to bring together research on trauma-informed yoga, creating our first set of Principles for Growth for our work with Yogis in Service, Inc. (see yogisinservice.org). These principles helped to inform the Principles of Embodied Growth and Learning created for this book. I can't wait to see what is next for these bright and motivated young women.

Thank you to Madison Weber, photographer, and Kayla Tiedmann, mindfulness and yoga model. I also extend a second note of appreciation to Lindsay Travers, who read each manuscript page, making sure we caught all of the typos and that the words made sense.

---

[1]"Be who God meant you to be," said Anglican Bishop of London Richard Chartres, citing St. Catherine of Siena in his address to the royal wedding couple Prince William and Kate Middleton at Westminster Abbey on April 29, 2011 (Bishop of London's amazing speech to William and Kate, Johannes 1721/YouTube, retrieved from https://www.youtube.com/watch?v=l1vh-zWt9h8).

I know teachers usually get the whole summer off. Thank you for spending your summer with this book.

To the Snyder Running Club, Yogis in Service, Inc., and all my yoga friends: Thank you for all your love and support. As you all know, I wrote this book without missing a run, a workout, or a yoga practice. Sustainability comes from good self-care and great friends. I am lucky to have both.

Last, I would like to note the substantial gratitude I feel for Dr. Wendy Guyker, who has joined my research team as a coleader. Her contributions and positive, creative energy have supported the team and me as I worked on this project. I am looking forward to a productive future with our Mindful Self-Care Scale (see Chapter 14) and all of our other exciting projects.

Thank YOU!

PART I

A MODEL FOR SELF-REGULATION AND ENGAGEMENT

CHAPTER 1

A CONCEPTUAL MODEL OF EDUCATING FOR SELF-REGULATION AND INTENTIONAL, REFLECTIVE ENGAGEMENT

Learning how to learn is the element that is always of value . . .
I am talking about LEARNING—the insatiable curiosity . . .
significant, meaningful, experiential learning . . .

When such learning takes place,
the element of meaning to the learner
is built into the whole experience.

—Carl Rogers, *Freedom to Learn* (1983, pp. 18, 19, 20)

FROM LEARNING TO LIFE

Think back to the moments you truly remember from school. For me, it was those moments when I was completely engaged in the process of learning. There was a first grade play that we, a committee of 6-year-olds, wrote and performed as our own production. I recall sketching the choreography on the chalkboard and working out each step, erasing and reworking as we created. I remember my mom helping me sew my costume, the satin fabric, her hand over mine as we stitched, our single-mindedness, breathing in concert as she guided my fingers, the needle, and thread. I have another memory of raising flour beetles in third grade. I observed them keenly, taking notes as they scrambled around in the bottom of a waxed-paper cup. Throughout their life cycle, from eggs to pupae to larvae to adults, our teacher thoughtfully guided us to notice each aspect of the beetles. We detailed their three-segmented antennae and notched eyes as they grew. In sixth grade, I was lucky enough to be considered gifted and talented and be assigned to an experimental classroom with a dark room, botany lab, engineering lab, and loft filled with musical instruments, sound system, and stage. The entire year was a practice in presence, focused attention, and integration of mind and body. Of all my years of school memories, this year is the richest. We wrote and bound our own books. A dear friend and I handcrafted puppets and were puppeteer MCs at the variety shows performed in our classroom. We learned about photography and developed our own photos in the dark room. I ran year-long trials exploring and recording the outcomes of various ways to grow basil effectively. We danced, sang, and argued about the myths of the Egyptian pyramids. What sets each of these experiences apart is the embodied mindfulness, pure observation, engagement of the senses, and construction of meaning. The many years of my education that followed pale in comparison to these crisp and clear memories. Years passed. I graduated from high school, college, and grad school. Not without bumps in the road. Nevertheless, I graduated.

At the age of 35, I took my first yoga class. It had been about 25 years since I had been in sixth grade, constructing my own learning, engaging in bare attention. As I left the yoga class, my heart was light, my head was clear, and I was full of ideas. There was something more. I could not put words to what I was feeling. I later realized that it was nostalgia. In yoga, I felt the mind and body connection, the joy that was part of my experience of self so many years ago. I wasn't sure when and how I had become disembodied. I tried to trace my life back to the point of separation when my mind and body began to exist in parallel ontologies. It seems that, at some point, there were two distinct aspects of self: the part of me that thought and processed information (e.g., school stuff), and the part of me that was in the experience (e.g., friendships, fun). I am certain this disconnection was the source of my disengagement from learning during my later middle and high school years. Moreover, it is what put me at risk for substance use, eating disorder, mood dysregulation, and anxiety. I had somehow made it through the cognitive achievements of my education without an authentic experience of embodied learning and most certainly without joy. The more I realized this, the more my nostalgia turned to a real sense of loss. It was then that I began researching yoga as a prevention intervention in schools. I was determined to give kids tools to stay connected and integrated before they lost a sense of themselves.

Over the years, owing to a multitude of influences, some valid and some less so, schools have become increasingly focused *solely* on the cognitive aspects of learning, the academics, test scores, and grades. Still, there has always been a voice—sometimes raised as a confident herald, loud in the forefront of the discussion, bolstered by supporters, and other times expressed as a quiet whisper in the back row—asking, "Why are we doing this?" and "What is our goal?" This voice has come from many: teacher, parent, student, lawmaker, and educational researcher. Perhaps harkening back to the roots of education in the United States, there is a growing consensus that school is about more than academics, and the charge is to prepare students not only for work, but for life—the embodied experience of life (Comer, Ben-Avie, Haynes, & Joyner, 1999; Dewey, 1938; Mondale & Patton, 2001).

I have spent most of my life thinking about and researching the social and emotional aspects of learning and school. I have read extensively on the history and theory of education and spent nearly half my life as a student. I grew up the daughter of an English teacher (my mother) and physics and Junior Reserve Officer Training Corps (JROTC) teacher (my father). My father also went on to be a vice principal, principal, and school superintendent. I have worked as a school psychologist and, for many years now, as a university educator, researcher, and mentor. I have distilled my countless readings and experiences down to this: Essentially there are three main goals of education: (a) impart academic knowledge (i.e., conceptual and procedural) and tools for learning, (b) teach students to be active architects of their own learning and well-being, and (c) prepare students to be collaborative problem solvers in service of societal well-being. To achieve these goals, education should be embodied, active, and filled with purpose. Aligned with Vygotskian theory (see Karpov, 2014), schools can be seen as mentorships for life (see Figure 1.1). Fittingly, given the complexities, dynamics, and rapid evolution of today's geopolitical and sociocultural landscape, it makes

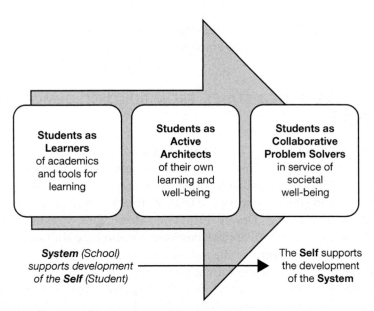

FIGURE 1.1 Effective schools as supportive mentorships.

sense that, in order to prepare students for life, we must teach students more than what we know—knowledge and skills, that is, academics and tools for learning. We must teach them how to know, how to apply knowledge and skills to build a good and healthy life, and, finally, how to use what they know to create, problem solve, and know more. As Comer et al. said in 1999, "And when this is the case for most people in society, that society has a reasonable chance to survive and thrive for a sustained period of time" (p. xx).

Ultimately, the goal is to help the student mature from the early developmental stages during which the school setting provides the support and structure for learning into an independent, whole, integrated, and creative problem solver who now helps to support and develop the structure from which he or she came (see Figure 1.1). There is a growing consensus that for school learning to be an effective mentorship for life, it should be *embodied*, filled with moments of sensory experience and bare attention. Academic learning is most certainly primary in this process. Also critical to the process is learning how to learn, self-regulate, care for your own needs, work with others, and contribute in an intentional and reflective manner. Within the process is an essential role for self-regulating tools (i.e., methodologies and practices) that help the students develop a measured and intentional way of being with their schoolwork, friends, families, and communities (Comer et al., 1999).

In this chapter, the conceptual model for the text is presented with a focus on the student as an effective learner who is mentored in the use of academic and self-regulatory tools that can be found in mindfulness and yoga practices. These tools facilitate the learner's ability to construct his or her own meaning and cultural impact. A brief history of the goals and values of education in the United States is offered as context. Connections to Social Emotional Learning (SEL), Service Learning (SL), and Contemplative Education (CE) are made. Next, based on the attuned representational model of self (ARMS; Cook-Cottone, 2006, 2015), the text reviews the Mindful and Yogic Self as Effective Learner (MY-SEL) model, as well as the theoretical underpinnings and empirical support underlying the development of a mindful and yoga-based approach to embodied self-regulation and well-being. Finally, the concept of teacher as learner and practitioner is emphasized.

EDUCATION IN THE UNITED STATES: FROM BUILDING DEMOCRACY TO ONTOLOGIES

The roots of formal school systems in the United States can be traced back to 1635 when a Latin grammar school was opened in Boston, Massachusetts, and a free school was opened in Virginia. Throughout the centuries that have passed, there has been a range of goals for education, including creating effective work and military forces as well as an educated, egalitarian, democratic community (e.g., Dewey, 1916, 1938; Meier, 2013; Mondale & Patton, 2001). Historically, American educational approaches have reflected the shifting balance between the needs of society and the needs of the individual during any given era. In the late 18th and early 19th centuries, during the formative years of the nation, thinkers like Thomas Jefferson advocated for public education to not only impart academic knowledge but also to support democracy (Mondale & Patton, 2001). Indeed, it was held that the main function of school in the early 1800s was to teach "correct" political principles to the young (Mondale & Patton, 2001, p. 2).

As the 19th century progressed, and the nation grew in numbers and diversity, educational thinking evolved. Founding ideals gave rise to the modern, public school system. Horace Mann, often called the Father of the Common School, believed that school should be free, embracing children of all backgrounds and means, and taught by well-trained, professional teachers. Central to his vision was this: that, above all, schools should build character and instill the values that, in turn, would shape a responsible, productive citizenry (Mondale & Patton, 2001). Later in the century and into the 20th century, this idea was endorsed and expanded by the progressive educational thinker, Dewey, saying (1916), ". . . a government resting upon popular suffrage cannot be successful unless those who elect and who obey their governors are educated" (p. 83). And, so, a fundamental link was established that informs education to this day: That school, in giving students the tools they need to reach their full potential, is vital to a stable democracy and strong social fabric.

Over the course of the 20th century, local schools grew and evolved along with their associated school districts as the national educational system was built. There were initiatives for smaller schools in the 1960s, advocacy and action for *cultural democracy* or equal rights and access for all to education, and calls for *economic democracy* in order to close the gap between districts of different income levels (Mondale & Patton, 2001). Many of these issues remain central to the educational discussion today. A review of the history of academics reveals that, at its roots, the U.S. education system was never solely about academics. The system was created to facilitate the development of citizens, voters, and skillful community members. For all of these hundreds of years, it has almost always been about preparing students for life and community, a process that includes academic learning, of course, as well as so much more (Comer et al., 1999). Notably, for much of this time, it has been a top-down, didactic process.

At the present moment, we are faced with challenges. To negotiate our future, we must not only be capable of the academic solutions, we must also manage the personal, social, and civic collaboration that will be required to effectively address the massive challenges we face as a nation. In this way, graduates need to be both educated, active problem solvers, as well as citizens capable of working as effective and collaborative members of the community. Again, they need to be able to do more than know all that we know. It is our collective hope that the future scientists who will cure the now incurable diseases; the environmental engineers who will figure out our massive waste management challenges; those who will solve the food, energy, and water crises to come; and the creators of literature and arts not yet imagined will be effectively prepared in today's schools. In essence, our way of life depends on the content and quality of the education provided to each child in this country (Comer et al., 1999). It cannot be more of the same. Today's students need to be innovators, creators, and destroyers of paradigms. For deep change, this cannot be taught top-down.

These challenges are complicated by a world with a rapidly changing landscape of obstacles, tools, and problems (Comer et al., 1999). As educators, we struggle to keep pace with sociocultural and technological changes that are undoubtedly shaping the brains and minds of students. The term *ontological development* describes the experiential shaping process in which the mind affects the world and the world affects the mind. The process of human development is an ongoing cycle of mutual and contingent influences creating a student body inherently different from school cohorts of past decades, even past years (Vygotsky, 1978). This process can be passive or active (Roeser & Peck, 2009). Today's students can, and perhaps must, learn to be active architects of their experiences both internal and external. In Siegel's (1999) groundbreaking book, *The Developing Mind: Toward a Neurobiological Understanding of Interpersonal Experience,* he discusses a phenomenon that can be referred to as *ontological sculpting* in which we have the opportunity to be the architects of our own neurobiological development. Accordingly, as educators, we can help to create a learning environment and experiences that support the positive, healthy development of our learners. Specifically, the term *ontological sculpting* recognizes that individual genetics and biology shape experience. Conversely and reciprocally, the environment (e.g., loved ones, friends, community, and culture) shapes us, the learners. Ontological sculpting occurs within lived experience and is an ongoing, recursive, iterative, process of mutual self/environment influence. Who is the sculptor? That is, in part, up to us. In a school in which we are educating for life and for the well-being of all, an empowered, effective student learns skills and gains the competencies needed to be the architect of his or her own learning and, ultimately, his or her own life experience (Roeser & Peck, 2009; Vygotsky, 1978).

The history of public education in the United States is the story of a gradual shift toward the learner as the maker of meaning (Karpov, 2014). Rechtschaffen (2014) explains that, before formal education, it was believed that we did not learn about experiences, we learned from them. In fact, he explain that the root of the word *learn* has the same etymological root as the words to *follow* or *track*. Rechtschaffen (2014) calls to mind how our ancestors may have learned. He paints the picture of a young student, guided by his or her mentor, tracking animals through the grass, streams, and forests, learning about the world through the senses—an experience-up process. He suggests that, at its roots, learning is a "purely sensory, relational, and wholly mindful experience" (p. 16). To be true constructors of meaning, students need an experiential process in which they can integrate what is explained to them and what they know in a felt sense. Consistent with what is known about neurobiology and learning, truth lies in the place between what is told to us and what we have lived. Echoing and extending Deweyian thinking (Dewey, 1938), today's schools should be places in which students can find their truth, liberation, and place within society through opportunities to both know and experience.

THE LARGER CONTEXT OF YOGA AND MINDFULNESS IN SCHOOLS: SOCIAL EMOTIONAL LEARNING, SERVICE LEARNING, AND CONTEMPLATIVE EDUCATION

As we have reviewed the progression of education and the learner, we are left with the notion that: (a) education is about preparing students for life, and (b) we are, in our essence, mindful and embodied learners. From this, SEL, SL, and CE initiatives emerged as efforts to offer embodied learning experiences that prepare students for life. It is not entirely clear exactly when these types of learning initiatives first formally entered public education. In the late 1960s, Comer initiated a school approach that would later be viewed as one of the early roots of SEL (Comer, 1988). His work centered on the theory that it was the contrast between a child's experiences at home and those in school that deeply affected the child's psychosocial development. Comer (1988) created the School Development Program in 1968, focusing on two poor, low-achieving, predominately African American elementary schools in Connecticut. These schools reported poor attendance and low academic achievement. Comer helped the schools to create an environment that integrated social and behavioral, school-wide goals and supports that changed the experience of the students. By the early 1980s, academic performance at the two schools was reported to exceed the national average, accompanied by a notable decrease in both truancy and behavior problems. His approach held central that effective schools do more than deliver academic knowledge. It was from this line of understanding education that the SEL movement began.

Social Emotional Learning

SEL competencies are believed to be important foundations for students' well-being (Ashdown & Bernard, 2012; Durlak, Weissberg, Dymnicki, Taylor, & Schellinger, 2011). There are many SEL definitions and foci to be found in the education, psychology, and political literatures. The SEL competencies vary by source and program and can include: emotion regulation, self-awareness, self-management, relationships and relationship skills, social awareness, and effective learning (Ashdown & Bernard, 2012; Collaborative for Academic, Social, and Emotional Learning [CASEL], 2003; Durlak et al., 2011; Elias et al., 1997; Philibert, 2016a, 2016b; Rechtschaffen, 2014). Across programs and approaches, you will nearly always find goals that address both the development of the capacity to form close and secure peer and adult relationships and the development of specific relationship skills (e.g., conflict resolution; Ashdown & Bernard, 2012; CASEL, 2003; Elias et al., 1997; Parlakian, 2003). Broadly, SEL approaches integrate the promotion of competence and youth development. These approaches accomplish this by developing protective mechanisms known to lead to and maintain positive adjustment as well as the reduction of risk factors (Durlak et al., 2011; Philibert, 2016a, 2016b). To promote resiliency, SEL programs provide direct instruction and actively practice social and emotional skills (Durlak et al., 2011). To reduce risk, many SEL programs apply skill development in the prevention of problem behaviors (e.g., substance use, bullying, and school failure; Durlak et al., 2011). Both of these foci may also include opportunities to be actively involved in whole-school initiatives and community building (Durlak et al., 2011). Example programs include the Inner Resilience Program (www.innerresilience-tidescenter.org/index.html) and the Collaborative for Academic, Social, and Emotional Learning (CASEL; www.casel .org). See also Philibert's *Everyday SEL in Elementary School: Integrating Social-Emotional*

Learning and Mindfulness Into Your Classroom, and *Everyday SEL in Middle School: Integrating Social-Emotional Learning and Mindfulness Into Your Classroom* (Philibert, 2016a, 2016b).

In an extensive meta-analysis of 213 school-based, universal, social and emotional learning programs involving 270,034 kindergarten through high school students, Durlak et al. (2011) found that, compared to controls, SEL participants demonstrated significantly improved social and emotional skills, attitudes, behaviors, and academic performance. Overall, many of the significant findings remained significant at the 6-month follow-up with a noted reduced magnitude in scores. Specifically, SEL programs have been shown to promote youth development, reduce negative behaviors, and increase social-emotional competence (i.e., positive self-orientation, positive other orientation, and positive work orientation) and social skills (i.e., cooperation, assertion, and self-control; Ashdown & Bernard, 2012; Durlak et al., 2011). Not surprisingly, in Durlak et al.'s (2011) meta-analysis, researchers found the largest effect size (mean = 0.69) in the focus area that included emotion recognition, stress management, empathy, problem solving, and decision making. Further, SEL programs enhanced student behavioral adjustment as shown by increased prosocial behaviors and reduced conduct and internalizing problems (Durlak et al., 2011). Perhaps of most interest to academics, DiPerna and Elliot (2002) reported that social-emotional and cognitive competence (i.e., reading, writing, and critical thinking skills) were found to be predictors of academic achievement. In fact, in Durlak et al.'s (2011) meta-analysis, an 11-percentile-point gain in achievement was found for those participants who engaged in school-based universal SEL compared to controls. It is important to note that many programs reviewed for this analysis did not collect academic data at posttest or follow-up.

In a cluster-randomized trial demonstrating SEL impact specifically on academic achievement among elementary school children, Schonfeld et al. (2014) found that the Promoting Alternative Thinking Strategies (PATHS) curriculum fostered acquisition academic proficiency, especially among youth attending high-risk school settings. The PATHS curriculum is a program for educators and counselors designed to facilitate the development of self-control, emotional awareness, and interpersonal problem-solving skills. The curriculum consists of six volumes of lessons designed for use with elementary school children. The specific intervention used for the Schonfeld et al. (2014) study included other intervention elements, such as additional training and support for teachers, that may have contributed to the positive impact. Specific findings include greater basic proficiency in fourth-grade reading and math, and in fifth- and sixth-grade writing, compared to the control group. Interestingly, the analysis of dosage effects provided additional support for intervention effects for both reading and math.

Overall, SEL programs are focused on the development of relationship and personal emotional competencies that help to promote well-being and positive school adjustment. Learning experiences are both didactic and experiential and can be individual, class wide, and school wide. Further, methodologies include the weaving of SEL goals and learning experiences into academic learning, as well as distinct SEL learning opportunities. Although many programs encourage active learning, the emphasis is on the development of psychosocial competencies and not necessarily the experiential or embodied nature of learning. Notably, self-awareness and intra- and interpersonal self-regulation are key competencies addressed in SEL.

Service Learning

SL is a pedagogical approach that integrates community service with academics (Celio, Durlack, & Dymnicki, 2011). SL theory is based on the beliefs that learning is best when students are involved in their own learning; learning is active and experiential; and the learning has a distinct service/civic purpose (Berman, 2015; Billig, 2000; Celio et al., 2011). Accordingly, SL typically involves active participation in organized experiences that focus on the needs of the community and the cultivation of a sense of caring for others (Billig, 2000). Berman (2015) holds that SL helps students understand their connectedness to their communities as they experience the role of a provider of services versus the role of consumer. Further, in service of the academic curriculum, there is an emphasis on the application of skills and knowledge and a commitment to extended learning opportunities (Billig, 2000). The National Youth Leadership Council (NYLC; http://nylc.org) provides a good illustration on their web page. They explain that picking up trash along a riverbank is *service*. Moreover, studying various water samples under a microscope is *learning*. SL occurs when environmental biology students collect and analyze water samples, document their results, and present findings to a community pollution control agency.

The roots of SL can be traced back as far as John Dewey and Jean Piaget (Billig, 2000; Giles & Eyler, 1994). Although Dewey did not specifically refer to what we now understand as SL, he and his colleagues established the intellectual foundations of SL (Berman, 2015). Dewey's principle of interaction holds that the internal and objective aspects of an experience interact to form a learning situation (Dewey, 1938; Giles & Eyler, 1994). Learning occurs within the transaction between the learner and the environment (Giles & Eyler, 1994). Within this philosophical context, SL provides the environment and accompanying, real-world challenges that cultivate learning situations. Key also is Dewey's notion of reflective thinking as central to the learning process (Giles & Eyler, 1994). Finally, Dewey wrote extensively on the connection between education, citizenship, community, and democracy (Giles & Eyler, 1994). In this way, pedagogy is more than a methodology used in schools; it is a means by which citizens become informed, communicate their interests, create public opinion, and make decisions (Giles & Eyler, 1994). Giles and Eyler (1994) suggest that schools go beyond preparing students for life, they model it: ". . . saturating [the student] with the spirit of service, and providing [the student] with the instruments of effective self-direction, we shall have the deepest and best guarantee of a larger society which is worthy, lovely, and harmonious" (Dewey, 1900, p. 44).

In 1961, President John F. Kennedy established the Peace Corps. In 1964, President Lyndon B. Johnson created the Volunteers in Service to America (VISTA). These programs were markers of the national commitment to service (Berman, 2015). The term *service learning* was coined in 1967 by Robert Sigmon and William Ramsey to imply a value consideration linking authentic community service, intentional academic learning, and reflection (Berman, 2015). In the 1970s, the National Student Volunteer Program was established and began publishing the *Syntegist*, a journal that emphasizes community service and learning (Berman, 2015). Since those early days, the field of SL has grown, adding journals, AmeriCorps (www.nationalservice.gov/programs/americorps), the National Service Learning Clearinghouse (https://gsn.nylc.org/clearinghouse), and national and internal conferences on SL. For more on the history of SL, see Berman (2015).

SL is believed to help develop higher order thinking, cultural awareness, personal and interpersonal development, motivation to engage in social issues, academic motivation, self-efficacy, and civic responsibility (Warren, 2012). In a meta-analysis of 62 studies involving 11,837 students in SL, Celio et al. (2011) found that, compared to controls, students participating in SL programs showed significant gains in five outcome areas: attitude toward self, attitudes toward school and learning, civic engagement, social skills, and academic performance, with mean effects ranging from 0.27 to 0.43. In a much smaller meta-analysis of 11 studies, Warren (2012) found that SL was associated with statistically significant and positive effects on student learning outcomes that were measured by both self-reported and concrete measures of learning (e.g., exams and student assignment scores).

The Celio et al. (2011) study also found that better SL outcomes were associated with: linking SL programs to academic curriculum; incorporating the youth voice in planning, implementing, and evaluating SL experiences; involving community partners in the creation of the elements and goals of SL projects; and providing opportunities for reflection (Celio et al., 2011). Interestingly, it is believed that the opportunity to reflect on the SL experience provides the link between the action of service and the ideas of learning (Celio et al., 2011). In fact, reflection was included in at least half of the studies reviewed by Celio et al. (2011). Overall, SL combines embodied, active learning through meaningful service projects as a methodology for integrating academic curriculum and real-world needs. A common thread through many SL models is an emphasis on reflective learning and practice. To learn more about SL, see the National Society for Experiential Education (www.nsee.org) and the Corporation for National Service (www.nationalservice.gov). For a list of standards for SL programs, see the NYLC (http://nylc.org).

Contemplative Education

Contemplative practices are those practices that require individuals (e.g., students and teachers) to practice intentional control over physical and mental activity (Mind and Life Education Research Network [MLERN] et al., 2012). Roeser and Peck (2009) offer a more comprehensive definition: Contemplative practices are "a set of pedagogical practices designed to cultivate the potentials of mindful awareness and volition in an ethical-relational context in which the values of personal growth, learning, moral living, and caring for others are also nurtured" (p. 127). Many see CE programs as complementary to SEL and SL programs (e.g., Roeser & Peck, 2009). As can be found in both SEL and SL methodologies, CE involves active student participation and a set of experiential learning opportunities provided to the student by a competent, contemplative instructor (Roeser & Peck, 2009). Unique to CE is the primary goal of helping students to develop the ability to access concentrated states of awareness within the context of open-mindedness, curiosity, and caring for others (Roeser & Peck, 2009; Waters, Barsky, Ridd, & Allen, 2015). Roeser and Peck (2009) describe CE learning opportunities as including: nature walks, art, tai chi, yoga, guided imagery, contemplation of existential questions, and practicing meditation. It is believed that the key mechanisms of growth are the presence of a disciplined practice and a one-pointed awareness that is cultivated and maintained over time (Roeser & Peck, 2009).

The Garrison Institute's report on CE (2005) describes three types of programs being offered in schools: small, voluntary programs; social and emotional learning programs that integrate mindfulness and yoga practices; and school-wide programs. Research on CE is in its early stages and has yet to organize a set of best practices (Lawlor, 2014). Often, research focuses solely on meditation, mindfulness, and/or yoga practices depending on the researcher's definition of CE (e.g., Waters et al., 2015). For the context of this text, we look specifically at mindfulness and yoga, along with the body of literature that accompanies each, as distinct sets of practices. For more about CE, see the Garrison Institute (www.garrisoninstitute.org/contemplation-and-education).

Yoga and Mindfulness as Contemplative Practices

Overall, SEL, SL, and CE share many key competencies as operational goals (e.g., the development of psychosocial skills, mindfulness, and active/embodied learning). Generally speaking, mindfulness and yoga are considered contemplative practices (Greenberg & Harris, 2012; MLERN et al., 2012). As sets of practices, mindfulness and yoga provide powerful tools fitted for each of the larger contexts of SEL, SL, and CE (Figure 1.2). Yet, mindfulness and yoga should not be minimized as simply activities or techniques. Beyond their obvious compatibility with SEL, SL, and CE, mindfulness and yoga are practices with their own unique histories and relevancies in research as well as in the larger culture, community, and in the schools (MLERN et al., 2012). They are described here briefly as a basic introduction and considered in detail throughout the text.

Mindfulness

The interest in mindfulness programs has grown rapidly within the last 15 years (Greenberg & Harris, 2012). Siegel, in his foreword for Jennings's (2015) book, *Mindfulness for Teachers: Simple Skills for Peace and Productivity in the Classroom*, defines mindfulness as a "... way of being aware of what is happening within us and around us with a clear focus of attention on moment-to-moment experience that enables us to be fully present for life" (p. xi). Mindfulness is the ability to guide and direct attention to the current experience as it unfolds, in the moment, with an open-minded curiosity and acceptance (Greenberg & Harris, 2012; Kabat-Zinn, 2013; Schonert-Reichl & Lawlor, 2010). The most accepted definition of mindfulness comes from *The Mindful Nation. U.K.* (MAPP, 2015): "Mindfulness means paying attention to what's happening in the present moment in the mind, body, and external environment, with an attitude of curiosity and kindness" (p. 14). Mindfulness is further described as the development of the

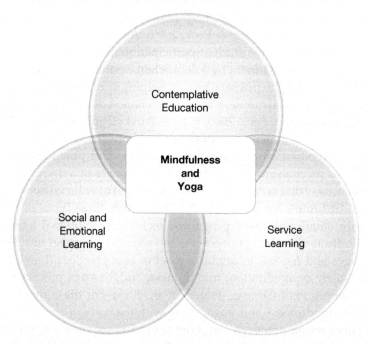

FIGURE 1.2 A context for mindfulness and yoga in schools.

ability to sense life deeply and to observe experience. Therefore, it is first the differentiation of sensing and observing, and next, the integration of or linkage of both the sensation and the observation of the experience (Siegel, 2015). Mindfulness has a deep and rich history, a growing body of research, and a range of practices. Mindfulness practices include entire programs such as mindfulness-based stress reduction (MBSR), and distinct practices such as walking and seated meditation (Cook-Cottone, 2015). There are also both formal (e.g., loving-kindness meditation) and informal (e.g., mindful eating) practices (Cook-Cottone, 2015).

Generally, mindfulness has been found to be associated with improved self-regulation, physical health, self-awareness, and reduced reactivity, worries, and anxiety (Weare, 2013). Mindfulness has also been utilized as an effective intervention for youth. To illustrate, a recent meta-analysis of 20 studies found that overall mindfulness interventions with youth are helpful and do not carry iatrogenic harm (Zoogman, Goldberg, Hoyt, & Miller, 2014). The primary omnibus effect size was small to moderate at 0.23 ($p < .0001$), indicating superiority of mindfulness interventions over active control comparisons. Further, a larger effect size was found for psychological symptoms and for studies drawn from clinical samples.

Given the variety of specific formal and broader informal mindful practices, as well as protocols specifically designed for implementation in schools, researchers have struggled to aggregate studies (Zenner, Herrnleben-Kurz, & Walach, 2014). Overall, findings on mindfulness in schools suggest effectiveness and promise. For example, Zenner et al. (2014) completed a systematic review and meta-analysis on mindfulness interventions in schools, finding positive effect sizes for cognitive performance, stress reduction, and resilience. Much more on mindfulness in schools—the research, applications, and school-based programs and activities—is provided in Chapters 4 to 7 of this text.

Yoga

Yoga is a set of practices designed to bring calm, alert awareness to the mind, and health and well-being to the body (Cook-Cottone, 2015). As practiced in schools, yoga consists of a set of physical postures called asanas, regulated breathing techniques called pranayama, relaxation, and meditation (Cook-Cottone, 2015; Hagen & Nayar, 2014). There is a growing body of evidence that suggests that yoga can help with the development of executive functions like self-control, self-discipline, and creativity (Diamond & Lee, 2011). Yoga works by helping the practitioner develop a calm yet highly alert awareness within the context of embodied action (Cook-Cottone, 2015). It is believed that calm and alert awareness helps school performance. To illustrate, both independent and collaborative learning require both *stirrha* (i.e., structure) and *sukkha* (i.e., ease). That is, there needs to be a balance of structure and ease. To be successful, students need to demonstrate self-control and discipline (stirrha), as well as the creativity and flexibility that come from ease with content and materials (sukkha; Diamond & Lee, 2011). There are a variety of formal yoga practices (e.g., asana [yoga poses], breath work, relaxation, and meditation), informal practices, and yoga protocols specifically designed for schools. These, along with yoga theory, a review of Eastern yoga roots and current practices, as well as a review of research, are discussed in Chapters 8 to 11 of this text.

THE MY-SEL: FROM ARCHITECT TO CONSTRUCTION OF MEANING

As introduced earlier, the Vygotskian framework of school-as-mentor holds that there are mentors and apprentices that are working to teach the learner a craft. In the case of the education system, the *craft* is the construction of meaning. To do this, our students need *psychosocial tools*, and they need to learn how to use them. Mindfulness and yoga are specific sets of tools that have been developed and proven for thousands of years to enhance individual efficacy (Roeser & Peck, 2009). Given that mindfulness and yoga share common values and methodologies with SEL, SL, and CE (Lawlor, 2014), they are increasingly popular and considered accepted and feasible psychosocial tools for the cultivation of SEL competencies (see Figure 1.2; Rechtschaffen, 2014). The next section details the model of the MY-SEL. You will see how these methodologies, practices, and techniques can enhance nearly any approach to student learning.

The MY-SEL

The MY-SEL can be represented as a system of both internal and external influences (see Figure 1.3). Within this context, the learner exists in a central position negotiating challenges and benefiting from both: (a) the internal and interacting influences of his or her body (i.e., genetics and current physiology and health), emotions (i.e., the internal emotion regulatory system), and thoughts (i.e., internal cognitive systems), and (b) the external and interacting influences of his or her family (i.e., microsystem), school and community (i.e., exosystem), and culture and society (i.e., macrosystem). At the center, the *self as effective learner* practices the integration and attunement of two critical aspects of being: (a) self-regulation and care, and (b) intentional, reflective engagement. In this way, the self as effective learner is the architect of his or her own learning and experience.

The Effective Learner as Central Architect

The learner is the effective, central actor in his or her own educational journey (Roeser & Peck, 2009). The effective action of the student is manifest in internal self-care and regulation and in the external school environment promoting a freedom to learn and perhaps even a

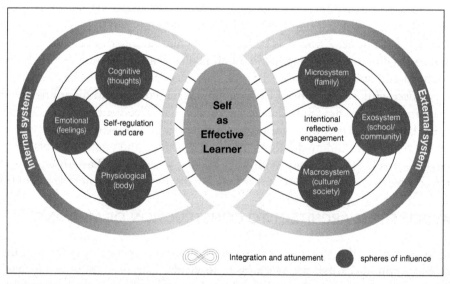

FIGURE 1.3 The mindful and yogic self as effective learner.

transcendence of formal education. It is important to note that, within the MY-SEL model, the dualistic notion of mind over matter holds. That means that the learners, you and me as students of life as well as the students in the classroom, have the ability to create our own learning experiences in a manner that is not solely determined by the apparent physical limitations of our brains. I tell the students with whom I work, "You are the boss of your brain. Don't let it tell you what is and is not possible." For example, when I am working with a child who has attention difficulties, I explain, "This is good information you now have about your brain. It is harder for your brain to pay attention than it is for a lot of other students' brains. Now, it is your responsibility to secure the tools that will help your brain attend and learn." I explain to them that I don't have a great sense of direction; for some reason my brain is not very effective at navigation. I ask them, "Does this mean I should stay home and not try to go anywhere because I might get lost?" They laugh. When I ask what I should do, they answer that I should use a GPS or a map. "Yes," I say, "I need tools." Better, I explain that there are cognitive tools that help me find my way around without a GPS or a map, and they too can learn about and practice their own cognitive tools for their challenges.

Similarly, Roeser and Peck (2009) explore self-regulated learning and motivation within the framework of the Basic Levels of Self (BLoS) model. This comparatively complex and compelling model of self differentiates the concepts of *I*, defined as both active and passive awareness, and *Me*, which reflects the sense of self we hold as our ideas about ourselves, our representation of self. According to Roeser and Peck (2009), the Me-self includes our self-narratives held in long-term memory, our temperamental characteristics, emotions and moods, our beliefs, as well as our implicit motives. For example, my Me-self can be reflected in my explanation that I am not a good navigator. That is how I see myself and part of my Me-story. Within their model, the I- and the Me-selves are differentiated by the stream of consciousness inclusive of a sense of self, self-awareness, and self-reflection (Roeser & Peck, 2009). The I-self is in the experience and in the awareness of experience. According to some theorists, the I-self is the active architect of that experience, allowing me to set-shift, regulate my focus, and manage myself as I work toward a goal (Roeser & Peck, 2009). For example, it is the I-self who is finding her way to her car in the parking lot, looking at the tree line, the cars in rows, feeling the wind on her face, and using the tools that I have developed over the years to support my lack of visual–spatial awareness. It is the I-self who is recalling that, when I parked, I said, "four and two," so that I would recall that I am four rows back and two cars in. It is the I-self who keeps me focused and out of rumination about my lack of visual–spatial skills. In its way, my I-self can volitionally control my Me-self (i.e., the self I know to lack navigation skills). See Roeser and Peck (2009) for a complete description of the BLoS model.

The MY-SEL model is consistent with the BLoS model. The MY-SEL model integrates the Me-self into the cognitive and emotional aspects of the internal side of the MY-SEL model. Next, the I-self and aspects of the stream of consciousness are consistent with the *self-as-effective-learner* represented centrally in the MY-SEL model (Figure 1.3). Finally, the MY-SEL model adds the external self-system as integral to the phenomenological experience of self. That is, within the MY-SEL model, the self does not exist distinct or wholly separate from its internal (i.e., body, emotions, and thoughts) or external context (i.e., external self-system; family, school/community, and culture). Further, as reflected in Figure 1.3, the lines that weave the internal and external aspects of self together reflect the integration and attun-ement that are required for effective functioning. Integration is the bringing together of each of the aspects of self, both in service of being in the present moment and in action within relationships and toward goals.

In his book, *The Mindful Therapist: A Clinician's Guide to Mindsight and Neural Integration,* Siegel describes the importance of differentiation before integration. I often explain to my students and patients that the human body is a beautiful example of differentiation and integration within an effective system. I explain that the liver, stomach, heart, and lungs are all made of tissue, human cells. If they were undifferentiated masses of cells, they could not perform their critical roles as organs in our body. We would have no filtering of the blood, storing of glycogen, digestion of food, or pumping and oxygenation of blood. Without differentiation, our organs and, by default, our bodies could not function. Also, we need our organs to work together, to integrate as an effective system. The integration is as critical as the differentiation. Analogously, each aspect of our psychosocial self works in this same way. We must be able to differentiate our cognitions, emotions, and physical self; the unique needs and demands of our families, friends, school community, and cultures, as well as our roles within them. The differentiation allows for effective integration of our own abilities and strengths within the context of our unique roles within the external systems.

Critically, attunement is the quality of effective integration within self and within the context of your relationships and external world. Attunement is the ability to experience reciprocal and supportive processes and interactions within, with those in our lives, and within the context of community and culture. As you see in the MY-SEL model (see Figure 1.3), the mindful and yogic self (center) is aware of each aspect of self and is the central architect of how these processes are integrated and attuned as the self develops and learns.

How we, as educators, view this process can play a substantial role in how students internalize their understanding of the centrality of their role in learning (see Figure 1.3; External System). We have known this for a long time. In his 1973 essay titled, "The Banking Concept of Education," Freire (2013) writes about a narrator concept of teaching in which the teacher talks about reality as if it were "motionless, static, compartmentalized and predictable," as if it were a commodity, money to be placed in a bank (p. 103). He explains that, within the context of the banking concept of education, teachers fill students with the content of their narration of words, words disconnected from reality, emptied of their concreteness and experienced as hollow and alienating (Freire, 2013). Education, then, becomes an act of depositing. Implicit in the banking concept of learning is the assumption of a dichotomy between human beings (e.g., students) and the world (Freire, 2013). In his words, "a person is merely *in* the world not *with* the world or with others; the individual is spectator and not a creator" (Freire, 2013). It is what I believed happened to me over the years of learning. I slowly left my embodied, active self and became a bank account in which I facilitated deposits of information. Consistent with the model of self as effective learner (MY-SEL; Figure 1.3), and what I hope for all students, Freire (2013) argues for students to be active subjects, not objects, in a conscious problem-posing education. In this way, we teach the students the content of academics and we give them tools (Karpov, 2014). Ultimately, the self as effective learner is viewed as the problem-solving architect of knowledge (Siegel, 1999).

Embodied Experience and Practices as the Facilitators of Learning

The MY-SEL model holds that embodied experiences and practices are the facilitators of learning (see Chapter 3). To educate students for work, civic engagement, and life, it is believed by many that students must acquire the collective, organized body of information, as well as actively practice the skills that allow them to comprehend and use the material (Dewey, 1938). If learning is the internalization of knowledge, skills, and tools, then what is the role of experience? Experience allows for an externalized practice in which students can eventually internalize psychological tools (Karpov, 2014). Experience and practice allow the learners to do in order to know. Karpov (2014) argues effectively that psychological tools cannot be taught in a lecture format. It is in the application of knowledge within the context of experience that the tools of self-regulation and care, as well as intentional reflective engagement, become critically important. As we apply what we know to real-world problems and challenges, not only must we deal with the limits of our concrete knowledge and set of skills, we must also negotiate the needs, strengths, and limitations of our bodies, our emotions, and our mental states. We need to teach academic tools as well as the tools that help us with our ways of being with the challenges we face (see Figure 1.4).

Noah was a first-grade boy with severe behavioral problems. He had many family issues that included drug and alcohol abuse, drug-related criminal mischief, and borderline neglect. Despite many visits from child protective services, he remained in his home, with few improvements. Noah brought all of his stress and anger to school with him each morning. One-on-one, he was insightful, reflective, and surprisingly thoughtful. He was able to problem-solve the behavioral difficulties he had experienced the previous day and plan for interpersonal challenges that would likely present in the classroom after our meeting. If this were the only assessment of his success, that is, his ability to know the information and list the skills he needed to use, he would have demonstrated a 100% success rate. However, it was the experience, the lived, in-the-moment behavioral choices that were his challenges. This well intentioned, insightful, stressed first grader was unable to utilize what he knew and the skills that he could articulately describe when he needed them most. In the lived experience, all he knew did not seem to matter. Noah needed real-time, active practice.

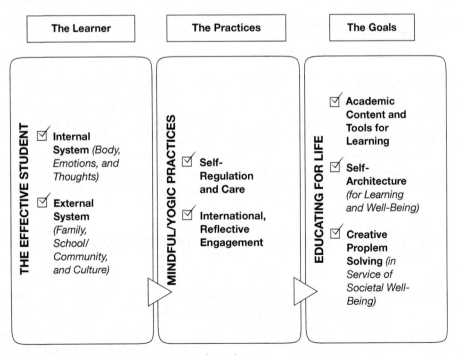

FIGURE 1.4 Learner, practices, and goals.

As part of an after-school program, Noah took part in a twice-weekly, 60-minute yoga session. The teachers noted that he really struggled to pay attention. In fact, there were times when they wondered if he heard anything they were saying. The class would be in tree pose, or deep breathing, and it seemed as though Noah was somewhere else. To be certain, he was rarely in tree pose. Before class, he would get into disagreements with others and needed constant redirection to get back on his mat during sessions. Each week, yoga class began with each student stating what they were working on. Each week, Noah told the group he was working on breathing and thinking before acting when he was mad. For the first few weeks, the teachers reported that, despite Noah's proclamations, he seemed to be struggling. Over time, the teachers began to notice something different. They noticed that he had begun to hold poses longer. His breathing had become part of his yoga practice as well. The teachers noticed that, in active and challenging poses like lunge, Noah appeared to be using his breathing and self-talk to persevere. During his active, embodied yoga practice, Noah was applying the very tools that could help him with peers and in class.

It was around the fourth week of yoga class that the yoga teachers noticed a shift. Noah had rolled out his mat and walked away to get a drink of water. Another student sat down on Noah's mat to begin class. Class started; Noah was just returning only to see another child on his mat. The teachers described how Noah clearly chose intentional, reflective thinking and breathing. He stood, perhaps for 10 seconds, staring at the little boy on his mat. Noah placed a hand on his own stomach and breathed. He walked over to where the yoga mats were stored, picked one up and rolled it out, noticeably far from his first mat and the little boy who had taken his spot. The teachers acknowledged his good choices as an example of using your yoga *off the mat* (see Chapter 10). Through embodied practice, Noah was able to bring skills to his social world and set himself up for even more learning. It was from this shift in his behavior that Noah was able to more successfully benefit from the academic aspects of his classroom. As shown in Figure 1.4, Noah demonstrated the *self-as-effective-learner* as he practiced the integration and attunement of two critical aspects of being, his own: (a) self-regulation and care, and (b) intentional, reflective engagement. In this way, Noah was an effective learner and an empowered architect of his own learning and experience.

Dewey (1938) argues, "there is an intimate and necessary relation between the processes of actual experience and education" (p. 20). There must be real-time opportunities for growth and learning. As the teachers and schools provide learning environments that facilitate the development of an engaged and active learner, the internal experience of the student is also central (see Figure 1.4). For Noah, there was no learning if there was no self-regulation. Further, there was no self-regulation without the opportunity to actively practice the skills on his yoga mat and then within the classroom.

CULTIVATING THE QUALITIES OF A MY-SEL: MINDFULNESS AND YOGA PRACTICES

The qualities of mindful and yogic learners can be viewed in terms of the self-system (i.e., internal or external) in which they are most actionable (see Table 1.1). First, some student learning occurs independently. Within the internal system of cognitions, feelings, and physiology, self-regulation is the key mechanism of effective functioning and facilitator of learning. Specifically, the independent activities of learning require the student

TABLE 1.1 Qualities of a Mindful and Yogic Learner

INTERNAL SYSTEM QUALITIES (SELF-REGULATION AND CARE)	EXTERNAL SYSTEM QUALITIES (INTENTIONAL, REFLECTIVE ENGAGEMENT)

Independent Learner Skills
 • Self-regulation
   – Self-awareness
   – Executive control
   – Emotion regulation
   – Stress regulation
   – Responsible decision making
 • Self-care
   – Mind–body awareness
   – Healthy behaviors
   – Self-compassion
	Collaborative Learner Skills
	 • Intentional, reflective engagement with others
	   – Social awareness
	   – Compassion for others
	   – Maintenance of close, secure, meaningful, and positive relationships
	 • Intentional, reflective engagement in learning and service
	   – Inquiry
	   – Active, intentional learning
	   – Civic contribution

Source: Ashdown and Bernard (2012), CASEL (2003, 2005), Diamond and Lee (2011), Durlak et al. (2011), Elias et al. (1997), Greenberg and Harris (2012), Parlakian (2003), Weare (2013), and Willard (2016).

to be self-regulated and engaged. That is, a well-regulated learner is able to demonstrate self-awareness, executive control, emotion and stress regulation, and responsible decision making. Further, he or she shows positive self-care skills that begin with mind and body awareness, health-promoting behaviors, and self-compassion. The learner has the psychological and self-care tools needed to be in the classroom ready to learn.

One of the most compelling reasons to bring mindfulness and yoga into the classroom is stress and trauma. Childress and Harper (2015), Willard (2016), and Steele and Malchiodi (2012) all underscore the unmatched stress and trauma exposure experienced by children today. The stress and trauma experienced is embodied and integrated as our students develop into adults (Damasio, 1999). In addition to the potential learning outcomes, a key benefit of implemented mindfulness and yoga programs is giving our children and youth tools to manage their stress and negotiate the effects of trauma as it presents in day-to-day life. Willard (2016) describes this generation of teens as the most stressed on record with high achievement demands, a seemingly unsteady economy, testing, domestic and foreign terrorism, and ongoing war. Many of our students have too few tools to deal with all they hear and see, including the stress in their own homes. A student with knowledge of breathing techniques, who can slow his or her breath, find grounding and stillness within his or her own body, and act with intention, even when triggered and upset, has a substantial advantage in today's schools.

Next, as much of learning is collaborative, the effective learner is also able to negotiate the external system in a manner that facilitates learning and creativity. Learning and the development of creative ideas are often the fruit of family, student–teacher, and peer relationships. Of course, self-regulation and management of the internal system is key. For example, it is readily accepted that self-regulation, especially emotion regulation, is required for a student to learn successfully within the context of relationships (Durlak et al., 2011). As the tasks of the internal self-system are managed, external engagement is enhanced. Further, the effective learner has the psychosocial tools and skills needed to present as intentional and reflective while engaged with others. These skills include social awareness, compassion for others, and relationship skills. Empowered with these tools and skills, the effective learner presents with a sense of inquiry, engagement in active and intentional learning, as well as a commitment to civic contribution and creation of meaning. From the regulation of the internal aspects of self to the active commitment to contributing to community and culture, the self-as-effective-learner is grounded in a solid sense of who he or she is, the strengths and challenges, and his or her valued place within the ecology.

Mindfulness and yoga-based methodologies are the psychosocial tools for these processes. As mindfulness and yoga are the foci of this text, they are introduced here briefly and expanded upon theoretically, empirically, and practically in the following chapters.

LEARN FOR YOURSELF: PRACTICE IS FOR STUDENTS AND TEACHERS

Ultimately, mindfulness and yoga practices ask you to learn from your own practice. In this way, you are the researcher. Mindfulness and yoga practices require the teacher to be the very things he or she hopes to teach the students. In order to teach these skills effectively, it is believed that you must understand the journey, the challenges, and the benefits. In her essay titled, "Success in East Harlem," Meier (2013) writes, "We have also become better observers of our own practice, as well as more open and aware of alternative practices" (p. 145). In Comer et al.'s groundbreaking book, Joyner (1999) writes, "To ask the best of children, we must ask the best of ourselves" (p. 277). The truth is modeling matters (Joyner, 1999). The teacher is a practitioner. David and Sheth (2009) suggest that gaining experience with practices such as mindfulness and yoga prepares you to teach these skills with authenticity. In the book, *Mindful Teaching and Teaching Mindfulness: A Guide for Anyone Who Teaches Anything*, David and Sheth (2009) describe the reciprocal relationship between mindful teaching, which nurtures the learner, and teaching mindfulness through direct instruction. As with other subjects, information and instruction is followed by practice (David & Sheth, 2009). I would argue that it starts with practice.

CONCLUSION

This chapter presented an overview of the historical pathway of education to the implementation of mindfulness and yoga in schools. The concept of the student as active architect of his or her own learning was emphasized within a Vygoskian constructivistic framework, with references to more recent neurobiological understandings of the brain, relationships, and learning. The specific tools of mindfulness and yoga within the context of SEL, CE, and SL were discussed. The MY-SEL model was introduced and reviewed, and the concepts of yoga and mindfulness were presented as technologies for learning. The shortcomings in the body of research in the field of mindfulness and yoga were reviewed to potentiate the reader to look critically at the evidence presented as techniques, tools, and protocols that are introduced in the forthcoming chapters. Last, the importance of the teacher's own practice was emphasized in accordance with an ongoing personal mantra of mine, which I believe makes me a better teacher and yogi: "We can't give what we don't have."

REFERENCES

Ashdown, D. M., & Bernard, M. (2012). Can explicit instruction in social and emotional learning skills benefit the social-emotional development, well-being, and academic achievement of young children? *Early Childhood Education, 39,* 397–405.

Berman, S. (2015). *Service learning: A guide to planning, implementing, and assessing student projects* (2nd ed.). New York, NY: First Skyhorse Publishing.

Billig, S. (2000). Research on K-12 school-based service-learning: The evidence builds. *Phi Delta Kappa, 81,* 658–664. http://digitalcommons.unomaha.edu/slcek12/3

Celio, A. I., Durlack, J., & Dymnicki, A. (2011). A meta-analysis of the impact of service learning on students. *Journal of Experiential Education, 34,* 165–181.

Childress, T., & Harper, J. C. (2015). *Best practices for yoga in schools.* Atlanta, GA: Yoga Service Council.

Collaborative for Academic, Social, Emotional Learning (2003). *Safe and sound: An educational leader's guide to evidence-based social and emotional learning (SEL) programs.* Chicago, IL: Author.

Collaborative for Academic, Social, Emotional Learning (2005). *Safe and sound: An educational leader's guide to evidence-based social and emotional learning (SEL) programs.* Chicago, IL: Author.

Comer, J. P. (1988). Educating poor minority children. *Scientific American, 259,* 42–48.

Comer, J. P., Ben-Avie, M., Haynes, N. M., & Joyner, E. (1999). *Child by child: The Comer process for change in education.* New York, NY: Teachers College Press.

Cook-Cottone, C. (2006). The attuned representational model for the primary prevention of eating disorders: An overview for school principals. *Psychology in the Schools, 43,* 223–230.

Cook-Cottone, C. (2013). Dosage as a critical variable in yoga therapy research. *International Journal of Yoga Therapy, 23,* 11–12.

Cook-Cottone, C. P. (2015). *Mindfulness and yoga for self-regulation: A primer for mental health professionals.* New York, NY: Springer Publishing.

Damasio, A. (1999). The feeling of what happens: Body and emotion in the making of consciousness. Fort Worth, TX: Harcourt College.

David, D. S., & Sheth, S. (2009). *Mindful teaching and teaching mindfulness: A guide for anyone teaching anything.* Boston, MA: Wisdom Publications.

Dewey, J. (1900). The school and society: The child and the curriculum. Chicago, IL: Centennial Publications of the University of Chicago Press.

Dewey, J. (1916). *Democracy and education.* New York, NY: The Macmillan Company.

Dewey, J. (1938). *Experience and education.* New York, NY: Simon & Schuster.

Diamond, A., & Lee, K. (2011). Interventions shown to aid executive function development in children 4-12 years old. *Science, 333,* 959–964.

DiPerna, J. C., & Elliot, S. N. (2002). Promoting academic enablers to improve student achievement: An introduction to the mini-series. *School Psychology Review, 31,* 293–297.

Durlak, J. A., Weissberg, R. P., Dymnicki, A. B., Taylor, R. D., & Schellinger, K. B. (2011). The impact of enhancing students' social and emotional learning: A meta-analysis of school-based universal interventions. *Child Development, 82,* 405–432.

Elias, M. J., Zins, J. E., Weissberg, R. P., Frey, K. S., Greenberg, M. T., Haynes, N. M., . . . Shriver, T. P. (1997). *Promoting social and emotional learning: Guidelines for educators.* Alexandria, VA: Association for Supervision and Curriculum Development.

Freire, P. (2013). The banking concept of education. In A. S. Canestrari & B. A. Marlowe (Eds.), *Educational foundations: An anthology of critical readings* (3rd ed., pp. 103–115). Washington, DC: Sage.

Giles, D. E., & Eyler, J. (1994). The theoretical roots of service-learning in John Dewey: Toward a theory of service-learning. *Michigan Journal of Service Learning, 1,* 77–85.

Greenberg, M. T., & Harris, A. R. (2012). Nurturing mindfulness in children and youth: Current state of research. *Child Development Perspectives, 6,* 162–166.

Hagen, I., & Nayar, U. (2014). Yoga for children and young people's mental health and well-being: Research review and reflections on mental health potential of yoga. *Frontiers in Psychiatry, 5,* 1–6. doi:10.2289/fpsyt.2014.00035

Jennings, P. A. (2015). *Mindfulness for teachers: Simple skills for peace and productivity in the classroom.* New York, NY: W. W. Norton.

Joyner, E. T. (1999). Epilogue: To ask the best in children, we must ask the best in ourselves. In C. P. Comer, M. Ben-Avie, N. M. Haynes, & E. Joyner (Eds.), *Child by child: The Comer process for change in education* (pp. 277–283). New York, NY: Teachers College Press.

Kabat-Zinn J. (2013). *Full catastrophe living.* London, UK: Piatkus.

Karpov, Y. V. (2014). *Vygotsky for educators.* New York, NY: Cambridge University Press.

Lawlor, M. S. (2014). Mindfulness in practice: Considerations for implementation of mindfulness-based programming for adolescents in school contexts. *New Directions for Youth Development, 2014,* 83–95.

Meier, D. (2013). Success in East Harlem: How one group of teachers built a school that works. In A. S. Canestrari & B. A. Marlowe (Eds.), *Educational foundations: An anthology of critical readings* (3rd ed., pp. 141–150). Washington, DC: Sage.

Mind and Life Education Research Network, Davidson, R. J., Dunne, J., Eccles, J. S., Engle, A., Greenberg, M., . . . Vago, D. (2012). Contemplative practices and mental training: Prospects for American education. *Child Development Perspectives, 6,* 146–153.

Mindfulness All-Party Parliamentary Group (2015). Mindful nation U.K. The Mindfulness Initiative. Retrieved from http://www.themindfulnessinitiative.org.uk

Mondale, S., & Patton, S. B. (2001). *School: The story of public education.* Boston, MA: Beacon Press.

Parlakian, R. (2003). *Before the ABCs: Promoting school readiness in infants and toddlers.* Washington, DC: Zero to Three.

Philibert, C. T. (2016a). *Everyday SEL in elementary school: Integrating social-emotional learning and mindfulness into your classroom.* New York, NY: Routledge.

Philibert, C. T. (2016b). *Everyday SEL in middle school: Integrating social-emotional learning and mindfulness into your classroom.* New York, NY: Routledge.

Rechtschaffen, D. (2014). *The way of mindful education: Cultivating well-being in teachers and students.* New York, NY: W. W. Norton.

Rogers, C. (1983). *Freedom to learn.* New York, NY: Merrill.

Roeser, R. W., & Peck, S. C. (2009). An education in awareness: Self, motivation, and self-regulated learning in contemplative perspective. *Educational Psychologist, 44,* 199–136.

Schonert-Reichl, K. A., & Lawlor, M. S. (2010). The effects of a mindfulness-based education program on pre- and early adolescents' well-being and social and emotional competence. *Mindfulness, 1*(3), 137–151. doi:10.1007/s12671-010-001108

Schonfeld, D. J., Adams, R. E., Fredstrom, B. K., Weissberg, R. P., Gilman, R., Voyce, C., . . . Speese-Linehan, D. (2014). Cluster-randomized trial demonstrating impact on academic achievement of elementary social-emotional learning. *School Psychology Quarterly, 30*(3), 406–420. doi:10.1037/spq0000099

Siegel, D. J. (1999). *The developing mind: Toward a neurobiological understanding of interpersonal relationships.* New York, NY: Guilford Press.

Siegel, D. J. (2015). Forward. *Mindfulness for teachers: Simple skills for peace and productivity in the classroom.* New York, NY: W. W. Norton.

Steele, W., & Malchiodi, C. A. (2012). *Trauma-informed practices with children and adolescents.* New York, NY: Routledge.

Vygotsky, L. S. (1978). *Mind in society: The development of higher psychological processes.* Cambridge, MA: Harvard University Press.

Warren, J. L. (2012). Does service learning increase student learning?: A meta-analysis. *Michigan Journal of Community Service Learning, 18*(2), 56–61.

Waters, L., Barsky, A., Ridd, A., & Allen, K. (2015). Contemplative education: A systematic, evidence-based review of the effect of meditation interventions in schools. *Educational Psychology Review, 27,* 103–134.

Weare, K. (2013). Developing mindfulness with children and young people: A review of the evidence and policy context. *Journal of Children's Services, 2,* 141–153.

Willard, C. (2016). *Growing up mindful: Essential practices to help teens and families find balance, calm, and resilience*. Boulder, CO: Sounds True.

Zenner, C., Herrnleben-Kurz, S., & Walach, H. (2014). Mindfulness-based interventions in schools—A systematic review and meta-analysis. *Frontiers in Psychology, 5,* 603. doi:10.3389/fpsyg.2014.00603

Zoogman, S., Goldberg, S. B., Hoyt, W. T., & Miller, L. (2014). Mindfulness interventions with youth: A meta-analysis. *Mindfulness, 6,* 290–302.

CHAPTER 2

DYSREGULATION TO DISORDER: DEVELOPMENT, RISKS, AND OUTCOMES RELATED TO A LACK OF SELF-REGULATORY SKILLS—A THREE-TIER APPROACH

The Africa Yoga Project teachers said
these were the three most important ways
yoga had changed their lives:

"I value my life more.
I trust myself more.
My life has more meaning and/or purpose."

—Klein, Cook-Cottone, and Giambrone (2015, p. 121)

In the mindful and yogic framework, there is an acceptance of vulnerabilities, challenges, and life events. These things are expected. Ultimately, *the practice* is in the effective manifestation of your life's work within the context of what life has presented to you. It is an empowering way to view the world and one's life. In this way, your work is not about fixing anything because nothing is considered broken. As you read, you may wonder how this framework fits within a school system that spends a lot of time assessing, tracking, diagnosing, and labeling children. The system of sorting children out by their needs and abilities is complex and multitiered. It is based on a long history of schools working to effectively manage the specific learning needs of each and every student. Accordingly, there is a body of literature and research supporting current school-based practices. Despite the many years of progress, there is always more to do as educators continue to face new and complex challenges.

Teaching for the 21st-century learner means looking beyond the concept of the whole child. The Association for Supervision and Curriculum Development (ASCD) and the Centers for Disease Control and Prevention (CDC) agree (ASCD, 2014): When a student does not have the skills or support to negotiate stressors and the trials of daily life, these challenges can interfere with learning as well as academic progress, and may cause additional struggles that preclude the completion of school (e.g., learning disabilities, attention deficits, substance use, student alienation, mental health issues, and violence; Greenberg et al., 2003).

Accordingly, educators have been working to address these challenges as well as to develop preventive strategies to develop resilience and health (Greenberg & Harris, 2012; Liew, 2012). Acknowledging that the process is about more than cognitive academic achievement, the CDC's latest definition of academic achievement includes academic performance (i.e., grades, test scores, and graduation rates), educational behavior (i.e., attendance, rates of dropout, and school behavioral problems), and cognitive skills and attitudes (i.e., mood, concentration, and memory; ASCD, 2014).

Together, the ASCD and the CDC created the Whole School, Whole Community, and Whole Child (WSCC) model, calling for a greater alignment, integration, and collaboration between education and health, "to improve each child's cognitive, physical, social and emotional development" (ASCD, 2014, p. 6). The WSCC model is an ecological approach directed at the whole school, acknowledging that the school draws its resources from the community in efforts to service the whole child. Consistent with the Mindful and Yogic Self as Effective Learner (MY-SEL) model (see Chapter 1, Figure 1.3), the ecological context and the health and well-being of the child are viewed as critical components of facilitating academic performance. When things are going well, the student's inner experiences (i.e., physiological, emotional, and cognitive) are integrated and attuned through a process of self-regulation and care. When a student is resilient and shows what people call grit, he or she is able to effectively negotiate external challenges and demands in order to experience everyday and long-term success (Duckworth & Gross, 2014).

A philosophy firmly grounded in the Social Emotional Learning (SEL) movement holds that a key challenge to 21st-century schools involves educating diverse students with varied abilities, neurological and behavioral readiness, and motivation for learning (e.g., Durlak, Weissberg, Dymnicki, Taylor, & Schellinger, 2011). Some believe the challenges students bring into school, accompanied by deficits in social–emotional competencies, create risk for a lack of connection with individual learning and school in general (Durlak et al., 2011). The MY-SEL model suggests that there is more to academic, school, and life success than intelligence and natural ability. There is a growing body of work suggesting that, through practices such as mindfulness and yoga, individuals can develop self-regulation, self-control, interpersonal effectiveness, and grit (e.g., Cook-Cottone, 2015; Duckworth & Gross, 2014; Duckworth, Peterson, Mathews, & Kelly, 2007; Duckworth & Quinn, 2009; Perkins-Gough, 2013). The MY-SEL model holds that these skills can be, and should be, taught and practiced in schools. As such, it also holds that, when these skills are not taught and practiced, students may languish or, worse, descend into school failure and disorder.

THE DYSREGULATED AND DISENGAGED STUDENT

The MY-SEL model illustrates the connection between self-regulation and care (see the internal system, Figure 1.3) and intentional, reflective engagement with school (see the external system, Figure 1.3). I remember when I was a graduate student in school psychology, and my mom, an English teacher, would try so hard to understand the *one thing* that was getting in the way of a particular student's learning. She would wonder if it is were trouble at home, anxiety, drug use, or fatigue from working late. You see, she thought that if it were just one thing, she could target it. I know for sure that my mom would have done anything she could have to fix anything that was holding her students back. I agree that, every so often, it is one thing. And every so often, we can identify that thing and support the student.

When we do, the pathway to learning is opened up. For example, a student might have an abusive parent in the home and, with support, the parent might get help. With the potential changes in the family, the student was freed from chronic stress and domestic violence and could focus on his or her studies. However, as I was beginning to learn in school, through my work in neighborhood centers and group homes, and would later experience directly in schools, school disengagement and failure are, more often than not, a complex mix of risk factors that present within the student, the school environment, family, and community. School is like life in this way. It's complicated.

For example, Alesha, age 16, dropped out of school because of obstacles that she believe she could not surmount. For Alesha, despite years of adequate academic progress in elementary school, a bumpy yet manageable middle school experience, 10th grade was more than she could handle. It wasn't *one thing*. There was trouble at home, and it was often difficult to study. Her older brother had dropped out and was in and out of trouble with the police. Alesha had always been an anxious child, following after her mother, and her worries about her brother and her parents got in the way of her ability to pay attention in class and persist in longer homework assignments. School felt frenetic, and many of the teachers seemed stressed and overworked. She was starting to struggle in the classes that required her to write papers. She felt overwhelmed by them and did not know where to start. She avoided the classes in which the outlines and drafts were due. She no-showed for afterschool help. It was difficult for her to get in to see the school counselor, school psychologist, or school social worker because they all worked across several buildings, and their schedules were difficult to access and figure out. There were teachers who cared and tried, but Alesha didn't trust them and often avoided the people who could have helped her. Alesha's response to all of it was to shut down emotionally, disengage socially, and sidestep her schoolwork. On the outside, this looked like resistance and lack of effort as her behaviors did little to engender the support that she needed. The school had long ago cut its social and emotional learning program and had only one part-time counselor to offer support to the hundreds of students in the building. Feeling a need to do something positive in her life, Alehsa got a job at a local salon helping out. She felt needed there, made some side money to help around the house, and felt part of a community. Whenever she thought about school, she was overwhelmed. Alesha had only a few positive coping skills and felt disarmed when it came to approaching academic challenges. There were no programs at school and no one at home to model them for her. Without intention and skills to help her handle her distress, her lack of attendance gradually transitioned to school dropout status.

Benjamin, age 15, experienced the challenges in a different way. He lived with his grandmother because his dad had been incarcerated, and his mom was engaged in an ongoing struggle with substance abuse. Child protective services had placed Benjamin in kinship care with his grandmother because his mother did not provide adequate supervision or food. Benjamin was the oldest and worked hard to try to keep his family together. His grandmother drank nightly, and, although she provided basic care, she often needed a lot of help to get dinner to the table and the younger kids to bed. Benjamin's grandmother was also actively dating and had her boyfriend, and sometimes his friends, to the house on school nights. By the time Benjamin got to school some mornings, he was exhausted and irritable. He had been behind in reading during his early elementary years and had been placed initially in academic intervention services and then special education. He also had a long list of discipline referrals. Benjamin did not respect adults, including adults at school. If you asked Benjamin, he would explain that his mother, grandmother, and father were all less committed to raising his young siblings than he was. Teachers did not like working with Benjamin as he seemed resistant and disinterested in class. Things took a turn for the worse when his mom began living at his grandmother's house. She was out of control with her substance use, creating a chaotic home environment when layered on top of the grandmother's drinking. Benjamin was terrified that child protective services would remove him and his siblings from the house and separate them. At school, he was increasingly distracted and irritable. This escalated into a confrontation with his teacher, which resulted in an in-school suspension. Like Alesha, Benjamin had no pathway for developing the coping skills that he needed to negotiate the stress at home and effectively manage the school environment.

For many students, intelligence and learning skills are only a small part of what they need to learn. Duckworth et al. (2007) suggest that there are two questions. Citing James (1907), the Duckworth team asks: (a) What are the human abilities? and (b) By what means can one unleash these abilities? (Duckworth et al., 2007). Yoga and mindfulness cannot increase IQ or innate abilities (i.e., the first question). They can, however, help students unleash their abilities. Helping students develop an effective sense of self is critical to long-term academic engagement and achievement. Risk and disorder commonly co-occur with ineffective self-regulation and care within the internal system (see Chapter 1, Figure 1.3, and Figure 2.1). Further, risk and disorder can be exacerbated by stress, trauma, reactivity, lack of support, and disengagement within the external systems. Often, there is also an absence of integration and attunement linking each of the aspects of self (e.g., cognition, emotional, physiological) and the external experiences of family, school, community, and culture. As illustrated in Figure 2.1, there is little differentiation between each aspect of the self and essentially no effective attunement and connection between them. There is no clear sense of self within the inner experience or within the context of the outer world. There is no perseverance, distress tolerance, self-regulation, or grit. The student feels overwhelmed within the academic environment and has no tools, as illustrated by Alesha and Benjamin.

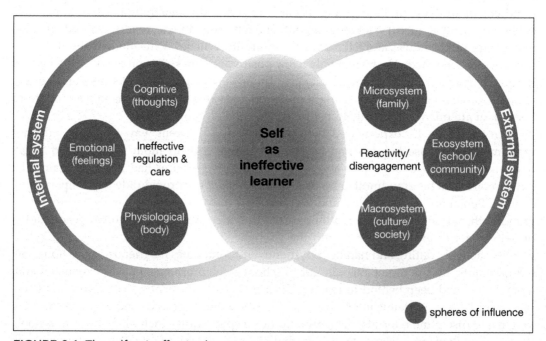

FIGURE 2.1 The self as ineffective learner.

TABLE 2.1 Qualities of the Ineffective Learner

INTERNAL SYSTEM QUALITIES (SELF-REGULATION AND CARE)	EXTERNAL SYSTEM QUALITIES (INTENTIONAL, REFLECTIVE ENGAGEMENT)

Independent Learner Skills
• Low levels of self-regulation
  – Reduced self-awareness
  – Low executive control
  – Reduced emotion regulation
  – Decreased stress regulation
  – Reduced responsible decision making
• Low levels of self-care
  – Reduced mind-body awareness
  – Fewer healthy behaviors
  – Limited self-compassion
	Collaborative Learner Skills
	• Lack of intentional, reflective engagement
	  with others
	  – Lower social awareness
	  – Limited compassion for others
	  – Reduced maintenance of close, secure,
	    meaningful, and positive relationships
	• Lack of intentional, reflective engagement in
	  learning and service
	  – Less inquiry
	  – Reduced active, intentional learning
	  – Limited civic contribution

To break down the challenges into accomplishable sets of skills and link the skills into unified sets of actions, a mindful approach is required. The skills required beyond academics include competencies such as the ability to self-regulate, balance self-care and effort, and work effectively with others (Karpov, 2014). Without the cognitive, emotional, and physiological tools for self-regulation or competencies for connecting with and gaining support from friends, teachers, other school personnel, family, and other external systems, students are at risk for a host of nonacademic challenges, as well as poor academic performance, school failure, and dropout.

You will see that, across all of the challenges and struggles described in the section that follows, there is a lack of development, or a disrupted development, of the qualities cultivated and practiced in the mindful and yogic learner described in Chapter 1. Table 2.1 reviews these qualities as seen in the ineffective learners. Students who struggle have lower levels of independent learning skills and self-care. Further, they often struggle to collaborate with other students, their teachers, and members of their family and community. Ultimately, those who are struggling are often so consumed with symptoms, relationship problems, and coping that being in inquiry, reflective learning, and service to others is not accessible.

THE THREE-TIER MODEL

The three-tier model of prevention and intervention is a classification system pertinent to the field of prevention and intervention within schools (see Figure 2.2). This model highlights the importance of promoting and maintaining health and well-being, rather than solely focusing on the prevention of disease and disorder (Cook-Cottone & Vujnovic, in press; Leavell & Clark, 1953, 1958, 1965). Schools work within this three-tier system to deliver programs based on the level of student need, the likelihood of impact, and the goals of the prevention and/or intervention program. Mindfulness and yoga programs for schools are best understood within this three tier model. Working within this model helps school personnel, not familiar with mindful and yoga approaches, see more clearly and explicitly how these programs can work within the current school intervention framework.

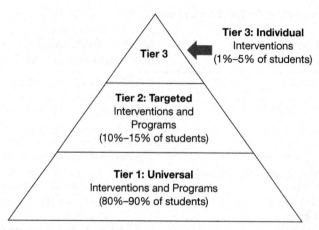

FIGURE 2.2 Three-tier model of interventions in schools.

The first tier is known as the primary prevention level, intended for the promotion of health and well-being and to provide specific protection against the onset of disease (Cook-Cottone & Vujnovic, in press). The primary prevention level includes the implementation of procedures (i.e., screening) to identify potential risk and to intercept such risk prior to the need for classification (Cook-Cottone & Vujnovic, 2016). Subsequently, secondary prevention is intended for early detection and timely treatment to prevent or limit prolonged disability, or lack of academic success for the individual (Cook-Cottone & Vujnovic, 2016). Finally, the tertiary level of prevention is considered for the treatment of symptoms, rehabilitation, and the reduction of further developmental disruption and disorder (Cook-Cottone & Vujnovic, 2016; Leavell & Clark, 1953, 1958, 1965). Notably, in the 1990s, the field of prevention adopted the terminology endorsed by the Institute of Medicine (IOM): universal, selective, and indicated (Cook-Cottone & Vujnovic, 2016).

Over the past few decades, the field of education has increasingly embraced the prevention model framework for a number of reasons, including the increased development of research documenting the efficacy of evidence-based interventions; an emphasis on the promotion of well-being; acknowledgment of the increasing levels of need among students; recognition of the limitation of resources; and a need for a cost-effective approach (Cook-Cottone & Vujnovic, 2016). In 2010, the three-tier model was outlined by the National Association of School Psychologists explicating a multitier model, school-based academic support and special education classification system (Cook-Cottone & Vujnovic, 2016; Shin & Walker, 2010). Applied within the school framework, the three-tier model is incredibly effective for providing services to all students, especially as school personnel are frequently the first line of defense against emerging academic, behavioral, and mental health problems (Cook-Cottone, Tribole, & Tylka, 2013).

Tier 1, the universal level, is conceptualized as the core instructional or social-behavioral program. Tier 1 programs are research supported and aim to meet the needs of 80% to 90% of students (Cook-Cottone & Vujnovic, 2016). Accordingly, the majority of students, including those who may be at risk for concerns, respond sufficiently to this level of programming (Stoiber, 2014). Tier 2 is the targeted level, intended to serve a smaller group of students who require increased support to enhance the core programs at the Tier 1 level (Stoiber, 2014). Tier 3 is the intensive level, designed to be individualized and strategically aligned with the needs of the individual student being serviced. This level is intended to be implemented for the smallest percentage of students, the 1% to 5% who continue to require supports beyond those in the first two tiers (Stoiber, 2014).

The process of moving a student from Tier 1 to Tier 3 intervention involves unsuccessful attempts at remediation at Tiers 1 and 2. The record of unsuccessful attempts at remediation in both Tiers 1 and 2 is termed the Response to Intervention (RTI) process. The RTI process is a problem-solving model that moves a student through the tiers of intervention in order to offer the student the least restrictive placement and academic program while still meeting the student's academic, emotional, and behavioral needs. Often, assessment is interwoven throughout the tiers so that the best fit can be made between the student's needs and the intervention of choice. For example, if a student was found to be struggling with self-regulation (i.e., Joey often does not think before he speaks or interacts with others, gets in fights with peers, and has a few discipline referrals), despite a school-wide SEL program, the student might be selected to partake in a smaller mindfulness and yoga group for students with impulsivity and anger management issues—designed to increased self-awareness and self-regulation. Joey might respond positively to such a program and no longer need support. Or Joey may not respond enough to the intervention (e.g., Joey is getting into fewer fights), warranting increase frequency, duration, or intensity of the program. If those changes do not support behavioral change, Joey might be assessed by the school psychologist for consideration for referral to another program or for a Tier 3 program that integrates more structure, a smaller class size, and continued work on self-regulation. Ultimately, the goal of the three-tier system and the individualized RTI model is to allow students like Alesha, Benjamin, and Joey to remain in the least restrictive learning environment with the most appropriate level of support.

Tier 1: Approaches for the Promotion of Self-Regulation and Care and Intentional, Reflective Engagement

Tier 1 approaches for health and well-being promotion are interventions at the universal level. In general, they are core instructional or social–behavioral programs that are implemented for all students within the school and likely to be sufficient in meeting the needs of the majority of students (Stoiber, 2014). For example, yoga might be offered school wide as part of a school district's social–emotional learning program. In this way, each student takes part in a yoga class two to three times per week as part of his or her routine academic schedule. There is a long-standing history in the provision of universal programs in education that illustrates the link between physical health and learning. For example, school lunch programs were among the first interventions provided within the school setting to address a foundational health need that was notably interfering with student learning (Cook-Cottone & Vujnovic, 2016; Cook-Cottone, Tribole et al., 2013). Since first initiated, school-based programs to promote nutrition and physical health have grown substantially. They now include large-scale, federally funded school lunch programs and integrated physical and health education. They also target all levels of well-being support from supportive counseling services to family support. Current implementation issues hinge on funding, challenges related to scheduling and time constraints, and finding evidence-based programs that meet school needs (Cook-Cottone & Vujnovic, 2016).

Beyond the provision of school lunches, there is emerging evidence that universal practices designed to promote well-being and health are effective in schools (Cook-Cottone,

Tribole et al., 2013; Shoshani & Steinmetz, 2013). However, research is in the early stages; much of the evidence is based on pilot studies or short-term controlled trials as opposed to more rigorous, randomized trials. At the universal level, there is a significant need for higher quality research with randomized controlled trials and assessment of long-term outcomes in areas such as yoga and mindfulness (Serwacki & Cook-Cottone, 2012; Shoshani & Steinmetz, 2013). Social–emotional learning programs may be having a documented effect. Reviews of available research related to universal programs have identified several key factors across programs that are believed to play a role in student well-being at the universal level, including the cultivation of positive emotions, gratitude, hope, goal setting, and development of character strengths (Shoshani & Steinmetz, 2013). Overall, research on SEL programs indicates that they result in an increase in student well-being (Ashdown & Bernard, 2012; Durlak et al., 2011). Benefits include increased emotional regulation, self-awareness, stress management, relationship skills, social awareness, and an impact on learning (Ashdown & Bernard, 2012; Durlak et al., 2011). These larger-scale, often school- and district-wide approaches provide a foundational context for more specific programs that focus on healthy eating and physical health promotion. Specific mindful and yoga protocols are reviewed throughout this book.

Tier 2: Approaches to Facilitate Self-Regulation and Intentional, Reflective Engagement

Tier 2 approaches are intended to serve a smaller group of students who require increased support to enhance the core programs at the Tier 1 level (Stoiber, 2014). Tier 2 programs often target a specific risk group (e.g., students scoring low on state exams) or students already showing risk factors (e.g., behavioral referrals) without manifesting full diagnostic criteria (Cook-Cottone & Vujnovic, 2016).

Programs such as *Girls Growing in Wellness and Balance: Yoga and Life Skills to Empower* (GGWB), which utilize yoga and a risk-reducing curriculum, can be used as a Tier 2 intervention for girls at risk for eating disorders. To participate, students may have been identified by a school screening program, the child study team, peer report, teacher observation, or parent report. Once referred, the student is invited to take part in the Tier 2 intervention. In this case, the student takes part in a 14-week program that integrates yoga, relaxation, and specific psycho-educational lessons and activities designed to reduce eating disorder risk factors and increase protective factors. The GGWB program has been found, in controlled trials, to reduce body dissatisfaction, increase self-care, and decrease drive for thinness (Cook-Cottone, Kane, Keddie, & Haugli, 2013; Scime & Cook-Cottone, 2008; Serwacki & Cook-Cottone, 2012). However, for this program and other Tier 2 programs, there is still much work needed before there is an evidence base built on randomized controlled trials. Mindfulness and yoga programs that meet Tier 2 intervention criteria are reviewed throughout this text along with current outcomes and the need for future research.

Tier 3: Assessing and Supporting Students in Self-Regulation and Intentional, Reflective Engagement

Once a student is showing symptoms of a disorder (e.g., anxiety, attention, substance use), he or she should be considered for a Tier 3 level of intervention (Cook-Cottone & Vujnovic, 2016). Tier 3 is the highest level of intensity, designed to be individualized and strategically aligned with the student's individual needs (Stoiber, 2014). Further, Tier 3 approaches often involve a coordination of care, aligning school efforts, and outside provider treatments (e.g., psychologist). For some students, Tier 3 interventions can be handled entirely within the school, while for others there is a sharing of treatment provision within the school and community.

The three-tier system, putting prevention first, is needed. The Youth Risk Behavior Surveillance System (YRBSS), which monitors six categories of priority health-risk behaviors among youth and young adults using the Youth Risk Behavior Survey (YRBS), found that many high school students (grades 9–12) are engaged in priority health-risk behaviors associated with the leading causes of death among persons aged 10 to 24 years in the United States (Kann et al., 2014). In a nationally representative face-to-face survey of 10,123 adolescents aged 13 to 18 years, Merikangas et al. (2010) found that approximately one in every four to five youth in the United States meets criteria for a mental disorder with severe impairment across their lifetimes. Their disturbing numbers were followed by a plea for the United States to engage in a shift from treatment to prevention and early intervention.

THE RISKS, CHALLENGES, AND DISORDERS RELATED TO DYSREGULATION AND DISENGAGEMENT

The range of difficulties is substantial. This is why the three-tier model is in place. A large proportion of students may be typically functioning, ready to benefit from instruction in skills such as those taught in mindfulness and yoga programs. Learning these skills can help them thrive and perform at their highest academic potential. As shown in the three-tier model, depending on the risks associated with poverty, resources, community violence, and a host of other environmental, socioeconomic, cultural, community, familial, and even genetic factors, upward of 50% of students in a given district can have substantial needs. Because of this complex mix of etiologies, students engage in behaviors (e.g., substance use, violence, smoking, bullying, and sex), or fail to engage in behaviors (e.g., self-care, sobriety, caring friendships, and studying), in ways that place them at risk for the leading causes of morbidity and mortality (Kann et al., 2014). In order to orient the reader and provide a brief review of the challenges for today's schools, the most prevalent disorders (e.g., anxiety, behavioral, substance use) and problem behaviors (e.g., bullying, peer victimization) are briefly described along with research detailing prevalence, risks, and challenges.

Attention and Impulsivity

Attention difficulties and impulsivity create risk for academic failure and disengagement as well as physical safety risk. When these problems occur at a clinical level, it is referred to as attention-deficit/hyperactivity disorder (i.e., ADHD). Specifically, ADHD manifests as a persistent pattern of inattention that may or may not be associated with hyperactivity and impulsivity (American Psychiatric Association [APA], 2013). Further, the attention, activity, and impulsivity symptoms interfere with school and daily functions (APA, 2013). Children and adolescents who have been diagnosed with ADHD fail to pay close attention to details; do not appear to listen when spoken to; do not follow through with instructions; struggle to organize tasks; resist tasks that require sustained mental effort; lose things; and can be easily distracted by extraneous stimuli (APA, 2013). The students who also experience hyperactivity and impulsivity squirm, tap their feet and hands, struggle to stay seated, may talk excessively, blurt out answers, and interrupt others (APA, 2013). Often these symptoms are associated with school failure and difficulties with peer relationships (APA, 2013). According to the APA (2013), the prevalence is about 5% among children. Interestingly, Merikangas et al. (2010) found the prevalence rate at ages 15 to 16 to be 8.6%. Beyond school challenges and peer relationship problems, there can be personal and public safety concerns. To illustrate the public safety dangers of attention and impulsivity difficulties, according to the YRBSS, during the 30 days before the survey, 41.4%, of the 64.7% of the students who drove a car reported texting or e-mailing while driving (Kann et al., 2014). A study by Winston, McDonald, and McGehee (2014) found that adolescents with ADHD were at significantly increased risk for negative driving outcomes. Although prevention is less likely to be an approach for a neurological-based condition, early and ongoing school interventions can help. Children with attention difficulties, impulsivity, and ADHD have been found to respond to mindful and yoga interventions (e.g., Serwacki & Cook-Cottone, 2012).

Anxiety

The leading condition experienced by children and adolescents, anxiety disorders have a cumulative prevalence among children at a rate of 32.1% by the ages of 15 to 16 (Merikangas et al., 2010). In a school of 1,000, that is 321 students. In its most common form, anxiety can be a feeling or experience that a student has about day-to-day challenges, such as taking a test, typical family problems, or speaking in front of the class. There is also a set of anxiety disorders that features persistent, excessive fear and anxiety, which is connected with behavior that can interfere with individual well-being, school success, and relationships (APA, 2013). Specific anxiety disorders include: separation anxiety (i.e., fear of being separated from those to whom one is attached), selective mutism (i.e., a consistent failure to speak in social situations such as school, in which one is expected to speak), specific phobia (i.e., fear regarding a specific object or situation), social anxiety (i.e., fear about social situations in which one feels he or she might be under the scrutiny of others), panic disorder (i.e., recurrent panic attacks), agoraphobia (i.e., fear associated with public transportation, open spaces, enclosed places, crowds, or being outside of the home alone), and generalized anxiety (i.e., excessive fear or worry without the sense that one can control it; APA, 2013). Current treatments are finding small-to-medium effect sizes when compared to controlled conditions (Reynolds, Wilson, Austin, & Hooper, 2012). Prevention and school support are our best line of action.

Posttraumatic Stress Disorder (PTSD)

Up to 5% of adolescents ages 13 to 18 report clinical-level PTSD, with higher rates among females (8.0%) than males (2.3%; Merikangas et al., 2010). Specifically, PTSD involves exposure to actual or threatened death, serious injury, or sexual violence, either by directly experiencing the event, witnessing the event, or learning of the event occurring to someone emotionally close (APA, 2013). Also, PTSD may be the result of repeated or extreme exposure to the details of a traumatic event (APA, 2013). Those who have clinical-level PTSD often have recurrent, intrusive, and distressing memories of the trauma. They may have trauma-related dreams. Those with PTSD may also have dissociative reactions and flashbacks—feeling disconnected from the present moment and as if they are experiencing the traumatic moment. Further, PTSD is associated with the persistent avoidance of trauma-reminiscent stimuli, negative moods and thoughts associated with the event, and notable alterations in arousal and reactivity associated with the traumatic event (APA, 2013). Students with PTSD may have behavioral problems, high levels of anxiety, attendance problems, and difficulty maintaining academic success (Cook-Cottone, 2004). The role of mindfulness and yoga in the treatment of PTSD is reviewed in forthcoming chapters of this book.

Mood Disorders and Suicidality

According to the YRBSS, during the 12 months before the survey, 29.9% of student nationwide had felt so sad or hopeless almost every day for 2 or more consecutive weeks that they stopped some of their usual activities (Kann et al., 2014). These rates varied by ethnicity and race and were substantially higher among females (39.1%; White females 35.7%; Black females 35.8%; Hispanic females 47.8%) than males (20.8%; White males 19.1%; Black males 18.8%; Hispanic males 25.4%; Kann et al., 2014). Mood disorders are the third most common mental health condition experienced by students (Merikangas et al., 2010). According to Merikangas et al. (2010), 8.4% of 13 to 14 year olds, 12.6% of 15 to 16 year olds, and 15.4% of 17 to 18 year olds experience a major depressive disorder or a milder form of the disorder. Depressive disorders are marked by the presence of a sad, empty, or irritable mood that is experienced along with cognitive and physical changes that significantly affect a student's ability to function (APA, 2013). There are several disorders in the depressive disorder category including: disruptive mood dysregulation disorder (i.e., severe recurrent verbal or behavioral outbursts, along with a persistent irritable mood), major depressive disorder (i.e., depressed mood; diminished pleasure in activities; physical changes in sleep and activity levels; worthlessness and/or excessive inappropriate guilt; difficulty concentrating; and thoughts of death or suicide), persistent depressive disorder (i.e., dysthymia, a milder, yet impairing form of depression), and premenstrual dysphoric disorder (i.e., depressive symptoms presenting in the final week of the menstrual cycle, prior to menses; APA, 2013). Depressive disorders can be life impairing and interfere significantly with school performance.

There are a substantial number of students who are at risk for suicide. According to the YRBSS, during the 12 months before the survey, 17.0% of high school students had seriously considered attempting suicide (Kann et al., 2014). These rates vary by race, ethnicity, and gender, with females showing higher rates (22.4%; White females 21.1%; Black females 18.6%; Hispanic females 26.0%) than males (11.6%; White males 11.4%; Black males 10.2%; Hispanic males 11.5%; Kann et al., 2014). Up to 13.6% of students surveyed had made a plan about how they would attempt suicide. According to the YRBSS, during the 12 months before the survey, 8.0% of high school students had attempted suicide (Kann et al., 2014).

School Disengagement and Dropout

Klem and Connell (2004) report that, by the time students reach high school, as many as 40% to 60% are chronically disengaged from school. To illustrate the pathway to dropout, in a study of 1,272 youth as they aged from 7th to 11th grade, Wang and Fredricks (2014) found that adolescents who had declines in behavioral and emotional engagement with school tended to have increased delinquency and substance use over time. Further, there was a bidirectional association between behavior and emotional engagement in school and youth problem behaviors over time. Finally, the researchers found that lower behavioral and emotional engagement and greater problem behaviors predicted a greater likelihood of dropping out of school. Researchers acknowledge that the risks and protective factors associated with early school leaving, or dropout, are complex, and there is still much to be understood about the problem (De Witte, Cabus, Thyssen, Groot, & van den Brink, 2013). As the following chapters in this book demonstrate, mindfulness and yoga intervention can play a role in the reduction of risk in school dropout, perhaps through a disruption in the pathway to risk.

Bullying and Violence

Despite our wish to see school as a safe haven, research tells us that schools can be a place of risk for bullying and violence (Hong & Espelage, 2012). Bullying and peer victimization are serious concerns for students, parents, teachers, and school officials (Hong & Espelage, 2012). These are system-wide as well as relational problems, with the factors associated with bullying and peer victimization present at all ecological levels (Hong & Espelage, 2012). According to the findings of the YRBSS, 7.1% of students had not gone to school on at least 1 day in the past 30 days before the survey because they felt they would be unsafe at school or on their way to or from school. This rate was higher among female (8.7%) than male (5.4%) students (Kann et al., 2014). According to the YRBSS, during the 12 months before the survey, 14.8% of high school students had been electronically bullied, and 19.6% had been bullied on school property (Kann et al., 2014). Of the students who completed the YRBSS, 17.7% had carried a weapon (e.g., gun, knife, or club), 5.5% had carried a gun, and 5.2% had carried a weapon on school property on at least 1 day during the 30 days before the survey (Kann et al., 2014). Nationally, 6.9% of high school students had been threatened or injured with a weapon on school property during the 12 months before the survey. Overall, 24.7% of students had been in a physical fight, and 3.1% reported being injured and needed treatment by a doctor (Kann et al., 2014). Of those completing the survey, 8.1% reported being in a physical fight one or more times on school property (Kann et al., 2014).

Sexual and dating violence is also an issue. Nationally, 7.3% of students reported being physically forced to have sexual intercourse when they did not want to, with rates being higher among females (10.5%) than males (4.2%; Kann et al., 2014). According to the findings of the YRBSS among the 73.0% of students who had dated or went out with someone during the 12 months before the survey, 10.3% had been hit, slammed into something, or deliberately injured with an object or weapon by someone who they were dating or going out with (Kann et al., 2014). Among that same group, 10.4% of students had been kissed, touched, or physically forced to have sexual intercourse when they did not want to by someone they were dating or going out with (Kann et al., 2014). Embodied practices can help. There is emerging evidence that yoga and mindfulness practice may be helpful in improving the school climate and working with traumatized youth (e.g., Spinazzola, Rhodes, Emerson, Earle, & Monroe, 2011; Wisner, Jones, & Gwin, 2010).

Oppositional Defiant and Conduct Disorders

The national study conducted by Merikangas et al. (2010) found that 19.1% of respondents reported a behavioral disorder, with 12.6% reporting symptoms of oppositional defiant disorder and 6.8% reporting conduct disorder. The *Diagnostic and Statistical Manual of Mental Disorders*, Fifth Edition (*DSM-5*) describes disruptive, impulse-control, and conduct disorders as conditions that involve problems in the self-control of emotions and behaviors (APA, 2013). They are unique in that the problems with emotional and behavioral control result in behaviors that violate the right of others or bring the student into significant conflict with authority figures or societal norms (APA, 2013). These disorders include: oppositional defiant disorder (i.e., angry irritable mood, argumentative and defiant behavior, and vindictiveness), intermittent explosive disorder (i.e., recurrent verbal or behavioral outbursts that reflect a failure to control inappropriate, aggressive impulses), conduct disorder (i.e., a pattern of behavior that violates the rights of others or societal norms), pyromania (i.e., deliberate, compulsive fire starting), and kleptomania (i.e., recurrent difficulty resisting impulses to steal; APA, 2013). As later chapters of this text reveal, mindfulness and yoga interventions have shown effectiveness in reducing behavioral problems in schools, detention centers, and prisons.

Eating Disorders and Obesity

A large number of students do not engage in healthy eating or exercise behaviors (Cook-Cottone, Tribole et al., 2013). Not surprisingly, then, the YRBSS found risk for obesity and eating disorder. According to the findings of the 2013 YRBSS, during the 7 days before the survey, 5.0% of high school students had not eaten fruit or drunk fruit juices, and 6.6% had not eaten vegetables (Kann et al., 2014). According to the findings of the 2013 YRBSS, 13.7% of students were obese, with higher rates in males (16.6%) than females (10.8%), and 16.6% were overweight (Kann et al., 2014). Overall, 47.7% of high school students reported that they were trying to lose weight (Kann et al., 2014). In terms of eating-disordered behavior, findings of the YRBSS indicated that 13.0% of students had not eaten for 24 or more hours in order to lose weight or to prevent weight gain during the 30 days before the survey (Kann et al., 2014). Further, 5.0% of students had taken diet pills, powders, or liquids without a doctor's advice to lose weight or to prevent weight gain during the 30 days before the survey. Nationwide, 4.4% of students had vomited or taken laxatives to lose weight or prevent weight gain with rates higher among females (Kann et al., 2014).

Given the risk, it is not surprising that Merikangas et al. (2010) found 3.8% of females and 1.5% of males to have clinical-level eating disorders. The three major eating disorders are anorexia nervosa (i.e., restriction of energy intake relative to energy needs, low body weight, intense fear of gaining weight, disturbed body image, and, for some, episodes of bingeing and purging), bulimia nervosa (i.e., recurrent episodes of binge eating associated with episodes of compensatory behaviors [e.g., purging, exercise], and self-evaluation unduly based on shape and weight), and binge eating disorder (i.e., recurrent episodes of binge eating, a sense of lack of control over eating, and distress regarding eating; APA, 2013). Further, prevalence studies show that rates of childhood obesity remain high, with 16.9% of 2 to 19 year olds meeting criteria for obesity (BMI ≥ 95th sex- and age-specific percentiles;

Ogden, Carroll, Kit, & Flegal, 2014). As shown in the Klein and Cook-Cottone (2013) review, there is evidence that yoga, as an embodied practice, can be helpful in preventing and treating disordered eating.

Sedentary Behavior

The need for physical activity among school-age children and adolescents is high (Cook-Cottone, Kane et al., 2013). According to the YRBSS, 15.2% of students had not participated in at least 60 minutes of any kind of physical activity that increased their heart rate and made them breathe hard some of the time on at least 1 day during the last 7 days before the survey (Kann et al., 2014). No physical activity was more prevalent among female (19.2%) than male (11.2%) students (Kann et al., 2014). Further, rates of sedentary behavior were higher among White females (16.1%), Black females (27.3%), and Hispanic females (20.3%) than White males (9.2%), Black males (15.2%), and Hispanic males (12.1%), respectively (Kann et al., 2014). Nationwide, 47.3% of students reported being physically active for 60 minutes a day on 5 or more days during the 7 days before the survey, with rates higher in male (57.3%) than female (37.3%) students. Further, rates of steady physical activity were higher among White males (59.6%), Black males (53.3%), and Hispanic males (54.4%) than White females (40.5%), Black females (29.3%), and Hispanic females (35.4%) (Kann et al., 2014). According to the findings of the 2013 YRBSS, 41.3% of high school students had played video or computer games, or used a computer for something that was not school work, for 3 or more hours per day on an average school day (Kann et al., 2014). Overall, 32.5% of students watched television 3 or more hours per day on an average school day (Kann et al., 2014).

The consequences of high levels of sedentary behavior are clear. To provide an example of the findings, in a review of studies of sedentary behavior among girls, Costigan, Barnett, Plotnikoff, and Lubans (2013) found strong evidence for a positive association between screen-based sedentary behavior and weight status. Further, positive associations were observed between screen time and sleep problems, musculoskeletal pain, and depression. Negative associations were identified between screen time and physical activity/fitness, screen time and psychological well-being, and screen time and social support. Yoga provides a way for students to regain a sense of physical embodiment and to turn their focus inward.

Self-Harm

Self-harm refers to intentional self-poisoning or self-injury, regardless of the motive or the extent of suicidal intent (Hawton, Saunders, & O'Connor, 2012). Self-harm is a substantial health problem among adolescents (Hawton et al., 2012); in fact, rates of self-harm are higher in the teenage years (Hawton et al., 2012). According to Hawton et al. (2012), genetic vulnerability and psychiatric, psychological, familial, social, and cultural factors may all play a role in risk for self-harm. Further, the effects of media, contagion, and the Internet also play a role. Research states that there is little evidence of effectiveness of either psychosocial or pharmacological treatment (Hawton et al., 2012). The rates of self-harm vary according to definition (i.e., nonsuicidal self-injury or deliberate self-harm) and the manner that it is assessed (i.e., single item assessments or behavioral questionnaire; Muehlenkamp, Claes,

Havertape, & Plener, 2012). For children and adolescents ages 11 to 18 years old, rates range between 16% and 24% (Muehlenkamp et al., 2012). With a disorder such as this, that often involves a struggle with self-regulation, yoga and mindfulness techniques may be helpful in treatment and prevention (Cook-Cottone, 2015).

Substance Use

Substance use and substance use disorders are a significant problem among students who are associated with other problem behaviors such as behavioral disorders, violence, school failure, and school dropout. Students engaged in substance use increase risk in their own lives, as well as present a public safety issue. Among the 64.3% of the students nationwide who drove a vehicle in the last 30 days before the survey, 10.0% had driven one or more times when they had been drinking alcohol (Kann et al., 2014).

Substance use rates are high. According to the YRBSS, 18.6% of students nationwide report having drunk alcohol (other than a few sips) for the first time before 13 years of age (Kann et al., 2014). Overall, most high school students (66.2%) have had at least one drink in their lives, with variability across race and ethnicity and rates higher among females (67.9%) than males (64.4%; Kann et al., 2014). According to the YRBSS, during the 30 days before the survey, 34.9% of students had drunk alcohol, and 23.4% had used marijuana (Kann et al., 2014). Overall, 20.8% of students had had five or more drinks of alcohol in a row on at least 1 day in the past 30 days, with 6.1% reporting more than 10 for the largest number of drinks they had had in a row in the past 30 days (Kann et al., 2014).

Nationwide, 40.7% of students reported that they had used marijuana one or more times during their life, and 8.6% reported that they had tried marijuana for the first time before 13 years of age (Kann et al., 2014). Among those surveyed, 23.4% of high school students had used marijuana one or more times during the 30 days before the survey (Kann et al., 2014). Other rates of substance use are also of concern, with 5.5% of students reporting to have used cocaine, 7.1% hallucinogenic drugs, 8.9% inhalants, 6.6% ecstasy, 2.2% heroine, 3.2% methamphetamines, 3.2% steroids without a prescription, and 17.8% other recreational drugs without a prescription (e.g., Oxycontin, Percocet, Vicoden, codeine, Adderall, Ritalin, or Xanax; Kann et al., 2014).

According to Merikangas et al. (2010), adolescents ages 13 to 18 reported clinical-level alcohol abuse/dependence (6.4%) and drug abuse/dependence (8.9%), while a total of 11.4% reported any substance use disorder. Substance use disorders are marked by a mix of cognitive, behavioral, and physiological symptoms that facilitate the continued use of a substance despite significant substance-related problems (APA, 2013). It is important to note that substance use disorders are characterized by an underlying change in brain circuits that are associated with relapse and craving present when the individual is not intoxicated (APA, 2013). To be diagnosed with a substance use disorder, the student must show a pathological pattern of behaviors associated with use of the substance, including impaired control over the substance, social impairment, and risky use of the substance (APA, 2013). A student may show unsuccessful attempts to cut down or quit using; a host of family and friendship difficulties related to use; and continued use even when previous use has created great risk and even injury. Researchers believe that mindful approaches may be helpful in the treatment of substance use among adolescents (e.g., Cohen, Wupperman, & Tau, 2013).

Engagement in Risky Behavior

Students report engagement in risky behaviors ranging from smoking, to sex, to failure to self-protect in risky situations. By way of example, during the 30 days before the survey, 21.9% of the students nationwide had ridden one or more times in a vehicle with a driver who had been drinking alcohol (Kann et al., 2014). For school-age children and adolescents, it can be very difficult to make the healthy decisions in the current moment. Indeed results from the 2013 YRBSS indicated that many high school students engage in behaviors that have been associated with chronic diseases (e.g., cardiovascular disease, cancer). For instance, during the 30 days before the survey, 15.7% of high school students had smoked cigarettes, and 8.8% had used smokeless tobacco (Kann et al., 2014). Nationwide, 9.3% of students reported that they had smoked a whole cigarette before the age of 13 years (Kann et al., 2014).

According to Kann et al. (2014), many high school students nationwide engage in sexual risk behaviors that contribute to unintended pregnancies and sexually transmitted infections (STIs), including human immunodeficiency virus (HIV). Specifically, nearly half (46.8%) of students have had sexual intercourse and 34.0% have had sexual intercourse, during the 3 months before the survey, with 5.6% reporting having had sexual intercourse before the age of 13 (Kann et al., 2014). Of the students surveyed, 15.0% reported having had sexual intercourse with four or more persons during their life (Kann et al., 2014). Also of concern, among the sexually active students, only 59.1% reported using a condom during their most recent sexual intercourse (Kann et al., 2014). Nationwide, 34.0% of students had had sexual intercourse with at least one person during the 3 months before the survey (Kann et al., 2014). Among these currently sexually active students, 22.4% had drunk alcohol or used drugs before their last sexual intercourse (Kann et al., 2014). Only 19.0% reported that they or their partner had used birth control during their most recent sexual intercourse (Kann et al., 2014). Nationwide, only 12.9% of students had ever been tested for HIV (Kann et al., 2014). Yoga and mindfulness practices are centered on calming the mind in the present moment so that students can have access to their wisest self when making decisions.

Note, due to the scope of this text, only the more prevalent challenges and disorders are included. There are, of course, children with other important challenges whom school personnel support, encourage, and educate daily. Please see the web pages for the National Association of School Psychologists (www.nasponline.org), the American School Counselors Association (www.schoolcounselor.org), the School Social Work Association of America (www.sswaa.org), and the Association for Children's Mental Health (www.acmh-mi.org/) for support, guidance, resources, and text recommendations.

CONCLUSION

In their study of lifetime prevalence of mental disorders among U.S. adolescents ($N = 10,123$ adolescents aged 13–18), Merikangas et al. (2010) found that 40% of participants met the criteria for a mental disorder. Further, of those, 22.2% described severe impairment and/or distress; 11.2% with mood disorders, 8.3% with anxiety disorders, and 9.6% with behavioral disorders. *Without including* those at risk—those who are smoking, having adolescent sex, are pregnant, dealing with unreported sexual assault and trauma, challenged with obesity and overweight— this is 400 students out of a district of 1,000. If we were to add in all of the other risk factors and risky behaviors, we would be hard pressed to find a child who did not present with some kind of obstacle to learning. To be sure, given simple everyday stressors, most would benefit from learning mindfulness and yoga skills to help with stress management, self-regulation, and coping.

Helping students develop an effective sense of self—as human beings and as learners—is critical to long-term academic engagement and achievement. For many students, intelligence and learning skills are only a small part of what they need in order to learn effectively. As Duckworth et al. (2007) and James (1907) suggest, there are two questions: (a) What are the human abilities? and (b) By what means can one unleash these abilities? To date, research suggests that yoga and mindfulness cannot increase IQ or innate abilities (i.e., the first question). However, there is a growing body of evidence that suggests they can help students handle stress, cope, and self-regulate. Perhaps these practices can help students unleash their abilities to their highest potential. For some, they may be the key to flourishing.

REFERENCES

American Psychiatric Association. (2013). *Diagnostic and Statistical Manual of Mental Disorders*, Fifth Edition. Arlington, VA: American Psychiatric Publishing.

Ashdown, D. M., & Bernard, M. (2012). Can explicit instruction in social emotional learning skills benefit the social emotional learning, well-being, and academic achievement of young children? *Early Childhood Education, 39,* 397–405.

Association for Supervision and Curriculum Development. (2014). *Whole school, whole community, whole child: A collaborative approach to learning and health.* Alexandria, VA: Author. Retrieved from http://www.ascd.org/programs/learning-and-health/wscc-model.aspx

Cohen, M., Wupperman, P., & Tau, G. (2013). Mindfulness in the treatment of adolescents with problem substance use. *Adolescent Psychiatry, 3,* 172–183.

Cook-Cottone, C. P. (2004). Childhood posttraumatic stress disorder: Ddiagnosis, treatment, and school reintegration. *School Psychology Review, 33,* 127–139.

Cook-Cottone, C. P. (2013). Dosage as a critical variable in yoga therapy research. *International journal of yoga therapy, 23,* 11–12.

Cook-Cottone, C. P., (2015). *Mindfulness and yoga for self-regulation: A primer for mental health professionals.* New York, NY: Springer Publishing.

Cook-Cottone, C. P., Kane, L., Keddie, E., & Haugli, S. (2013). *Girls growing in wellness and balance: Yoga and life skills to empower.* Stoddard, WI: Schoolhouse Educational Services, LLC.

Cook-Cottone, C. P., Tribole, E., & Tylka, T. (2013). *Healthy eating in schools: Evidence-based interventions to help kids thrive.* Washington, DC: American Psychological Association.

Cook-Cottone, C. P. & Vujnovic, R. (2016). *The healthy student: Schools, eating, and health psychology encyclopedia of health psychology.* New York, NY: Wiley.

Costigan, S. A., Barnett, L., Plotnikoff, R. C., & Lubans, D. R. (2013). The health indicators associated with screen-based sedentary behavior among adolescent girls: A systematic review. *Journal of Adolescent Health, 52,* 382–392.

De Witte, K., Cabus, S., Thyssen, G., Groot, W., & van den Brink, H. M. (2013). A critical review of the literature on school dropout. *Educational Research Review, 10,* 13–28.

Duckworth, A., & Gross, J. J. (2014). Self-control and Grit: Related but separable determinants of success. *Current Directions in Psychological Science, 35,* 319–325.

Duckworth, A. L., Peterson, C., Mathews, M. D., & Kelly, D. R. (2007). Grit: Perseverance and passion for long-term goals. *Journal of Personality and Social Psychology, 92,* 1087–1101.

Duckworth, A. L., & Quinn, P. D. (2009). Development and validation of the short grit scale (Grit-S). *Journal of Personality Assessment, 91,* 166–174.

Durlak, J. A., Weissberg, R. P., Dymnicki, A. B., Taylor, R. D., & Schellinger, K. B. (2011). The impact of enhancing students' social and emotional learning: A meta-analysis of school-based universal interventions. *Child Development, 82,* 405–432.

Greenberg, M. T., & Harris, A. R. (2012). Nurturing mindfulness in children and youth: Current state of research. *Child Development Perspectives, 6,* 162–166.

Greenberg, M. T., Weissberg, R. P., O'Brien, M. U., Zins, J. E., Fredericks, L., Resnik, H., & Elias, M. J. (2003). Enhancing school-based prevention and youth development through coordinated social, emotional, and academic learning. *American Psychologist, 58,* 466.

Hawton, K., Saunders, K. E., & O'Connor, R. C. (2012). Self-harm and suicide in adolescents. *The Lancet, 379,* 2373–2382.

Hong, J. S., & Espelage, D. (2012). A review of research on bullying and peer victimization in school: An ecological systems analysis. *Aggression and Violent Behavior, 17,* 311–322.

James, W. (1907, March 1). The energies of men. *Science, 25,* 321–332.

Kann, L., Kinchen, S., Shanklin, S. L., Flint, K. H., Kawkins, J., Harris, W. A., . . . Zaza, S. (2014). Youth risk behavior surveillance—United States, 2013. *Morbidity and Mortality Weekly Report, Surveillance Summary, 63,* 1–168.

Karpov, Y. V. (2014). *Vygotsky for educators.* New York, NY: Cambridge University Press.

Klein, J., & Cook-Cottone, C. (2013). The effects of yoga on eating disorder symptoms and correlates: A review. *International Journal of Yoga Therapy, 23,* 41–50.

Klem, A. M., & Connell, J. P. (2004). Relationships matter: Linking teacher support to student engagement and achievement. *Journal of School Health, 74,* 262–273.

Leavell, H. R., & Clark, E. G. (1953). *Textbook of preventive medicine.* New York, NY: McGraw-Hill.

Leavell, H. R., & Clark, E. G. (1958). *Preventive medicine for the doctor in his community* (2nd ed.). New York, NY: McGraw-Hill.

Leavell, H. R., & Clark, E. G. (1965). *Preventive medicine for the doctor in his community* (3rd ed.). New York, NY: McGraw-Hill.

Liew, J. (2012). Effortful control, executive functions, and education: Bringing self-regulatory and social-emotional competencies to the table. *Child Development Perspectives, 6,* 105–111.

Merikangas, K. R., He, J. P., Burstein, M., Swanson, S. A., Avenevoli, S., Cui, L., . . . Swendsen, J. (2010). Lifetime prevalence of mental disorders in US adolescents: Results from the National Comorbidity Survey Replication–Adolescent Supplement (NCS-A). *Journal of the American Academy of Child & Adolescent Psychiatry, 49,* 980–989.

Muehlenkamp, J. J., Claes, L., Havertape, L., & Plener, P. L. (2012). International prevalence of adolescent non-suicidal self-injury and deliberate self-harm. *Child and Adolescent Psychiatry and Mental Health, 6,* 1–9.

Ogden, C. L., Carroll, M. D., Kit, B. K., & Flegal, K. M. (2014). Prevalence of childhood and adult obesity in the United States, 2011–2012. *Journal of the Medical Association, 311,* 806–814.

Perkins-Gough, D. (2013, September). The significance of grit: A conversation with Angela Lee Duckworth. *Educational Leadership, 17,* 14–20.

Reynolds, S., Wilson, C., Austin, J., & Hooper, L. (2012). Effects of psychotherapy for anxiety in children and adolescents: A meta-analytic review. *Clinical Psychology Review, 32,* 251–262.

Scime, M., & Cook-Cottone, C. (2008). Primary prevention of eating disorders: A constructivist integration of mind and body strategies. *International Journal of Eating Disorders, 41,* 134–142.

Serwacki, M., & Cook-Cottone, C. (2012). Yoga in the schools: A systematic review of the literature. *International Journal of Yoga Therapy, 22,* 101–110.

Shin, M., & Walker, H. *Interventions for Achievement and Behavior Problems in a three-Tier Model Including RTI.* Bethesda, MD: National Association of School Psychologists.

Shoshani, A., & Steinmetz, S. (2013). Positive psychology at school: A school-based intervention to promote adolescents' mental health and well-being. *Journal of Happiness Studies, 15,* 1289–1311.

Spinazzola, J., Rhodes, A. M., Emerson, D., Earle, E., & Monroe, K. (2011). Application of yoga in residential treatment of traumatized youth. *Journal of the American Psychiatric Nurses Association, 17*(6), 431–444. doi:1078390311418359

Stoiber, K. C. (2014). A comprehensive framework for multitiered system of support in school psychology. In A. Thomas & J. Grimes (Eds.), *Best practices in school psychology* (5th ed.). Bethesda, MD: National Association of School Psychologists.

Verde, S. (2015). *I am yoga.* New York, NY: Abrams Books for Young Readers.

Wang, M., & Fredricks, J. A. (2014). The reciprocal links between school engagement, youth problems behaviors, and school dropout during adolescence. *Child Development, 85,* 722–737.

Winston, F. K., McDonald, C. C., & McGehee, D. V. (2014). Adolescents with ADHD demonstrate driving inconsistency. *The Journal of Pediatrics, 164,* 672–676.

Wisner, B. L., Jones, B., & Gwin, D. (2010). School-based meditation practices for adolescents: A resource for strengthening self-regulation, emotional coping, and self-esteem. *Children and Schools, 32*(3), 150–159.

CHAPTER 3

THE MINDFUL AND YOGIC LEARNER: 12 EMBODIED PRACTICES FOR SCHOOLS

Man is not fully conditioned and determined but rather determines himself
whether he gives into conditions or stands up to them.
In other words, man is ultimately self determining.
Man does not simply exist but always decides what his existence will be,
what he will become in the next moment.

Viktor Frankl, *Man's Search for Meaning* (1959, p. 131)

BETWEEN STIMULUS AND RESPONSE

"The way that you confront a challenging yoga pose is maybe the way you do the rest of your life. The way you read a book, or the way you solve a math problem, or the way you talk to your brother or sister," explains Kellie Love in a recent piece for *Healthline* (Radcliffe, 2016). Kellie Love is a yoga teacher at Girls Preparatory School in the Bronx, New York. I first met Kellie at the inaugural Yoga in the School Symposium at Kripalu Center for Yoga in Health. She is passionate about bringing mindfulness and yoga to schools. Over the years of her work, she has witnessed the shift that occurs within students as they become increasingly competent in managing themselves and their stress. What happens for these students is beyond an increase in self-esteem. It is competence, assuredness, self-trust, self-compassion, and strength. When practicing mindfulness and yoga in school, students learn more than how to manage themselves on their yoga mats and when meditating. They learn powerful self-regulation skills that they can generalize in their lives off the mat, in the world that exists outside of yoga and mindfulness sessions.

Mindfulness and yoga techniques embrace the tenet that we, as humans, are self-determining (Cook-Cottone, 2015). In my own work in both school- and community-based yoga, one of my central organizing quotes comes from Dr. Viktor Frankl (1959). A summary of his thinking, this quote gives us the essence of his book, *Man's Search for Meaning* (Frankl, 1959), as well as speaks to the embodied self-regulation that can be developed with mindful and yoga practices (Branson & Gross, 2014; Childress & Harper, 2015; Cook-Cottone, 2015; Frankl, 1959; Grabovac, Lau, & Willett, 2011; Herrington, 2012; Jennings, 2015; Rechtschaffen, 2014):

> *Between stimulus and response there is a space.*
> *In that space, is your power to choose a response.*
> *In your response, is your growth, freedom, and possibility.*

As beautifully summarized in this quote, the power of mindful awareness and embodied action is in the profoundness of the moment-by-moment choices we all make. Frankl (1959), a former Jewish prisoner of war in Nazi Germany, offers that, in every moment, if we slow down and look, we have choice. This is the level of self-awareness that allows students to make the best choices and to be in positive action interpersonally and academically. In fact, perhaps the most gratifying gift of teaching mindfulness and yoga to students is the ability to be witness to a student's dawning awareness that he or she has choice in how he or she might respond to a trigger, provocation, or idea. You realize, at the moment of awareness, you have seen a student move toward a very empowered place in his or her unfolding life.

It is to the moment-by-moment experience and the notion of choice in self-regulation that this text now shifts the focus. This chapter serves to transition you to the following chapters that address mindful and yoga approaches and the provision of mindfulness in schools. In Chapters 1 and 2, you were introduced to the Mindful and Yogic Self as Effective Learner (MY-SEL; Chapter 1) and the ways in which students can become at risk for a variety of difficulties associated with dysregulation and ineffective learning (Chapter 2). These chapters explicated how the integrated model of self (MY-SEL) reflects an ongoing process of attunement, integration, and construction of the self. Further, we saw in Chapter 2 that when there are challenges, obstacles, or dysfunction in either an internal or external domain, the regulation of the self can be disrupted or complicated. We now explore how the process of embodied self-regulation is preventive for all students and prescriptive for both students at risk and those who are in need of intervention and support. Further, for students who are doing well, the MY-SEL approach provides opportunities for them to do better, experience less stress, and refine their self-regulation and interpersonal skills. Recall that, within the MY-SEL model, our goals as educators are to (a) impart academic knowledge and teach tools of learning, (b) teach students to be active architects of their own learning and well-being, and (c) prepare students to be collaborative problem solvers (see Figure 3.1).

As you can see in Figure 3.1, as the students learn they, become increasingly competent as architects in their own learning and active solvers of their own problems. It is true for both mindful and yoga traditions that the experience of self as learner is considered *self-determined* and *embodied through practice* (Ajaya, 1983; Herrington, 2012; Jennings, 2015; Prabhavananda & Isherwwood, 2007). Mindful and yoga practices help create the *space and opportunity* required to cultivate an experience of self that will serve the student and his or her large learning goals. As students engage in mindful and yogic practices, they will become increasingly aware, cultivate inquiry and understanding, and create an intentional experience of self through choice.

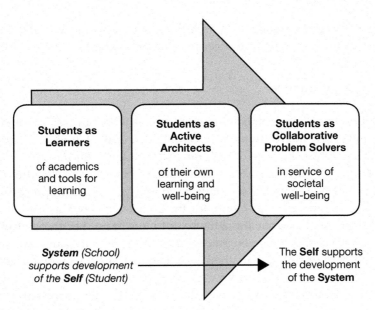

FIGURE 3.1 Reminder of our goals as educators.

MECHANISMS OF MINDFULNESS AND YOGA IN SCHOOLS

I believe that mindful and yoga approaches uniquely help students work toward a self-determined, embodied presence in their schoolwork and relationships. The research on mindfulness and yoga in schools is in the early stages. That is, there is a lot more to learn about the key mechanisms of change for these practices and how yoga and mindfulness uniquely and respectively contribute to student well-being and engagement. Most agree, mindfulness and yoga are distinct. Accordingly, forthcoming chapters in this book address the unique bodies of research. It is also a given that the practices share historical roots and core practices (e.g., meditation, relaxation, mindfulness). Here we explore the shared benefits, practices, and principles.

Finding the space between stimulus and response through the process of mindfulness and yoga is aligned with and builds on positive psychology constructs that are currently being studied among youth populations. These constructs include growth mindset, grit, self-compassion, and self-care. These approaches all point to the ability to be fully aware, engaged, and self-determining. That is, *who we really are*, who a student is becoming as a person, need not be dependent on internal experiences (i.e., feelings, thoughts, and bodily sensations) or external triggers (e.g., relationships, environmental factors; Cook-Cottone, 2015). That is, despite of, or without regard for, internal or external contingencies, consequences, or rewards—we can create who we are. We can construct the experience of self (Cook-Cottone, 2015).

How is that done? For years, we have argued nature versus nurture, and this line of thinking suggests that the self-need not rest solely in the hands of either. For all of us, teachers and students, the active process of constructing, experiencing, and regulating the self involves awareness, inquiry, active engagement, self-regulation, and intentional effort. Further, the practice must be embodied, lived. This chapter addresses some of the key mechanisms of change that can help us understand what mindfulness and yoga practice has to offer students. These include a positive, embodied practice, grit and perseverance, and a growth mindset.

Positive, Embodied Practice

Advances in neuroscience have helped illuminate exactly what our way of being and behaving is doing to our brain (Cook-Cottone, 2015; Siegel, 2015, 2010). I think this is best explained in a book that is an all-time favorite of my university students: *Buddha's Brain: The Practical Neuroscience of Happiness, Love, and Wisdom*. The authors, Hanson and Mendius (2009), make a compelling case for how you can use your mind and your thought processes to change your brain, and your experience of living, for the better. This book artfully, and in a very accessible way, explains how your thoughts sculpt your brain. For those of us who work with kids, it makes sense that what you practice gets stronger. In the same way that students work to develop good writing and math skills, creating a healthy, happy sense of self can happen with positive practice. There is now neurological evidence to support what Aristotle is believed to have said many years ago, "We become what we repeatedly do." In other words, what you practice you become. Over time, you and your students can develop a reliable, positive, and supportive inner coach that helps you when things get tough, be it math, physics, composition, oral presentations, or relationships. Accordingly, positive, embodied practice is the essence of this text. There is much more on mindfulness, as well as a set of practices, in Chapters 4 through 7. Further, for an easy-to-understand review of the neuroscience underlying the changes seen in mindfulness practices, see Hanson and Mendius (2009). To understand more about the neuroscience of the developing brain, see Siegel (2015).

Grit and Perseverance

In an effort to understand what factors lead to academic and life success, Angela Duckworth, at the University of Pennsylvania, has been studying grit for many years (Perkins-Gough, 2013). Her work on grit has garnered great interest. She is a winner of a MacArthur Fellowship for her work studying grit (MacArthur Foundation, 2016). Her captivating TED talk on grit can be found on the website: www.ted.com/talks/angela_lee_duckworth_the_key_to_success_grit?language=en. Duckworth became interested in the concept of grit after working as a teacher in a challenging urban setting. She defines grit as something more than resilience (Perkins-Gough, 2013). Duckworth argues that grit is a specific definition of resilience that is connected to a sense of optimism, the ability to come from an at-risk or challenging situation and thrive nevertheless (Perkins-Gough, 2013). Duckworth explains that what resilience and grit have in common is the positive response to failure and adversity (Perkins-Gough, 2013). In her measures of grit, about half of the questions are about responding resiliently to situations of failure and adversity and about being a hard worker (Perkins-Gough, 2013). The remainder of the questions is about having persistence toward a goal, consistent interests, and focused passion (Perkins-Gough, 2013).

Duckworth and colleagues devised empirical measures of grit and self-control for both children and adults. The scales are available here: www.sas.upenn.edu/~duckworth/gritscale.htm. Using these measures, Duckworth's team found that these traits predict objectively measured success outcomes, even when controlling for cognitive ability (MacArthur Foundation, 2016). For example, in prospective longitudinal studies, grit predicted final ranking of specific, actual participants at the Scripps National Spelling Bee, persistence at the U.S. Military Academy at West Point, and graduation rates from Chicago public high schools (MacArthur Foundation, 2016). These findings held true over and beyond standardized achievement test scores (MacArthur Foundation, 2016). The findings ultimately indicate that self-control predicts report-card grades and improvements in report-card grades over time, better than measured intelligence (MacArthur Foundation, 2016).

Mindfulness and yoga provide active practice in, and the tools needed for, grit and perseverance. Both practices give students ample opportunity to feel frustrated and to practice persevering. You can argue that sports like soccer, swimming, and running offer opportunities for grit and perseverance. I agree, they do. However, what is unique about mindful and yoga practices is that they provide accessible tools (e.g., breath work, positive self-talk, self-reflection) that support the development of grit and perseverance. To illustrate, Sue is a 10th-grade runner on the track team. The coach needed someone to run the 2-mile this year. She selected Sue. Sue was not happy about this; she felt as if she hardly made it through the 1-mile last year. However, something was different this year. This year, she has been practicing yoga as an elective at her school. Sue's yoga teacher had taught the students how to stay focused on the task at hand (e.g., plank pose) by continuously noticing the physical sensations and redirecting their thoughts in a positive and empowering manner. Next, she taught them how to breathe and to become aware of exactly what was happening in the present moment (e.g., her hands are pressing into the mat; her muscles are working; for both legs she is hugging the muscles onto the bone). In yoga, Sue was learning how to *not* add more negative thinking to the process (e.g., "I can't do this," or "Plank pose is hard"), which creates distress rather than empowers. Last, Sue's yoga teacher taught her how to be a positive coach for herself in challenging poses with empowering self-talk (e.g., "Sue, you have this;" "You are stronger than you think you are;" "Sue, you are worth the effort;" and "Your breath is your most powerful tool, Sue").

Sue had been practicing these techniques for many months when spring track season arrived. She decided to take on the challenge of the 2-mile race. Sue used her yoga skills of mindful awareness, breathing, ignoring and stopping negative self-talk, and creating a positive inner coach. Although Sue had never been known for her speed, she showed up very differently in track this year. The coach noticed. Her parents noticed. In each race, she had a strong steady pace. Sue's attitude was different as she brought a quiet strength to one of the hardest races in track. Sue explained, "You can do yoga, even when you're running the 2-mile, because yoga isn't a pose. Yoga is the way you approach your challenges." Sue used her yoga and mindfulness skills, and what showed up was grit and perseverance.

Growth Mindset

Mindfulness and yoga also give students lived opportunities to develop a growth mindset. Yeager and Dweck (2012) ask the question, "When students struggle with their schoolwork, what determines whether they give up or embrace the obstacle and work to overcome it?" (p. 302). Dweck's work on the growth mindset evolved from her effort to answer such questions. Her team suggests that the development of a growth mindset promotes student resilience. A growth mindset is a mindset, or way of understanding things, that incorporates a core understanding that people can change and grow. Yeager and Dweck (2012) explain that students can be taught to see intelligence as malleable and that effort, help, and strategies can improve academic outcomes. This shifts student goals from looking smart to learning. A growth mindset shifts response from a tendency to give up, to working harder and smarter, and ultimately results in improved academic performance. Mindful and yoga practices embrace a growth mindset and emphasize effort and presence over ability. Mindfulness and yoga offer what Yeager and Dweck (2012) suggest:

> As students move through our educational system, all of them will face adversity at one time or another, whether it is academic or social in nature. A central task for parents and educators is to prepare students to respond resiliently when these inevitable challenges arise. (p. 312)

THE MINDFUL AND YOGIC LEARNER (MY-SEL)

The MY-SEL model holds that mindfulness and yoga approaches and practices can help students cope, engage, and learn by helping them develop a sense of what we call *mindful grit* (i.e., positive embodiment and hard work toward long-term goals with an eye to self-care, compassion, and sustainability) and *mindful growing* (i.e., a growth mindset supported by mindfulness and yoga tools). The 12 embodied practices reflect the body of work on yoga in schools. Note, several of these principles were developed as part of work with Yogis in Service, Inc., and with research assistants Melissa LaVigne, Lindsay Travers, and Erga Lemish as part of curriculum development for a trauma-informed, growth-oriented yoga intervention developed in partnership with the Africa Yoga Project. Figure 3.2 illustrates how the 12 principles are points of action helping the student manage internal triggers and challenges as well as external stressors and obstacles (Cook-Cottone, 2015).

As a member of the school faculty, staff, or administration wanting to integrate mindful and yoga approaches, you may feel overwhelmed by the thought of having to select and review all the books on kids' yoga, as well as the research articles on yoga in schools. This text is organized to distill these readings, traditional to the recent, into a practical set of 12 essential practices to facilitate embodied self-regulation, self-care, and intentional, reflective engagement for you and your students. The 12 embodied practices are briefly reviewed

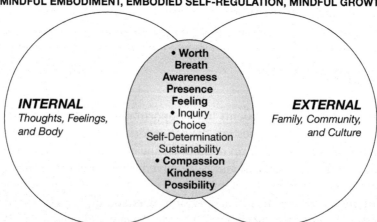

FIGURE 3.2 The MY-SEL as 12 embodied practices.

Note, several of these principles were developed as part of work with Yogis in Service, Inc., and with Melissa LaVigne Lindsay Travers and Erga Lemish, as part of curriculum development for a trauma-informed, growth-oriented yoga intervention developed in partnership with the Africa Yoga Project.

TABLE 3.1 The 12 Principles for Embodied Growth and Learning

Mindful Embodiment

1. WORTH: I am worth the effort
2. BREATH: My breath is my most powerful tool
3. AWARENESS: I am mindfully aware
4. PRESENCE: I work toward presence in my physical body
5. FEELING: I feel my emotions in order to grow and learn

Embodied Self-Regulation

6. INQUIRY: I ask questions about my physical experiences, feelings, and thoughts
7. CHOICE: I choose my focus and actions
8. SELF-DETERMINATION: I do the work
9. SUSTAINABILITY: I find balance between effort and rest

Mindful Growth

10. COMPASSION: I honor efforts to grow and learn
11. KINDNESS: I am kind to myself and others
12. POSSIBILITY: I work toward the possibility of effectiveness and growth in my life

here (see Table 3.1). For ease of understanding, the 12 principles of embodied growth and learning are further broken down into three mechanisms of action: (a) mindful embodiment, (b) embodied self-regulation, and (c) mindful development.

Mindful Embodiment

Mindful embodiment is the skill of being aware of and inhabiting the body as you engage in your tasks and relationships throughout the day (Cook-Cottone, 2015). In our cognitive (i.e., thinking) and technology-oriented school culture, it is easy for students to lose a sense of being connected to and aware of their bodies. Accordingly, the 12 principles begin with tools for mindful embodiment. These include: worth, breath, awareness, presence, and feeling.

Principle 1: Worth: "I am worth the effort"

Research suggests that engagement in mindfulness and yoga practice enhances self-efficacy and self-esteem among students (e.g., Berger, Silver, & Stein, 2009; Case-Smith, Shupe Sines, & Klatt, 2010). In school, students are continuously in the growth zone, a place that is outside of their comfort zone. By definition, things are uncomfortable, difficult there. Vygotsky (1978) called this the zone of proximal development, the zone in which students are challenged; learning to do things they have not mastered; expected to fail to some degree as they work; and likely to need teacher support or tools of learning. Similarly, in mindfulness and yoga practice, the growth zone is viewed as the place where the most robust learning occurs. To be in a growth zone and remain effective, students need to be reminded that they are worth the effort. As well articulated by Hanson and Mendius (2009), the human brain tends to scan for what is wrong and not working when we are challenged. To combat this natural human tendency during mindfulness and yoga practice, students work with the mantra (i.e., mind tool), "I am worth the effort." When practice becomes difficult, it is especially important to remind students that they are worth the effort. Reminding students that they are worth the effort helps them pair challenge and difficulty with thoughts of self-worth rather than excuses or reasons to quit. Try this in your mindfulness work, yoga class, or classroom today. It will not take long before you notice the children internalizing this empowering tool. In our work with school-age children, we have observed them reminding each other, "Hey Joey, remember you are worth the effort," during interpersonal and academic situations.

Principle 2: Breath: "My breath is my most powerful tool"

Breath is an essential component of mindful embodiment. Breath work comes primarily from yogic traditions. Breath is so important to yoga practice, it has been said, "If there is no focus on breath, there is no yoga." Breath is the bridge between the body and the mind. Breath is central to yoga teachings, and you can find instruction on breath work in the traditional yoga texts (Cook-Cottone, 2015). For example, Yoga Sutra 1.34 reads, "The mind may also be calmed by expulsion and retention of the breath" (Prabhavananda & Isherwood, 2007, p. 70). Decades of research tell us that breath is an antidote to the stress response, as well as a potent tool in emotional regulation.

Breath is the access point to the relaxation response first described by Benson in 1976. Specifically, your breath aligns with your internal activation, your feelings state, and your state of arousal. You have control of both your voluntary breath and involuntary, automatic breath (Harper, 2013; Simpkins & Simpkins, 2011). This fundamental truth of voluntary and involuntary breath control is the source of the power of intentional breath (Cook-Cottone, 2015; Harper, 2013; Simpkins & Simpkins, 2011). For students, skill development in breath control can help them learn how to voluntarily shift out of psychological activation, down regulate the chronic stress response, and move themselves into the relaxation response (Simpkins & Simpkins, 2011; Weintraub, 2012). This means that they can learn to calm themselves down by simply breathing. In these ways and more, the breath is very powerful. It is so powerful, that my research team has given it the label of the *most powerful tool*.

Principle 3: Awareness: "I am mindfully aware"

Mindful awareness is a way of being—"a way of inhabiting one's body, one's mind, one's moment-by-moment experience" (Shapiro & Carlson, 2009, p. 5). More obviously central to mindfulness-based practice, mindful awareness is also fundamental to yoga (Cook-Cottone, 2015). In fact, the yoga sutras' first teaching is, "Yoga is the control of the thought-waves in the mind" (Yoga Sutra 1.2; Prabhavananda & Isherwood, 2007, p. 14). Students, even many adults, do not have a developed skill of noticing the mind. Harper (2013) refers to this skill as keeping the "*thoughtful brain*" in charge (p. 13).

Mindful awareness is the state of being attentive to and aware of what is taking place in the present (Brown & Ryan, 2003). More specifically, students who are mindfully aware learn how to notice when their minds begin wandering and are able to bring them back (Harper, 2013). Siegel (2010) describes mindful awareness as a conscious and intentional approach to what we do, allowing us to be creative with possibilities. It involves an awareness of the present moment without judgment. It has been described as a flexible, receptive, and open presence (Brown & Ryan, 2003; Siegel, 2010). Mindful awareness and focus are skills that students can learn and then practice (Harper, 2013). Recent research has found mindful awareness to be associated with a variety of positive outcomes, including a sense of well-being and increased self-knowledge (Brown & Ryan, 2003).

Principle 4: Presence: "I work toward presence in my own body"

Like breath, the physical experience must also be honored as critical to healing and preventing struggle (Cook-Cottone, 2015; McCown, Reibel, & Micozzi, 2010). The experience of the physiological self is as relevant to mental health as are the cognitive and emotional aspects of self (Cook-Cottone, 2006; 2015). Embodied approaches to self-regulation view the role of physical practice as key to well-being and emotional growth (Cook-Cottone, 2015). Experiencing body sensations as they arise and pass away, without judgment, helps us to untangle, or defuse, our immediate experience from our stories about the experience (McCown et al., 2010). This happens in two steps (Baptiste, 2016). First, students practice bringing their focus to the physical experience of a pose. They can notice the sensations of their feet or hands on the mat, the work being done by their muscles and lungs, and their heartbeats. The goal here is to focus only on the physical sensations. Next, students notice their reactions to the physical sensations. Do they think the sensations are good or bad? Do they think the pose is hard or easy (Baptiste, 2016)? As students practice, the teacher helps them discern between their physical sensations and their reactions to them or stories about them.

Over time, a practice of bringing awareness to the body and away from the "privileged cognitive domain" helps lead us to new possibilities unencumbered by limited beliefs and past impressions (McCown et al., 2010, p. 145). This practice is believed to help facilitate creativity and a sense of freedom in learning (Baptiste, 2016). Emphasis on embodiment brings awareness to internal sensation (i.e., interoception) and can deepen a sense of resonance with others (Cook-Cottone, 2015; McCown et al., 2010). Without embodied practice, there can be no real change or growth (Cook-Cottone, 2015).

Principle 5: Feeling: "I feel my emotions in order to grow and learn"

Emotions are a composite of cognitive and physiological experiences. They live in the mind and body. Emotional memories are seated both in the brain and remembered in the body (Cook-Cottone, 2015). To access and process emotions, the body must be part of the focus and practice. Anchoring feelings where they reside within the physical self enhances self-awareness, leading to the greater likelihood of effective self-regulation (Cook-Cottone, 2015). That is, the body is key to effectively processing and regulating emotional experience (Bennett, 2002; Siegel, 2010). Together, steady, physical practice and awareness, and active processing of the physiological aspects of emotional experience create a physical foundation for self-regulation (Cook-Cottone, 2015). When a student knows that he or she can fully feel, process, and withstand any emotion, he or she is empowered. There is no need for emotional avoidance or control.

To illustrate, Zuri, a 13-year-old girl, sometimes struggles to be present to her feelings. Her mom is an alcoholic, and Zuri worries about her constantly. Her counselor at school, Mrs. Markham, has helped her to understand alcoholism and has encouraged her to go to support meetings to learn more about the disease. Mrs. Markham also helped Zuri sign up for the afterschool yoga program with Miss Amanda. Zuri often tells Mrs. Markham that she thinks that her mom's drinking is her fault. She comes to this thought as a result of her lived experience. She explains that her mom often tells her that, if she and her brothers were better behaved, she wouldn't need to drink so much. In fact, Zuri explains, when her mom leaves to go to the bar, she often does it right after she gets mad at Zuri and her brothers. Zuri explains that she becomes so anxious when her mom leaves that she can barely breathe. She says, "I am scared." She thinks, "Mom left because I am bad." She thinks she will not be okay if her mother is not there to make things okay. She tries to not feel anything and that does not work. Then, she becomes completely overwhelmed.

Mrs. Markham utilizes the aspects of mindfulness to help Zuri self-regulate. First, as Zuri tells Mrs. Markham, "I am scared," Mrs. Markham reflects, "You are feeling a lot of anxiety," immediately shifting identification as the feeling (e.g., "I am _____") to a process of observing the experience of feeling a strong feeling (e.g., "I am feeling _____"). Next, she asks Zuri to tell her about the anxiety, when it happens, how it happens, and how the anxiety feels in her body (e.g., Does your heart rate increase? Are there sensations in your body? Does your breath change?). Focus on the body and on experience increases connection for Zuri between body and mind (McCown et al., 2010), while allowing an experience of interpersonal attunement as Mrs. Markham shares a focus on Zuri's experience and validates Zuri's anxiety. Embracing the notion that all things, especially feelings, come and go, Mrs. Markham asks Zuri to allow the feeling of anxiety to just be there. She then asks Zuri to slow her breath and count to four as she inhales and to five as she exhales. They practice this together. She asks Zuri to notice how her body may feel different (e.g., heart rate, breath, sensations in her belly). Mrs. Markham helps Zuri understand that feelings come and go (i.e., impermanence), and that anxious feelings seem to be triggered when Zuri's mom leaves—which makes total sense. It is scary when your mom leaves, mad, to go out drinking. Her work with Zuri is designed around giving Zuri tools to manage her emotional experience. Appropriately, Mrs. Markham validates Zuri's feelings, gives her tools to cope with them, and encourages her to allow them. Zuri's mom still drinks; this is a problem outside of Zuri's control. Still, Zuri has learned tools to cope with her emotions that she can use from this point forward in her life. (Note, as any good school counselor would do, Mrs. Markham explores any child neglect issues, etc. These techniques are embedded within standard good practices.)

Embodied Self-Regulation

Embodied self-regulation is distinct from typical self-regulation processes and theories (Cook-Cottone, 2015; Schultz & Ryan, 2013). Typical self-regulation involves cognitive-driven emotional and behavioral regulation with an emphasis on motive, drive, and achievement (Cook-Cottone, 2015; Schultz & Ryan, 2013). The endpoint of traditional self-regulation is the achievement of goals. The scope of focus, or context, is the individual experience (Cook-Cottone, 2015; Schultz & Ryan, 2013) whereas embodied self-regulation targets mind and body integration within the context of active practice (e.g., mindfulness practice or yoga). The emphasis of embodied self-regulation is on honoring the process and the journey rather than on an endpoint (Cook-Cottone, 2015). The endpoint, or outcome, for embodied self-regulation is not the achievement of goals. Rather, it is balanced and sustained self-mastery. Finally, the scope goes beyond the individual and involves attunement within the self and among others (Cook-Cottone, 2015). The principles for embodied self-regulation are grounded in the mindful embodiment principles (i.e., worth, breath, awareness, presence, and feeling) and include inquiry, choice, self-determination, and sustainability. Notably, they lead to the mindful development principles (i.e., compassion, kindness, and possibility). For more reading on embodied self-regulation, see Cook-Cottone (2015).

Principle 6: Inquiry: "I ask questions about my physical experiences, thoughts, feelings, and actions"

Being in inquiry means always being curious about the present-moment experiences in all domains—physical, emotional, and cognitive. Yoga and mindful practices view life as the journey of the seeker of knowledge (Cook-Cottone, 2015; Wallace, 2011). Knowledge is not viewed as coming only from books, teachers, or study guides. Mindfulness and yoga traditions hold that knowledge comes from experience. That is, each moment in the classroom, you and your students are on a path of self-inquiry (Bennett, 2002). Wallace (2011) reminds us that, "The search for insight and wisdom is not done for the sake of knowledge itself; it is a search to deepen our experiential understanding" (p. 5). In this view of inquiry, students are asked to drop what they think they already know and become present to the current context (Baptiste, 2016). In this way, to be in inquiry means to come from a place of not knowing (Cook-Cottone, 2015; McCown et al., 2010). That is, as an educator, you want the student to get curious about the presemantic, before words and concepts, and experience the present moment (McCown et al., 2010). Each present-moment experience is an opportunity to learn and grow.

Inquiry stems from both yoga and mindful traditions. The Sanskrit word *Svadhyaya* means self-study as a path to deeper self-knowledge (Weintraub, 2012). Inquiry and curiosity cultivate an attitude of openness and nonjudgment (Cook-Cottone, 2015). Curiosity moves you away from a withdrawal and defense mode of processing and toward engagement and approach (Cook-Cottone, 2015; McCown et al., 2010). Presemantic (i.e., before words) inquiry questions would sound like this: "What am I noticing in my body?" or "What am I noticing in the current moment?" Inquiry questions can help guide behavior as well. For example, Shapiro and Carlson (2009) ask us, as adults, to inquire, "What is most conducive to my own and others' well-being?" (p. 6), or "What would best serve my intentions right now?" For older students, we ask, "How can I be more effective in my work right now?" "Am I reacting to the present moment or a story I am telling myself?" "If I focused only on the here and now, would I think about this differently?" For younger students, "What do I see and notice?" "Where is my focus?" "How is my breathing right now?" In this way, the process of growth is fluid, creative, responsive, nonjudgmental, ongoing, and open (Cook-Cottone, 2015).

Principle 7: Choice: "I choose my focus and actions"

In yoga and mindfulness practices, students are taught to be active decision makers. As well articulated in the Viktor Frankl quote at the beginning of this chapter, between stimulus and response there is a space and in that space is our ability to choose our response. Physical presence, breath, and awareness allow students access to the space between stimulus and response. The next step is for them to actively choose their intentional thought and action. As described by Kellie Love at the beginning of this chapter, students often want to choose to focus and attend but do not know how. Yoga and mindful practices teach students how to focus and choose behaviors. Better, these methodologies teach students how to be aware and focus, and then have them practice these skills in an embodied and active manner either on their yoga mat or in meditation. Research, thus far, has been corroborative, with students reporting increased self-awareness and ability to focus as a result of engaging in yoga (Serwacki & Cook-Cottone, 2012; Wisner, 2014).

Principle 8: Self-Determination: "I do the work"

There is an oft-repeated quote attributed to the yoga teacher, Sri K. Pattabhi Jois, "Do your practice and all is coming." The yoga teacher trainer, Baptiste (2016), cites this quote at the beginning of a book chapter titled, "Do the Work" (p. 97). Baptiste (2016) describes the process of doing the work as distinct from "wishing things to be different" (p. 98). Doing the work means getting into the physicality of the yoga or mindful practice, as well as bringing real action into your life. Doing the work is self-determination in action.

School students can sometimes have high aspirational goals. These goals sometimes manifest along with a substantial gap between what is wanted and hoped for, and what the student is actually doing. For example, Robert, a third-grade student, tells his teacher that he wants to be a medical doctor and work in the emergency room helping people, just like the doctor who helped save his dad when he fell from a ladder and fractured his spine. However, despite Robert's passion to help and his dream of being a spinal surgeon, he does not study for his science or math classes. In fact, he rarely does his homework. The school mindfulness and yoga teacher, Mr. Stevens, noticed this big gap between Robert's wishes and his day-to-day behavior. Robert told Mr. Stevens that he wanted to do a handstand. This was an aspirational pose for Robert, to be sure. Mr. Stevens guided Robert to begin his work at a simple standing pose (i.e., Tadasana). Robert found this pose boring and rested. Mr. Stevens held firm, saying, "Robert, if you want the big dreams you must do the work." Once Robert mastered the fine details of the standing pose, Mr. Stevens allowed him to work his way through a series of supported and unsupported plank poses. This took time. Robert's resistance lessened as he began to see the results of his work. Mr. Stevens continued to reinforce the notion of doing the work as the pathway to getting what you wish and hope for. The two had many long talks connecting handstand, a very hard pose, yet much more accessible than medical school, and what it takes to get there. Mindfulness and yoga practice are embodied methodologies for teaching students about the benefits of doing the work. They can experience with a felt sense the results of the practice.

Principle 9: Sustainability: "I find balance between work and rest"

Sustainability is found in a balance between effort and rest. Finding this balance can be difficult for students. Younger students are often guided by their teachers and parents in terms of how long to do their homework and how much studying is appropriate. As students become more self-guided in their learning, finding the right balance between effort and rest can be difficult. Further, in a culture that celebrates achievement and financial and material wealth, teaching about rest can feel like a defiant act.

As a psychologist in private practice working with older adolescents, I frequently see students stressed by the workload inherent in three to four advanced placement courses along with their other classes. Talking a student, and his or her parents, into a more reasonable and sustainable work load can be difficult as they struggle with the fears of not getting into the "right" college or university. As another example, a colleague, Dr. Wendy Guyker, and I are working with medical schools to help residents begin a practice of self-care so that they can develop a sustainable, professional practice. We find the same thing to be true for medical residents as we do for pressured high school students. The residents are working so hard to be effective practitioners, that they are not willing to take a break for self-care. The results? In their highly cited study, Shanafelt, Bradley, Wipf, and Back (2002) found that, among the medical residents surveyed, 76% met criteria for burnout and, among those, a significant portion reported engaging in suboptimal patient care. Without a commitment to balance and sustainability, people get hurt.

Balance, or equanimity, is a key principle of yoga practice originating from the early traditions of yoga (Cook-Cottone, 2015). Equanimity is an even, steady presence with what is—without the default to rumination, emotional overwhelm, or attachment. Hanson and Mendius (2009) describe equanimity as the mental mudroom, the entry room of the house where people place their muddy boots, rain coats, and lacrosse sticks. It is with equanimity that your initial reactions to things (e.g., I like that, I don't like that) are left in the mudroom so that the inside of your home, your mind, remains clean and of peaceful clarity (Hanson & Mendius, 2009). In yoga class, I remind students, "After great effort, take great rest." By letting go of the extremes and finding equanimity, a sustainable practice and way of being can be found. Teaching this skill is critical for our students today.

Mindful Development

Mindful development builds on mindful embodiment and embodied self-regulation. The focus is on creating a growth trajectory that is built on the principles of compassion, kindness, and possibility. The metaphor of a kind and compassionate coach comes to mind. This type of coach sees the student with an eye for the next possibility in the student's development. The words the coach uses are kind, no matter the performance of the student. When the student fails, the coach uses compassion. Despite failure and unsuccessful attempts, the coach still sees the possibility in each and every student. This is the essence of mindful development. The goal is to work toward students internalizing this kind and compassionate coach as a companion for life effort.

Principle 10: Compassion: "I honor efforts to grow and learn"

Embrace all that arises (Cook-Cottone, 2015; Shapiro & Carlson, 2009); compassion for self and others—these are key teachings of mindfulness and yoga. Compassion has to do with understanding the cause of human suffering. This dates back to the traditional texts and the origins of mindfulness practice. In mindfulness traditions, it is believed that we suffer not from what is happening but from our relationship with what is happening (Shapiro & Carlson, 2009). Teacher Shinzen Young (1997) created a mathematical equation to explain the relationship between suffering and resistance (Bien, 2006; Cook-Cottone, 2015; Shapiro & Carlson, 2009):

$$Suffering = Pain \times Resistance$$

Pain is all that we cannot control. It can be many things—a physical sensation, a relational loss, or a material loss. Pain can be small (a delay at the grocery store, a friend in trouble) or overwhelming (the loss of a loved one). The resistance to the pain is what we, and our students, can control. As the equation illustrates, if the resistance is ours to manage, so is the suffering (Cook-Cottone, 2015). For example, if a student misses the bus and must walk to school (low level of pain), yet the student manifests large amounts of resistance, he or she can experience a great amount of suffering while walking to school. Conversely, the student may experience substantial pain (e.g., not getting accepted to the college of one's choice or having an alcoholic parent) yet allow what has happened, or is happening, to be, and acknowledge it for what it is. In this case, despite the hardship, the student will experience manageable discomfort (Cook-Cottone, 2015; Shapiro & Carlson, 2009).

It is believed that the practices of mindfulness and yoga help students develop compassion for self toward others (e.g., Saksena & Sharma, 2016). Self-compassion is: (a) the ability to be kind and understanding toward oneself during instances of pain and failure rather than being harshly self-critical, (b) seeing one's experiences as part of the bigger human experience and not isolating, and (c) holding painful thoughts and feelings in mindful awareness rather than over-identifying with them (Neff, 2003). Being able to self-regulate and grow mindfully requires skill in both compassion and self-compassion. Mindfulness and yoga practices give students many opportunities to experience errors and failure, engage in compassion and self-compassion, and get back to good effort.

Principle 11: Kindness: "I am kind to myself and others"

In yoga tradition, kindness is considered one of a pair of practices—loving-kindness. Loving-kindness helps develop the capacity for empathy and connection (Cook-Cottone, 2015). Loving-kindness involves attending to self and others with a quiet and open heart (Cook-Cottone, 2015; Wallace, 2011). Siegel (2010) defines loving-kindness as the feeling of compassionate concern for, genuine interest in, and engagement with another. Kindness is distinct from compassion (Cook-Cottone, 2015). For example, Hanson and Mendius (2009) note, "If compassion is the wish that beings not suffer, kindness is the wish that they be happy" (p. 157). In her principles for teaching yoga in schools, Lisa Flynn of Yoga 4 Classrooms asks teachers and students to surround themselves with kindness by practicing gentleness and peacefulness in thoughts and actions (Flynn, 2013). Kindness can be expressed in self-talk, words used to communicate with others, and actions.

Principle 12: Possibility: "I work toward the possibility of effectiveness and growth in my life"

In 2013, my research team went to Nairobi, Kenya, to study the Africa Yoga Project. We used a method called concept mapping, a mixed-method approach using brainstorming, survey data collection, multidimensional scaling, and hierarchical cluster analysis. Among our many findings was this: Those who were teaching and practicing with the Africa Yoga Project reported that yoga helped them see possibility on their mats and in their lives (Klein, Cook-Cottone, & Giambrone, 2015). Mindfulness and yoga offer students opportunity, in active practice, to play with possibility in a safe and supportive environment. One of my most cherished experiences is seeing a young yoga student achieve a pose that he or she has been working on. I love that look in the student's eyes that says, "If I can do this, what else is possible?"

Mindful Grit and Mindful Growing

The principles of embodied growth and learning capture the essence of *mindful grit* and *mindful growing*. Mindful grit is a new term that builds on Duckworth's (2016) work that defines grit as passion and perseverance. Mindful grit holds space for positive embodiment and hard work toward long-term goals with an eye on self-care, compassion, and sustainability. In private practice, at the university, and in my personal life, I have seen the negative effects of passion and perseverance in the absence of sustainability and self-care. Mindful grit allows for sustainability and balance while still honoring work toward possibility.

Mindful growing is also a new term that builds on Dweck's work on growth mindset (e.g., Rattan, Savani, Chugh, & Dweck, 2015). In mindful growing, there is a focus on a mindset of possibility within the context of inquiry, choice, self-determination, and sustainability. Further, the movement toward possibility (i.e., mindful development) occurs within the context of the mindfulness and yoga tools of compassion and kindness. See Figure 3.3 for an overview of how mindful grit and mindful growing relate to the 12 principles of embodied growth and learning. The figure also illustrates how the 12 principles inform mindful and yoga practices and the key mechanisms of action (e.g., self-regulation, self-care, and intentional, reflective engagement). Finally, Figure 3.3 illustrates how these practices inform the goals and mission of education—that is, to support student learning of content and learning tools; help students become personal architects of their own learning and well-being; and graduate students who are creative and collaborative problem solvers ready to work together and manage the issues facing our people and planet.

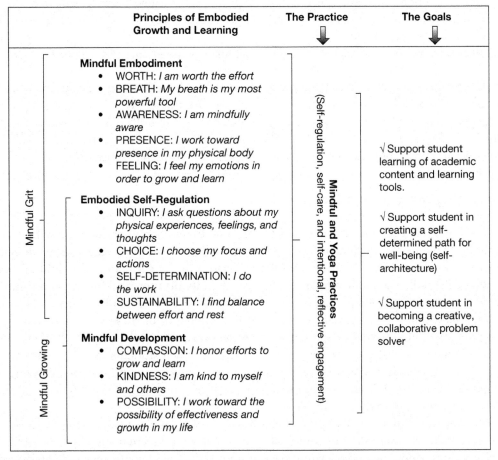

FIGURE 3.3 Overview of mindful grit, mindful growing, and the 12 principles in context.

TEACHING MINDFULNESS AND YOGA PRACTICES

School personnel reading this book likely have a broad range of mindfulness and yoga integration from none to whole-district programs, infused curriculum, and stand-alone classes. School-based mindfulness and yoga programs have been around long enough for experienced providers to offer tips as to how to do it best. Childress and Harper (2015) provide a wonderful list of how to effectively work with your school and district to facilitate a program.

- Communicate with your school (e.g., prioritize transparency; provide information on class content, schedule, and teachers; detail frequently asked questions; collaborate; and provide contact information and a tool for feedback and response; Childress & Harper, 2015).
- Account for your school and district needs (see Childress & Harper, p. 15).
- Consider education standards (see Childress & Harper, p. 20).
- Offer secular programs (see Childress & Harper, p. 21).
- Hire quality instructors (see Childress & Harper, p. 34).
- Know school rules, policies, and procedures (see Childress & Harper, p. 44).
- Be sure to obtain releases, permission, required certificates, liability insurance, first aid training, and professional screening (e.g., criminal check, FBI screening, etc.; see Childress & Harper, p. 46).
- Collaborate and prepare ahead for logistical challenges (see Childress & Harper, p. 48).

The forthcoming chapters detail much more about implementing a program. You are encouraged to seek a program designed for schools with trainers who have dual education backgrounds or staff that reflects experience and training in both mindfulness/yoga and education. This section addresses diversity and inclusion and who can teach mindfulness and yoga in schools, as well as emphasizes how much your own practice matters.

Addressing Diversity and Inclusion

Diversity and inclusion are critical issues to consider. In his chapter on working with diversity and inclusion, Rechtschaffen (2014) reminds us that diversity includes race, ethnicity, socioeconomic status, the location and characteristics of your school and neighborhood, ability levels, skills and challenges, sexuality, gender identity, personal history and trauma, religion, body size and shape, family and neighborhood values, family educational backgrounds, and many other variables and qualities. Given all of these variables, "You can never assume that you know what lies in the inner world of a child" (Rechtschaffen, 2014, p. 109). Remember first to listen and create a space in which students feel they can have a voice. It should be clear, when a student enters our classroom and school, that diversity is valued and celebrated. Your mindfulness and yoga programs should be aligned with the broader commitment to those priorities.

Overall, mindfulness and yoga practice should be taught in a manner that includes all students, makes adaptations and modifications; uses clear and secular language; and reflects secular values. Know when you might need training in cultural competence, diversity, and inclusion. If you are not sure, you probably need training. There are many online training programs for the workplace and educators. See the National Education Association's (NEA)

Diversity Toolkit: Cultural Competence for Educators (www.nea.org/tools/30402.htm). Finally, Childress and Harper (2015) offer a wealth of guidance in areas including: supporting positive body image development (pp. 26–27); working with disabilities (pp. 38–39); seeing all behaviors as communication (pp. 55–56); committing to inclusivity (pp. 57–58); creating equitable relationships (pp. 59–60); recognizing trauma's effects on students (pp. 65–66); considering social and emotional needs (pp. 82–83); creating a safe space (pp. 102–103); and addressing students' needs (pp. 104–105).

Who Can Teach Yoga and Mindfulness in Schools?

There is no consistent set of standards for the hiring of instructors that can be applied nationally, across states and school districts, at this time. Further, the fields of mindfulness and yoga have evolved both together and distinctly, along with two separate histories for standards of practice (Cook-Cottone, 2015). Be sure to check with your school district and consult the state regulations relevant to the school within which you would like to implement mindfulness and yoga instruction.

According to Rechtschaffen (2014) in his book, *The Way of Mindful Education: Cultivating Well-Being in Teachers and Students*, and Childress and Harper (2015) in *Best Practices for Yoga in Schools*, training in mindfulness and/or yoga, ongoing study (i.e., continuing education), and personal practice are encouraged and required. Essentially, given appropriate training, active practice, and the correct teaching credentials for your school district and state, anyone can teach mindfulness and yoga. In some schools, like Kellie Love's in New York, there is a dedicated yoga or mindfulness teacher. The students attend class just as they would attend a health, physical education, or math class. In other schools, physical education and health-and-wellness teachers are trained to provide mindfulness and yoga instruction to students. Still in other districts, classroom and subject teachers train in mindfulness and/or yoga and actively interweave mindfulness and yoga into their curriculum and throughout the school day. Currently, researchers are exploring which models work best, and there are no published studies that indicate one option is more effective than another.

When I began my yoga teaching, I was early in my career as a professor. I had just received my license as a psychologist in New York State and was eager to conduct research on using yoga to prevent eating disorders among young girls. For several years, I hired yoga teachers with training and certifications appropriate for New York State to teach yoga for my research studies in schools. You see, I saw teaching yoga as something that other people could do. As I observed the yoga classes, I was so inspired by what I was seeing among the students participating in my research, I decided to enroll in yoga teacher training myself.

As I learned, I began integrating what I was learning into my curriculum at the university. Over time, I added mindfulness and yoga components to my coursework on counseling with children and adolescents, and developed my own courses on mindful therapy and yoga for health and healing. Eventually, I created an Advanced Certificate in Mindful Counseling for Wellness and Engagement (gse.buffalo.edu/programs/adv-cert/counseling). We now offer additional courses in mindful coaching, evidence-based interventions for using mindfulness and yoga, and a course on balancing self-care and service. Taking the principle of possibility very seriously and personally, I founded and am president of a not-for-profit called Yogis in Service (www.yogisinservice.org) that offers yoga to those who would not otherwise have access. I also continue my research on self-regulation, self-care, and yoga.

I offer my own story to suggest that you can do this too. Along with what is required for your district and state, you need three things: (a) ongoing, active practice; (b) good foundational training; and (c) continuing education to keep your skills sharp and your knowledge current.

The Mindfulness and Yoga Teacher as a Practitioner

If you ask yoga teachers like me, Kellie Love, or Sarah Herrington (author of *Om Schooled: A Guide to Teaching Kids Yoga in Real-World Schools;* 2012), "Should teachers of mindfulness and yoga practices be required to have an established, steady personal practice?," you will get a resounding, "YES!" For thousands of years, teaching mindfulness and yoga has been a mentoring process in which a well-practiced mentor passes down knowledge and practices to the mentee. More, beyond being a tradition, it is a form of self-care (Cook-Cottone, 2015; Herrington, 2012; Rechtschaffen, 2014; see Chapter 14 of this text for more on self-care). In Herrington's book (2012), she describes how important it is to live your yoga off the mat while teaching yoga on the mat. She explains that teaching yoga in schools can be stressful, takes a lot of energy, and requires you to be steady and fully present no matter what kind of energy, feelings, and struggles the children and adolescents bring into the yoga space. Herrington, like many others, found that maintaining her own practice was essential. She found that, in her daily practice, she was inspired and restored: "I was viscerally reminded of the gifts of yoga; I could release, relax, regain myself, and start the next day from a point of center" (Herrington, 2012, p. 143).

As you read through the following chapters, I ask you to contemplate your own experience and your own practice. I use case studies and examples to illustrate points and challenges. As we move to Parts II and III of this text, we also shift to seeing the mindfulness and yoga teacher as an additional source of wisdom and insight. That is, you and your experience with mindfulness and yoga are integrated into your teaching of these methodologies (Cook-Cottone, 2015). As a mindfulness and/or yoga teacher using these techniques, you can speak from an authentic experience of practice and struggle (a part of practice; Cook-Cottone, 2015). As a result of your practice, when you speak, you speak from a knowing of this journey and the challenges it holds (Cook-Cottone, 2015). McCown et al. (2010) call this authority. This authority comes from a living it, loving it, and knowing it that can only come from dutiful practice (Cook-Cottone, 2015).

What does this mean in your day-to-day life? It means that you have a commitment to consistent, formal practice that mirrors the frequency, intensity, and duration you would hope for from your students (Cook-Cottone, 2015; McCown et al., 2010). It is important to note that there may be a dose-related response to these practices. That means that in order to get the full benefits of meditation, mindfulness, relaxation, and yoga practice, you may need to practice every day. For example, it is believed that in order to glean the therapeutic benefits of yoga practice, one should practice three times a week for a duration of at least an hour for a period of more than 6 weeks (Cook-Cottone, 2013). To teach yoga, certification is recommended with a foundation of steady practice of 2 years (Cook-Cottone, 2015). See Yoga Alliance (www.yogaalliance.org) for questions about yoga certification and registration as a yoga instructor. Yoga Alliance also sets standards and provides for yoga teachers and teacher-training programs. To effectively teach mindfulness and meditation, one should engage in some form of meditation or formal mindfulness practice daily for at least 90 days prior to teaching meditation or speaking about it from any sense of authority (Cook-Cottone, 2015; McCown et al., 2010).

CONCLUSION

The mindful and yogic learner is not a thing, or an object, but is a person in process (Cook-Cottone, 2015). This process requires a set of skills that make up what I call mindful grit and the capacity for mindful growing. These skills can be summarized in a set of 12 embodied practices: worth, breath, awareness, presence, feeling, inquiry, choice, self-determination, sustainability, compassion, kindness, and possibility. These practices integrate a large body of knowledge passed down from both mindful and yogic traditions, as well as a large and growing body of research on mindfulness and yoga in schools.

The following chapters break down mindful and yoga conceptualizations and detail specific practices referring back to these 12 practices as central organizing themes. Consider this your starting place. Continued study of the research, theoretical texts, and practical texts on mindfulness and yoga in schools is encouraged as you continue your path of self-development and refine your work with your students. Welcome to the journey.

REFERENCES

Ajaya, S. (1983). *Psychotherapy east and west: A unifying paradigm.* Honesdale, PA: The Himalayan International Institute.

Baptiste, B. (2016). *Perfectly imperfect: The art and soul of yoga practice.* Carlsbad, CA: Hay House.

Bennett, B. (2002). *Emotional yoga: How the body can heal the mind.* New York, NY: Fireside.

Benson, H. (1976). *The relaxation response.* New York, NY: Harper Torch.

Berger, C., Silver, E., & Stein, R. (2009). Effects of yoga on inner-city children's wellbeing: A pilot study. *Alternative Therapies in Health and Medicine, 15,* 36–42.

Bien, T. (2006). *Mindful therapy: A guide for therapists and helping professionals.* Somerville, MA: Wisdom.

Branson, C. M., & Gross, S. J. (Eds.). (2014). *Handbook of ethical educational leadership.* New York, NY: Routledge.

Brown, K. W., & Ryan, R. M. (2003). The benefits of being present: Mindfulness and its role in psychological well-being. *Journal of Personality and Social Psychology, 84,* 822–848.

Case-Smith, J., Shupe Sines, J., & Klatt, M. (2010). Perceptions of children who participated in a school-based yoga program. *Journal of Occupational Therapy, Schools, & Early Intervention, 3,* 226–238.

Childress, T., & Harper, J. C. (2015). *Best practices for yoga in schools.* Atlanta, GA: Yoga Service Council.

Cook-Cottone, C. P. (2006). The attune representational model for the primary prevention of eating disorders: An overview for school psychologists. *Psychology in the Schools, 43,* 223–230.

Cook-Cottone, C. P. (2013). Dosage as a critical variable in yoga research. *International Journal of Yoga Therapy, 2,* 11–12.

Cook-Cottone, C. P. (2015). *Mindfulness and yoga for self-regulation: A primer for mental health professionals.* New York, NY: Springer Publishing.

Duckworth, A. (2016). *Grit: The power of passion and perseverance.* New York, NY: Simon & Schuster.

Flynn, L. (2013). *Yoga for children: 200+ yoga poses, breathing exercises, and meditation for healthier, happier, more resilient children.* Avon, MA: Adams Media.

Frankl, V. (1959). *Man's search for meaning.* Boston, MA: Beacon Press.

Grabovac, A. D., Lau, M. A., & Willett, B. R. (2011). Mechanism of mindfulness: A Buddhist Psychological Model. *Mindfulness, 2*(3), 154–166. doi:10.1007/s12671-011-0054-5

Hanson, R., & Mendius, R. (2009). *Buddha's brain: The practical neuroscience of happiness, love, and wisdom.* Oakland, CA: New Harbinger Press, Inc.

Harper, J. C. (2013). *Little Flower Yoga for Kids: A yoga and mindfulness program to help your children improve attention and emotional balance.* Oakland, CA: New Harbinger.

Harrington, S. (2012). *Om schooled: A guide to teaching kids yoga in real-world schools.* San Marcos, CA: Addriya.

Jennings, P. A. (2015). *Mindfulness for teachers: Simple skills for peace and productivity in the classroom.* New York, NY: W.W. Norton.

Klein, J. E., Cook-Cottone, C., & Giambrone, C. (2015). The Africa yoga project: A participant-driven concept map of Kenyan teachers' reported experiences. *International Journal of Yoga Therapy, 25,* 113–126.

MacArthur Foundation. (2016). *Angela Duckworth, research psychologist.* Retrieved from https://www .macfound.org/fellows/889/#sthash.9QxSD1Qj.dpuf

McCown, D., Reibel, D., & Micozzi, M. S. (2010). *Teaching mindfulness: A practical guide for clinicians and educators.* New York, NY: Springer.

Neff, K. (2003). The development and validation of a scale to measure self-compassion. *Self And Identity, 2,* 223–250.

Perkins-Gough, P. (2013, September). The significance of grit: Conversation with Angela Lee Duckworth. *Educational Leadership, 71,* 14–20.

Prabhavananda, S., & Isherwood, C. (2007). *How to know God: The yoga aphorisms of Patanjali.* Hollywood, CA: Vedanta Press.

Radcliffe, S. (2016). Meditation and yoga joining arithmetic and reading in U.S. classrooms. *Healthline.* Retrieved from https://www.healthline.com/health-news/meditation-and-yoga-joining -arithmetic-and-reading-in-us-classrooms-011216#5

Rattan, A., Savani, K., Chugh, D., & Dweck, C. S. (2015). Leveraging mindsets to promote academic achievement policy recommendations. *Perspectives on Psychological Science, 10,* 721–726.

Rechtschaffen, D. (2014). *The way of mindful education: Cultivating well-being in teachers and students.* New York, NY: W. W. Norton.

Saksena, T., & Sharma, R. (2016). Yoga as a predictor of self-compassion in adolescents: Endeavors for positive growth and development. *The International Journal of Indian Psychology, 3,* 85–96

Schultz, P. P., & Ryan, R. M. (2005). The "why," "what," and "how" of healthy self-regulation: Mindfulness and well-being from a Self-Determination Theory perspective, In B. D. Ostafin, M. D. Robinson, & B. P. Meier (Eds.), *Handbook of mindfulness and self-regulation* (pp. 81–94). New York, NY: Springer.

Serwacki, M., & Cook-Cottone, C. P. (2012). Yoga in the schools: A systematic review of the literature. *International Journal of Yoga Therapy, 22,* 101–110.

Shanafelt, T. D., Bradley, K. A., Wipf, J. E., & Back, A. L. (2002). Burnout and self-reported patient care in an internal medicine residency program. *Annals of Internal Medicine, 136,* 358–367.

Shapiro, S. L., & Carlson, L. E. (2009). *The art and science of mindfulness: Integrating mindfulness into psychology and the helping professions.* Washington, DC: American Psychological Association.

Siegel, D. J. (2010). *The mindful therapist: A clinician's guide to mindsight and neural integration.* New York, NY: W. W. Norton.

Siegel, D. J. (2015). *The developing mind: How relationships and the brain interact to shape who we are.* New York, NY: Guilford Press.

Simpkins, A. M., & Simpkins, C. A. (2011). *Meditation and yoga in psychotherapy.* New York, NY: Wiley.

Vygotsky, L. S. (1978). *Mind in society: The development of higher psychological processes.* Cambridge, MA: Harvard University Press.

Wallace, B. A. (2011). *Minding closely: The four applications of mindfulness.* Ithaca, NY: Snow Lion.

Weintraub, A. (2012). *Yoga skills for therapists: Effective practices for mood management.* New York, NY: W. W. Norton

Wisner, B. L. (2014). An exploratory study of mindfulness meditation for alternative school students: Perceived benefits for improving school climate and student functioning. *Mindfulness, 5(6),* 626–638.

Yeager, D. S., & Dweck, C. (2012). Mindsets that promote resilience: When students believe that personal characteristics can be developed. *Educational Psychologist, 47,* 302–314.

Yoga Alliance. Retrieved from https://www.yogaalliance.org

Young, S. (1997). *The science of enlightenment* (Audio Cassettes). Boulder, CO: Sounds True.

PART II

MINDFULNESS IN EDUCATING FOR SELF-REGULATION AND ENGAGEMENT

CHAPTER 4

THE MINDFUL LEARNER: THE ROLE OF MINDFULNESS IN EDUCATING FOR SELF-REGULATION AND ENGAGEMENT

Learning to listen to [and see] ourselves
is a way of learning to love ourselves

Joan Borysenko (Goldman, 2009, p. 104)

This chapter introduces you to the basic principles of mindfulness as they can be applied to student self-regulation and engagement in schools. Mindfulness is conceptualized as a central feature of contemplative education (see Chapter 1; Waters, Barsky, Ridd, & Allen, 2015). Mindfulness is central to each of the 12 principles of embodied growing and learning (see Chapter 3). The first principle, worth (i.e., I am worth the effort; see Chapter 3, principle 1), is a good starting point, maybe even the most important starting point. A student that does not believe that he or she is worth the effort will be very difficult, if not impossible, to motivate in the classroom. In our fast-paced, achievement-oriented culture, it can be easy to lose a sense of inherent self-value. Our students spend their waking day listening and watching as mass and social media tell them what is important, attractive, and valuable. They get "liked," "reposted," "retweeted," and "shared" for being attractive or externally conspicuous in some way. Worse, the social media acknowledgments are all counted and compared in an empirical manner (i.e., they can do the math to find out how seemingly socially valued they are). It is a virtual world in which a video of self-induced vomiting may appear to, in terms of shares and likes, be more valued than an act of kindness. I used to be shocked when I would see the explicitly sexual and overtly provocative material posted by some of the most kindhearted dedi-cated, and sensitive students. However, these types of posts are so common now that I no longer find them surprising. The pressure seems to be so great that the students, even very young ones, spend a substantial amount of time in creation of a social media iden-tity to secure social capital (i.e., perceived social value), leaving the embodied, sensing, and learning self behind.

For many students, the focus on external value is echoed across their interpersonal and social experiences. At school, although we likely worry less about their appearance and social capital, we tell them what we (e.g., the school district curriculum team, the state, and the education department) think is important to know and learn. More, their coaches focus on showing them how to perform and the critical skills needed to win the game. In choir, band, and orchestra, the students play the songs we give them, performing how we tell them to—all to the exact and external manifestation of what others think they should be. Of course, there are so many teachers, like my mom, who value and encourage inner seeing and knowing, as well as foster constructive creativity within the context of teaching a rigorous curriculum. Nevertheless, we all appreciate that, in some classrooms and schools, the preceding description rings true. It is no surprise that our students lose a sense of their personal value as they are praised for, and their attention is turned to, their appearance, performance, and compliance over and over again for much of the day, almost every day. A felt sense of who they are and what they want to know and learn, along with an organic excitement about learning, can be lost in the centrifugal forces of expectations and societal trends. Ironically, this external focus on achievement, appearance, and social capital can appear as if the student is overly self-involved. It is important to make a distinction here. For many students, self-involvement is *not* an internal, embodied, integrated involvement. Rather, it is a fear- or anxiety-based, externally motivated focus. We want our students to have an inward focus on the self. We want them to be self-aware, self-knowing, and emotionally competent. This relationship with and connection to the self is one which involves compassion, kindness, and a healthy form of self-love and love of learning that actually expands students' capacity for empathy and connection with others.

So how do we shift the focus and self-value inward in an integrated and healthy manner? How do we create opportunities for students to experience their thinking (e.g., cognitive processes), to be in inquiry about what works best for them, and become architects of their own attentional focus and effort? Mindfulness practice offers a set of tools to help students turn inward, seeing and valuing their individual experience, allowing them to integrate who they are inside with who they are being outside. The results of this type of integration are self-regulatory.

Many of the quotes I have placed at the introduction of the chapters in this book come from the hundreds of quotes my mother used as journaling prompts when teaching her seventh-grade and freshman English classes. In the pile of dog-eared book pages, colorful quote lists torn from magazines, and hand-drafted notes-to-self, I found this quote, "Learning to listen to [and see] ourselves is a way of learning to love ourselves." I added to see in order to highlight the mindful part of each of us that can see, or witness, our thoughts, feelings, and actions. Ask yourself, when the voice in your head is talking, "Who is listening and seeing?" This is the mindful part of you, and it is present in each of us. This mindful witness has the capacity to notice all of the wide range of experiences in our lives. The mindful witness notices when we are attending or not, being rude or hurtful, having fun or checking out, and engaging in or ignoring our own self-care. The mindful witness is a powerful aspect of the self to access.

Take a moment and consider the people you really care about. You likely take the time to earnestly listen to them. You compassionately see them in all of their victories, failures, and times of emotional stability, as well as the times they might feel as if they are falling apart. This process of mindfully attending to, or seeing, those you care for is one of the many ways that you show them that you love and value them. The challenge is to be able to see and care for yourself in the same way. For me, the Borysenko quote speaks to the inherent self-valuing that occurs when we teach mindfulness in the classroom. In mindful practice, we take a break from the external and allow time to notice, listen to, and *see* our own internal workings. The process of mindful attention is an embodied valuing of our experiences. As educators, creating these moments of self-valuing for students is an essential aspect of helping them understand, in a felt sense, that they are worth the effort as well as a methodology for developing their own set of self-regulatory skills in order to more effectively engage in academic tasks.

This chapter explicates the definition of mindfulness and how mindfulness works in the classroom to help increase self-regulation and active engagement in learning throughout the school day. The basic characteristics of mindfulness are explored. Finally, the stage is set for Chapters 5 to 7, which detail the formal mindfulness practices, informal mindfulness practices, and the school-based mindfulness protocols that have empirical support.

MINDFULNESS

There are many definitions of mindfulness, a complexity in the field that can be traced back to the field's origins (Lutz, Jha, Dunne, & Saron, 2015). Mindfulness techniques are believed to steady the mind and help train attentional capacity, while increasing breadth of focus (Weare, 2013; Zenner, Herrnleben, & Walach, 2014). Lutz et al. (2015) have reviewed the literature in the field of mindfulness and psychology. They found that mindfulness is generally used with three meanings. These are (a) a soteriological or spiritual path (i.e., a story of salvation) contextualized in therapeutic health-promotion terms, (b) a mental trait, and (c) a single cognitive process commonly trained across multiple human activities (Lutz et al., 2015).

Mindfulness as a Story

First, in a broad sense, mindfulness has been referred to as a soteriological or transcendent path from suffering to well-being (Lutz et al., 2015). Early Sanskrit references to mindfulness use the term *smrti*, which has semantic overtones with the English word memory, or to remember (Lutz et al., 2015). I often think of it as remembering my practice or commitment. When I am not being mindful (i.e., the state-like use of the term), I *remind* myself to reconnect. In a sense, mindfulness can be seen as a commitment to a way of being, or a stance toward life that goes beyond any particular technique (Lutz et al., 2015). Many people, like myself, view mindfulness and yoga practices as a key factor in a shift in our way of being, bringing increased mental health and ease—and decreased suffering, bad habits, and/or pathology. There is a body of research that tells that same story. That is, if you engage in mindfulness practices you will feel, and be less addicted, depressed, dysregulated, compulsive, and so on (Cook-Cottone, 2015).

Along this line of thinking, Shapiro and Carlson (2009) provide a helpful distinction between big /M/ *Mindfulness* and little /m/ *mindfulness*. According to them, big /M/ Mindfulness is the fundamental way of being, of inhabiting your body and moment-by-moment experience (Shapiro & Carlson, 2009). Big /M/ Mindfulness is a path or journey. Little /m/ mindfulness involves the practices, or the way in which one intentionally pursues the path of big /M/ Mindfulness (Shapiro & Carlson, 2009). Some suggest that mindfulness may be an antidote to consumerism, messages from the media, and social media pressures and influences (e.g., Cook-Cottone, 2015; Rosenberg, 2004). This contention has been supported by reviews of the literature that indicate that mindfulness has been associated with well-being, voluntary simplicity, and a lifestyle shaped around intrinsically satisfying pursuits and expressions of self, away from material goals (Brown & Kasser, 2005). In other words, mindfulness has been associated with a healthy, internal sense of self.

Mindfulness as a Trait

Second, mindfulness is sometimes operationalized as a stable mental trait that can be measured by scales assessing disposition (Lutz et al., 2015). This can be problematic, as even those who study mindfulness as a trait do so within the context of measuring mindfulness with trained practitioners, suggesting that skill acquisition is involved (see Lutz et al. [2015] for a review). Further, given the current state of the research in this area, outcomes based on trait measures are difficult to interpret. In their review, Lutz et al. (2015) cite contradictory findings in studies that use trait mindfulness measures. They also note that studies using self-reported, trait mindfulness measures as an outcome of a mindfulness intervention does little to inform the field of mechanisms of action or shifts in clinical vulnerabilities, cognitive, affective, or social outcomes that might also be affected by the training (Lutz et al., 2015). Accordingly, the view is that mindfulness as a trait does not have empirical or theoretical support at this time.

Mindfulness as a Cognitive Process

Last, mindfulness is used as a term that describes a core cognitive process that is cultivated via various mindfulness-based practices (Lutz et al., 2015). Mindfulness is a particular way of paying attention in the present moment (Felver, Doerner, Jones, Kaye, & Merrell, 2013; Lutz et al., 2015; Weare, 2013; Zenner et al., 2014). Lutz et al. (2015) argue that there are shared contextual features across mindfulness practices. For instance, some physical postures are believed to be more conducive to cultivating mindfulness during formal meditation than others (Lutz et al., 2015). Another feature is a nonaversive affective tone (Lutz et al., 2015). This has been operationalized as an accepting, friendly, kind, compassionate, and even loving affective tone (Lutz et al., 2015). Also, most mindfulness practices share a goal or motivation to reduce suffering (Lutz et al., 2015). It is important to note that this conceptualization of mindfulness can be subtly different depending on the tradition or practice used or studied (e.g., Mindfulness-Based Stress Reduction or Transcendental Meditation; Lutz et al., 2015). As such, differences in conceptualization, even if they are small, as well as the use of a broad conceptualization of mindfulness, can affect the ability to formulate mechanistic hypotheses in research and practice (Lutz et al., 2015). When referring to mindfulness as a cognitive process, researchers and practitioners are typically referring to the following aspects of the term: (a) present moment awareness, (b) bare attention, (c) release of judgment, and (d) the focus of attention (see Figure 4.1).

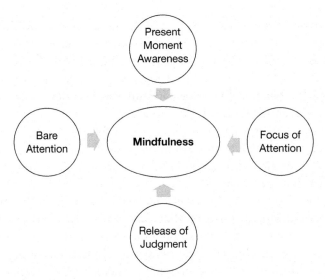

FIGURE 4.1 Components of mindfulness as a cognitive process.
Source: Lutz et al. (2015).

Present moment awareness is a necessary component of mindfulness (Felver et al., 2013; Lutz et al., 2015). Generally speaking, mindfulness concerns clarity of awareness of one's inner and outer worlds in the right now and right here of experience (Cook-Cottone, 2015; Brown, Ryan, & Creswell, 2007). Present moment awareness of the inner and outer worlds includes one's thoughts, emotions, and actions, as well as one's surroundings (Felver et al., 2013). Present moment awareness in mindfulness is a unique quality of consciousness, a receptive awareness of ongoing internal states, behavior, and external realities (Brown et al., 2007). Even more specifically, present moment awareness involves the conscious registration of stimuli associated with the five senses, kinesthetic senses, and the functions of the mind (Brown et al., 2007). Note that, in mindfulness tradition, the mind is viewed much like the other sense organs (e.g., ears, eyes, skin; Olendzki, 2012). Each of the senses, including the mind, has an object. For example, the nose is smelling scents, and the eyes are seeing things. In this way, the mind is thinking, which is considered knowing with the mind (Olendzki, 2012). The objects of the mind include anything that can be cognized, such as thoughts, images, and memories (Olendzki, 2012).

Mindfulness involves *bare attention* or an open and distortion-free perception of what is (Brown & Kasser, 2005; Brown et al., 2007; Lutz et al., 2015). In order to develop bare attention, we must acknowledge that we are of the tendency to quickly conceptualize what is happening. We construct, interpret, evaluate, assess, and connect what is happening with what we know (Brown et al., 2007). In mindfulness practice, there is an effort to decouple the nearly automatic tendency to intertwine attention and cognition (Brown et al., 2007). When the mind is in the mindful mode of processing, it does not compare, judge, categorize, evaluate, contemplate, reflect, introspect, or ruminate on experiences based on what is known (Brown et al., 2007; Cook-Cottone, 2015). Rather, with bare attention, the mind is open and present to input manifested by a simple noticing of what is happening (Brown et al., 2007; Cook-Cottone, 2015).

Mindfulness involves the *release of judgment*. It entails an unconditional presence and unconditional openness (Brown et al., 2007). This means that, when you are engaged in mindfulness, you are not deciding if you like something or not, or if it is good or bad. Rather, you are in inquiry about it. You are curious, exploratory, and present (see Chapter 3, principle 6, inquiry). It is believed that once you shift into judgment, you are no longer being mindful. This is true even for your mindful awareness of your own mindfulness. That is, as you notice yourself losing focus and moving to judgment, "My breathing is horribly uneven," or "I struggle so much to pay attention," you do not judge yourself for judging. You simply notice, "I see I am judging," and shift your focus back to your object of attention, your breath, or your simple awareness.

Mindfulness may also include a *focus of attention*. Lutz et al. (2015) identified common dimensions of the mindfulness construct that exist across many styles of mindfulness as related to object orientation. This is the "phenomenal sense that an experience or mental state is oriented toward some object or class of objects" (Lutz et al., 2015, p. 639). That is, the person practicing mindfulness is aware of some particular thing via perception, memory, or imagination. Further, the critical phenomenological feature is that there is a focus on an object, no matter how strongly or weakly, intellectually or unintentionally, the mind is focused on an object (Lutz et al., 2015).

The Practice of Mindfulness

Mindfulness is also a set of practices (Weare, 2013; Zenner et al., 2014). Typically, in mindful practice, students are instructed to focus attention; if the mind drifts away, the focus is gently brought back to the present moment experience. There are various ways to practice mindfulness in terms of the object of focused attention. These are represented well among the various styles of meditation described in Chapter 5. In some cases, the practitioner is actively practicing focused attention. In other cases, the practitioner is engaging in an open monitoring of the mind (Lutz et al., 2015). Specifically, in focused attention, there is an intention to focus on an object. The person practicing works to be in bare awareness of the object with good intensity. He or she may notice that attention of focus has waned and then bring awareness and attention back to the object. Distinctly, in open monitoring practice, the individual may deliberately reduce any intentional focus on objects. In this case, he or she simply observes the mind and the mental processes of awareness (Lutz et al., 2015). There are more how-tos to come. Chapters 5 to 7 focus on the practical application of mindfulness in schools.

HISTORICAL ROOTS OF MINDFULNESS TO MINDFULNESS IN SCHOOLS

According to Brown et al. (2007) and Zenner et al. (2014), mindfulness has its origins in Buddhist psychology. These models of the mind are thought to have developed in northern India in the fifth through third centuries BCE (Olendzki, 2012). Buddhist psychology, in its essence, is focused on the subjective perception of experience (Olendzki, 2012). The focus on the attentional and awareness aspects of consciousness is conceptually similar to ideas advanced by several other philosophical and psychological traditions. These include: ancient Greek philosophy, phenomenology, existentialism, transcendentalism and humanism in America, and naturalism as it was manifest in later Western European thought. McCown, Reibel, and Micozzi (2010) trace the European connection to Eastern spiritual thought and practice back to ancient Greece circa 327-325 BCE. In 1784, British scholars and magistrates of the Asiatic Society of Bengal authored the first translations of Hindu scriptures from Sanskrit to English (McCown et al., 2010). As these scriptures became more widely available, they dovetailed with and influenced other movements rising up on both sides of the Atlantic. In early 19th-century Europe, for instance, Romanticism brought an intensely emotional and visionary character to the arts—marking a break from the calm restraint of Classicism. And, often, the Romantics looked to the East for exotic, faraway themes and spiritual inspiration (Cook-Cottone, 2015; McCown et al., 2010). Concurrently, in New England, transcendentalism arose—shaped and driven by such notable thinkers as Ralph Waldo Emerson and Henry David Thoreau. As it sought to elevate the individual's relationship to the world and to existence, transcendentalism likewise tapped into Eastern teachings (Cook-Cottone, 2015; McCown et al., 2010).

Beginning in the 1950s, Daisetz Teitaro Suzuki, a Zen scholar, as well as a scholar of Western philosophy and psychology, was influential in bringing Zen to the United States and to the field of psychoanalysis (Harrington & Dunne, 2015). For Suzuki, "Zen was a radically antiauthoritarian practice and philosophy that was concerned, not with textual authority and scholastic training, not with ritual, dogma or even ethics, but with the transformative effects of experiencing the world as it really was" (Harrington & Dunne, 2015, p. 623). The "Zen Boom" of the 1950s and 1960s permeated both academic studies and popular culture (McCown et al., 2010). In a twist of fate that Harrington and Dunne (2015) describe as "Simply put, the sixties arrived" (p. 625), the Harvard LSD studies marred the narrative of mindfulness interventions (McCown et al., 2010), and Zen was appropriated by a counter culture movement in psychotherapy (Harrington & Dunne, 2015). Ultimately, mainstream integration of Zen declined substantially (Harrington & Dunne, 2015).

The 1980s and 1990s are considered the "painful passage into maturity" as mindful practices were scientifically assessed and accepted by academics, practitioners, and the mainstream public (McCown et al., 2010, p. 54). What has transpired over these many years is considered the movement toward a universalizing and secularizing discourse in order to create accessibility (McCown et al., 2010). Tension continues as the practices and traditions are extruded through Western constructs, such as the scientific method and practical and medical applications (Cook-Cottone, 2015). Some refer to the use of mindfulness in treatment as the medicalization of the practices, and some see it as further appropriation of valued traditions (Harrington & Dunne, 2015). In my personal practice, I am working to understand and know the heritage of the practices that have brought me great peace and happiness. However, in practice, especially in schools, it is important to maintain a clear distinction between historical traditions, mindfulness philosophy, and mindfulness practices that have been shown to be effective for student learning and well-being (e.g., Rechtschaffen, 2014; Waters et al., 2015).

The Evolution of Secular Mindfulness Practice

Felver et al. (2013) state that it is a misconception to identify mindfulness as a form of Eastern religion. They acknowledge that mindfulness and many of the mindfulness techniques have their roots in Eastern religion and philosophical schools of thought (Felver et al., 2013). However, they make a clear distinction between the concept of mindfulness and its applications, which, as delivered in schools, are completely secular in nature (Felver et al., 2013). They offer the metaphor of fasting. Although fasting is part of many world religions, fasting in and of itself is not a religious practice (Felver et al., 2013).

Let us ask the right question. Linehan (1993) teaches her patients that a focus on morality, or right or wrong, is not necessarily a useful line of inquiry. Linehan asks her patients to look to what is effective (Linehan, 1993). Current definitions of mindfulness and mindful practices are derived from (a) traditions, (b) tensions that arise from the application of practices with a long and rich tradition in school settings, and (c) an effort to create accessibility, or an opening to a whole new way of self-regulating and engaging for all students (Cook-Cottone, 2015). Purposefully, there is a Vygotskian scaffolding (Vygotsky, 1978) of Western language and culture integrated into the delivery of mindful practices in order to provide a comprehensible methodology for use in schools. Following Linehan's lead, this text seeks to detail what is effective for students.

In October of 2015, the *American Psychologist* published its 70th volume, 7th edition as a special issue titled, "The Emergence of Mindfulness as a Basic and Clinical Psychological Science," marking the official commencement of these practices into the treatment of psychological disorders. Some argue that the traditional ethical elements have been left behind as practitioners focus on the mindful practice (Harrington & Dunne, 2015). They ask if mindfulness was intended to be used for weight loss, helping children perform better in school, increasing employee productivity, or optimizing effectiveness of soldiers in war (see Harrington & Dunne [2015] for a full review).

MECHANISMS OF MINDFULNESS PRACTICES

Mindful practices are believed to strengthen the functioning of the prefrontal orbital cortex (PFC), which is known for executive control, inhibition, decision making, and purposeful intention (Hanson & Mendius, 2009). These practices strengthen access to the parasympathetic nervous system recognized for calming the body and mind (Hanson & Mendius, 2009). They also help to cultivate positive emotional experience from the limbic system, the emotional center of the brain (Hanson & Mendius, 2009). Finally, these practices help create neurological integration within the brain, allowing for increased feelings of inner and outer harmony and attunement (Siegel, 2010).

In private practice, when working with children in later elementary school and adolescents, I often use Daniel Siegel's *River of Integration* to explain what living in a regulated manner might be like (see Siegel, 2010). I grab a blank piece of paper and a pen and draw two lines from top to bottom and then make wavy lines running vertically between the two lines. This is the river. I write, along the center of the river, the word *INTEGRATION*. I explain that it is here that we feel our healthiest, make our best decisions, and connect most effectively with those in our lives. It is here that we can be truly present for ourselves and for others. I show the patient the two lines that demarcate the banks of the river of integration. I explain that there are ways to know that we are starting to fall out of integration or getting close to one of these banks. Our thoughts, emotions, and behaviors are our signs. If we become too close to the bank on the right, we are moving into *CHAOS*. I write the word—chaos—as I explain. Here we see substance use, out-of-control eating, emotional extremes, and increases in interpersonal struggles. Essentially, things begin to feel out-of-control. We have trouble with organization, details, and thoroughness. On the other bank, lies *RIGIDITY*. We can tell when we are close to this bank because we become over controlled; there is possible food restriction, and/or withdrawal from others or a need to control others. Thinking becomes overly rule governed, and we struggle to be flexible in problem solving. Many of my patients with eating disorders like to call these types of rigid behaviors "being perfect." I explain that calling these behaviors perfect is *romanticizing rigidity* (Cook-Cottone, 2015, p. 85).

On one occasion, after explaining the river of integration (Siegel, 2010) to a patient in late adolescence who was on the path toward recovery from a long history of anorexia nervosa (AN), I asked her what she thought of the model (Cook-Cottone, 2015). How did it relate to her life? She smiled as she explained to me that the model made a lot of sense to her. She explained to me how for years she had careened from one bank to the other, never experiencing integration (Cook-Cottone, 2015). When looking at the model, she could see how, over the years of her adolescence, she had moved from chaos to over-control and back to chaos, with neither experience being tolerable for too long (Cook-Cottone, 2015). She said, "I never touched a foot into the river of integration. I just zip-lined from one bank to the other" (Cook-Cottone, 2015, p. 86). For many years now, I have shared this anecdote with the psychologists-in-training at the university with my client's blessing. This anecdote speaks to so many of us—practitioners, teachers, administrators, and students. That is, we either take on rigid, unmanageable plans for self-regulation or careen into chaos because we are unable to tolerate our own unreasonable dictates (Cook-Cottone, 2015). Mindful and yoga practices can be approached in a gentle, manageable manner as a way to find the centerline of neurological integration (Cook-Cottone, 2015). In fact, yogic and mindful practices were born out of a search for a more centered and integrated way of being (Cook-Cottone, 2015).

BRIEF REVIEW OF MINDFULNESS OUTCOMES

There is a growing body of research on the positive effects of mindfulness practices. Mindfulness practices are associated with many positive outcomes including increased ability to self-regulate and be in effective, active engagement, as documented in empirical research and literature reviews (e.g., Brown et al., 2007; Brown & Ryan, 2003; Cook-Cottone, 2015; Duckworth, Grant, Loew, Oettingen, & Gollwitzer, 2011; Shapiro & Carlson, 2009; Siegel, 2010; Waters et al., 2015; Weare, 2013; Zenner et al., 2014). Specific processes that are enhanced include: cognitive performance; clarity of awareness; nonconceptual, nondiscriminatory awareness; flexibility in awareness and attention; an empirical stance toward reality; present-oriented consciousness; stability and continuity of attention and awareness; resilience; and enhanced self-regulation (Brown et al., 2007; Cook-Cottone, 2015; Weare, 2013; Zenner et al., 2014). In addition, these types of practices are negatively associated with psychopathology, alexithymia, neuroticism, disorders of self-regulation, and overall psychological distress (see Brown et al., 2007 and Cook-Cottone, 2015). With mindfulness practice, there is an increased sense of well-being, stronger affect regulation tendencies, greater self-awareness and understanding of emotions, and an increased ability to adjust unpleasant mood states (Brown & Ryan, 2003; Cook-Cottone, 2015).

Brown et al. (2007) explain that the disentanglement of consciousness from cognitive content may allow you and your students to think with greater effectiveness and precision. For example, when being mindful, the activity of conceptual thought can be purposefully engaged and disengaged by choice (Cook-Cottone, 2015; Brown et al., 2007). Shapiro and

Carlson (2009) refer to this as a shift to conscious responding versus automatic reactivity. In mindful traditions, suffering is thought to arise from the habitual ways in which we react and the seemingly automatic grip our mental habits have on us (Shapiro & Carlson, 2009). With mindfulness, one can be aware of thoughts as just thoughts, aware of emotions as simply emotions (Kabat-Zinn, 2013; Brown et al., 2007). See Chapter 3 for principles 3 (i.e., I am mindfully aware), 4 (i.e., I work toward presence in my physical body), and 7 (i.e., I choose my focus and actions) of the 12 principles for growth and learning.

In a systematic evidence-based review of the effects of meditation interventions in schools, Waters et al. (2015) analyzed 15 peer-reviewed studies of school meditation programs. They looked specifically at well-being, social competence, and academic achievement. Within the 15 studies, the overall number of participants in the effect size analysis was 1,797. The studies yielded 76 distinct results where the effect size could be effectively calculated (Waters et al., 2015). Overall, the researchers found that 61% of the results were statistically significant; 76% of the results had small effects; 24% of the results had medium effects; and 9% showed a large effect of meditation on student outcomes (Waters et al., 2015). Some types of meditation appeared to show better results. For example, Transcendental Meditation (i.e., silently repeating a word or mantra [meaningful phrase] to achieve a meditative state, with an ongoing redirecting of attention back to the word or mantra when distracted) showed a higher percentage of significant effects than other types of meditation programs (Waters et al., 2015). The authors note that these findings need to be further validated as the results could be due to characteristics related to the settings and program delivery rather than the meditation program itself (Waters et al., 2015). Overall, the authors report that meditation positively influences student success by improving cognitive functioning and emotion regulation (Waters et al., 2015). See Chapter 7 for more on the specific findings of the study.

To illustrate, Samuel, a third-grade student, took part in the school meditation program. This program included a loving-kindness meditation in which the students were instructed to focus their attention on themselves and then on other people in their lives with compassion, warmth, and care (see Waters et al., 2015; see also Chapter 5). Samuel came into the program challenged by peer relationships. He often struggled to be friendly to kids who had previously hurt his feelings. He kept a mental list of the kids he did not like anymore. Even if they were nice to him presently, he refused to engage in free-time activities with anyone on his mental list. If he was forced into paired work with any of the kids on his growing list, he was rude, often refused to effectively collaborate, and argued with his peers. During the loving-kindness meditation, Samuel was asked to call to mind someone whom he did not get along with well. This was easy for him as Mark, the boy whose desk was right next to Samuels's, came quickly to mind. The teacher asked Samuel, and all of the students in class, to wish for the person to be happy, to be healthy, to feel peaceful, and to feel relaxed and at ease.

The first few times the class did this meditation, Samuel shared with the class that he found this to be very hard to do. He said he was too mad at some people (i.e., Mark and the other kids on his list) to wish good things for them. His teacher told him that was okay and asked Samuel to keep trying and see what happens. Samuel kept practicing. He noticed that the anger he felt could be strong, or it could fade a bit if he focused on something else. After a while, he noticed that sometimes his anger went away altogether. As the weeks went by, Samuel's teacher noticed a softening in Samuel's peer interactions. She even noticed an improvement in his partner work in the classroom. When she checked in with him, he explained that, in order to wish Mark well, he had to stop paying so much attention to his anger. In essence, he said he had to let the anger go in order to think positive thoughts about his peers. Samuel said that, when he did this, it made it easier for him to be friends with Mark and some of the others kids he used to be mad at all the time.

THE WISDOM OF MINDFULNESS

A drive for wisdom comes from the intention to be effective in your life. Mindfulness combined with wisdom serves personal effectiveness. Mindful wisdom can be viewed from a few different perspectives.

Wisdom is the integration of thinking and feeling to make decisions and guide your actions (Cook-Cottone, 2015). When working with middle school, fifth-grade female students in a yoga-based program designed to increase self-care and decrease eating disorder risk, we introduce the thinking and feeling brain as a central teaching of the program (i.e., Girls Growing in Wellness and Balance: Yoga and Life Skills to Empower; Cook-Cottone, Kane, Keddie, & Haugli, 2013). The children are taught about the feeling part of their brains (i.e., the limbic system) and the thinking part of their brains (i.e., the prefrontal cortex). We use a drawing of a brain to show them the connections (see Figure 4.2). The thinking and feeling parts of the brain work together to make the best decisions. Real wisdom, equanimity, and neurological integration come from using both the thinking and the feeling parts of the brain together (Cook-Cottone et al., 2013). This program is described in greater detail in Chapter 11 of this text.

Hanson and Mendius (2009) call mindful wisdom "applied common sense" in which you come to understand what hurts and what helps. Wisdom in action can be viewed as the letting go of what hurts and strengthening what helps (Cook-Cottone, 2015; Hanson & Mendius, 2009). Sternberg (2012) makes a distinction between abstract wisdom and personal wisdom. Abstract wisdom is knowing of the conceptual, theoretical, and even empirical spheres of knowledge. Personal wisdom is an attitude toward life. It is the openness to learning about yourself and how you react to and are in your world. Concentration and

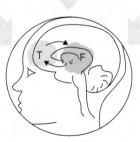

Equanimity and Integration
The brain works best when we use the **Thinking and Feeling** parts of the brain together to make choices.

The **Thinking** parts of our brain help us understand and make sense of things, put things in order, connect ideas, and make plans. Breathing helps us pay attention to this part (even when we are upset).

The **Feeling** part of our brain is the emotional part of our brain. It allows us to feel our feelings and is strongly connected to our bodies. Breathing helps this part calm down.

FIGURE 4.2 The thinking and feeling brain.

mindfulness turn into the practice of wisdom, or insight, when the focused mind is used to penetrate the illusions that create obstacles to insight (Olendzki, 2012). For Samuel, wisdom would be found in his insight regarding how the loving-kindness meditation was helping him let go of his anger and be a better friend to his peers.

The wisdom of mindfulness can also be cultivated by considering experience from both the internal and external perspective. When we do this, we notice the interaction and interdependency of the two (Cook-Cottone, 2015). That is, experience is constructed from what is presented to us on the outside and our processing of it on the inside (Olendzki, 2012). For Samuel, it was the way he was handling his peer relationships that was causing him trouble. By holding onto his list of hurts and seeing peer interactions as potentially hurtful, he was creating a way of being with his classmates that was fulfilling his internal belief system. Conversely, by practicing the loving-kindness meditation for Mark, his most challenging peer, Samuel was able to experience the powerful interaction of his inner and outer worlds. When he let go of anger and interacted with Mark in a positive manner, he had more effective partner work in the classroom.

THREE CHARACTERISTICS OF MINDFULNESS: IMPERMANENCE, NONATTACHMENT, AND NOT-SELF

Mindfulness can also be viewed within the context of three central characteristics: impermanence, nonattachment, and not-self. Grabovac, Lau, and Willett (2011) describe these as the three characteristics of mindfulness common to all experiences (i.e., sense impressions and mental events).

Impermanence

Despite what we would like to think, everything changes (Bien, 2006; Kabat-Zinn, 2013; Shapiro & Carlson, 2009). Interestingly, for children everything changes all the time—which is problematic given their strong need for structure and stability. When I teach Counseling with Children and Adolescents at the university, I spend time at the beginning of the semester reminding my students how children and adolescents are in a constant process of change. Their clothes fit differently from day to day. The can grow 5 to 7 inches in a school year. They don't know how to subtract one month, and some are multiplying in a few months. Their parents divorce or move. We tend to resist the impermanence of this nature. More than you and I, who wear essentially the same size, have stable jobs, and have finely tuned skill sets for years and decades, they know change. Perhaps it is because of all the change inherent in being a child or adolescent that they thrive on permanence and structure. Dealing with impermanence can be especially challenging for our students.

Having a sense of impermanence can be critical in self-regulation. A difficult situation at school or with peers manifests, becomes uncomfortable, and resolves. We tend to forget the impermanence of this nature. It is the nature of things to arise and pass away (Cook-Cottone, 2015). In terms of self-regulation, all sense impressions and mental events are transient in that they arise and pass away (Grabovac et al., 2011). Mindfulness scholars explain that we do not suffer because of all things being impermanent. We suffer because we resist or forget this fact (Bien, 2006; Kabat-Zinn, 2013). When things are pleasurable, safe, and good, we cling. When things are difficult and challenging, we want to avoid. The same is true for the times in between the good and the difficult. Those times pass, too. I like to show students how this is true, the waxing and waning of the good and the challenging. For example, if students are stuck waiting in line, ask them to notice how long it lasts.

Students can also be taught impermanence in meditation practice by watching, as witness to their thoughts, the arising and passing away of all phenomena (i.e., thoughts, feelings, and information coming to them through their senses; Olendzki, 2012). By witnessing over and over, time and time again, they begin to notice that everything is impermanent (Cook-Cottone, 2015). In the example with Samuel, he was able to see that anger was something that could fade and even diminish into nothing as he watched.

Like Samuel, students can also come to understand how impermanence shows up differently when something is uncomfortable, challenging, or distressing (Cook-Cottone, 2015). When something is uncomfortable, it is easy to react as if it is never going to end. Hence, being reminded of impermanence offers relief. When I am doing a difficult yoga pose or feeling resistance in meditation, I remind myself that the emotion or reaction I am feeling will arise and pass away. Similarly, Linehan (1993) asks her patients to notice impermanence when they are working to tolerate distress. They are asked to watch an urge or an uncomfortable emotion arise and pass away, not reacting, not allowing the sensation to trigger symptoms of dysregulation (Cook-Cottone, 2015). After a test, you can bring them to awareness of how the test came and went. With a classroom mindfulness practice, you can remind them how they used their tools (e.g., breathing [principle 2], staying aware and present [principles 3 and 4], being self-determined [principle 8], and creating possibility [principle 12]). All of that good work, while the test approached, was there for them, and then was done.

Nonattachment

Nonattachment is the process of not attaching to or attempting to avoid thoughts, feelings, emotions, people, things, and so on (Cook-Cottone, 2015). It begins at the most basic of levels. Each sense impression (e.g., smell or sound) or mental event is reflexively paired with a feeling-tone of positive, negative, or neutral (Grabovac et al., 2011). All of us, including our students, naturally feel drawn to the positive or pleasurable feeling-tones and are compelled to avoid the negative or aversive feeling-tones (Cook-Cottone, 2015).

Over time, habitual reactions, such as attachment and aversion to the feelings associated with a sense impression or mental event, as well as a lack of awareness of these processes, can lead to suffering (Grabovac et al., 2011). Mindfulness practice can help us to be present in each moment of experience without clinging or craving (Olendzki, 2012). Olendzki (2012) eloquently describes the heightened awareness that comes with mindfulness as a pry bar that gets under the common assumptions and habitual responses that we bring to each moment. With this pry bar, we are able to loosen the attachment to them (Olendzki, 2012). Helping students notice what they are drawn to and what they try to avoid is important in building their self-regulation skills. For Samuel, completing the loving-kindness meditations was hard at first. Still, his teacher encouraged him to keep trying. She encouraged him not to avoid the meditation just because it was challenging. She reminded him of principle 1, "Samuel, you and your classmates are worth the effort" (see Chapter 3), and "Samuel, you can do the work" (principle 8, self-determination).

Not-Self

Not-self is sometimes considered to be one of the most difficult mindful teachings for Westerners to understand (Shapiro & Carlson, 2009). Specific to self-regulation, both sense impressions and mental events do not contain anything that could be called a self (Grabovac et al., 2011). This concept is very hard for children and many adolescents to grasp. It requires a level of formal operative thought (i.e., the ability to think in abstractions and conceptualizations) that does not typically arise until the middle school years and, for some students, not until high school.

There are lots of ways students identify with what is happening as self. For example, I often meet adolescents in private practice who have identified wholeheartedly with a particular disorder (Cook-Cottone, 2015). For example, They might say, "I am anorexic," or "I can't control myself." I watch their language for these statements to reveal a sense of a nonchanging, permanent self that is serving their disorder or struggle (Cook-Cottone, 2015). When I hear a statement like this, I tell them what I noticed and ask them to reword the sentence in an empowering, *malleable* manner. For example, an adolescent can change "I am anorexic" to "I have struggled with food restriction when I feel overwhelmed." Another example is changing "I can't control myself" to "In the past, I didn't notice that I was triggered by clothing advertisements to shop."

Younger students often say things like, "I am mad," "I can't do that," or "I am bad." Here, mindfulness gives us the place to reframe these notions of self. This is important because, if a student views himself or herself as mad, there is little room for modification of the state. If a student views himself or herself as incapable, there is little room for progress. Last, if a student sees himself or herself as bad, cultivating positive experiences is dissonant from who they think they are. For students who identify as a feeling (i.e., "I am mad"), the teacher can help them reword, "Samuel, you are feeling angry right now." For students who are making brief statements regarding their capabilities (e.g., "I can't do that"), the teacher can help them reframe their statement: "Samuel, being kind to people who have hurt you can be very challenging. Let's practice and see how you do." Last, for students who conceptualize themselves as bad or unworthy of effort, a phenomenon that can be a risk factor for depression, the teacher can validate their experience and help them reframe: "Samuel, when you have engaged in behaviors that are against the rules, it feels bad. Still, what you do—and who you are—are two different things." In these ways, we don't need to explicitly teach the concept of not-self. Rather, we teach them how to create space between what they are feeling and challenged by and who they are. Chapter 3, principle 6, inquiry, speaks directly to this process. Ask students to ask questions about the space between what is happening and who they are.

ALLOWING WHAT IS

Allowing is a term that I find easier to negotiate than acceptance (Cook-Cottone, 2015). It is a subtle semantic difference. Yet, I believe it is an important one. Acceptance is intended to mean an acknowledgment of or a cessation of resistance to something (Cook-Cottone, 2015). However, in Western culture, acceptance has a connotation of agreement. Whereas, allowing suggests a clearer boundary between what you or I might consider acceptable and what is happening (Cook-Cottone, 2015). Allowing suggests that, although you or

I are not going to resist this happening, thing, feeling, experience, or person, we are also not of acceptance with it. Allowing is the antidote to resistance, a feeling that our students know well. It is resistance that adds suffering to pain (Kabat-Zinn, 2013; Shapiro & Carlson, 2009). That which is already painful can become seemingly unbearable when resistance is added. We explore allowing in Chapter 5, in specific activities (e.g., soften, soothe, allow).

CONCLUSION

Many of the students that I have worked with have spent years reacting to complicated family experiences, difficult neighborhoods, achievement expectations, and other challenging risks (see Chapter 2). Without knowing or having other tools, these students have done the best that they could to make it through the day (Cook-Cottone, 2015). With mindfulness practices, students have a chance to learn a healthy and effective set of ways of seeing themselves, their environments, and the world. Mindfulness practices promote well-being, neurological integration, as well as connection, attunement, and community with others (Cook-Cottone, 2015). These mindful conceptualizations have been refined, practiced, and passed down for thousands of years and then adapted for students in today's schools. They offer a secular set of healthy techniques for understanding and coping (Cook-Cottone, 2015; Weare, 2013; Zenner et al., 2014). Referring back to the quote at the start of this chapter, mindfulness offers practice in learning to listen to and see ourselves as a way of learning to love ourselves.

REFERENCES

Bien, T. (2006). *Mindful therapy: A guide for therapists and helping professionals.* Boston, MA: Wisdom.

Brown, K. W., & Kasser, T. (2005). Are psychological and ecological well-being compatible? The role of values, mindfulness, and lifestyle. *Social Indicators Research, 74,* 349–368.

Brown, K. W., & Ryan, R. M. (2003). The benefits of being present: Mindfulness and its role in psychological well-being. *Journal of Personality and Psychological Well Being, 84,* 822–848.

Brown, K. W., Ryan, R. M., & Creswell, J. D. (2007). Addressing fundamental questions about mindfulness. *Psychological inquiry: An international Journal for the Advancement of Psychological Theory, 18,* 272–281.

Cook-Cottone, C. P. (2015). *Mindfulness and yoga for self-regulation: A primer for mental health professionals.* New York, NY: Springer Publishing.

Cook-Cottone, C. P., Kane, L., Keddie, E., & Haugli, S. (2013). *Girls growing in wellness and balance: Yoga and life skills to empower.* Stoddard, WI: Schoolhouse Educational Series.

Duckworth, A. L., Grant, H., Loew, B., Oettingen, G., & Gollwitzer, P. M. (2011). Self-regulation strategies improve self-discipline in adolescents: Benefits of mental contrasting and implementation intentions. *Educational Psychology: An International Journal of Experimental Educational Psychology, 31,* 17–26.

Felver, J., Doerner, E., Jones, J., Kaye, N., & Merrell, K. (2013). Mindfulness in school psychology: Applications for intervention and professional practice. *Psychology in the Schools, 50,* 531–547.

Goldman, C. (2009). *Healing words for the body, mind, and spirit: 101 words to inspire and affirm.* Harrisburg, PA: Morehouse Publishing.

Grabovac, A. D., Lau, M. A., & Willett, B. R. (2011). Mechanisms of mindfulness: A Buddhist psychological model. *Mindfulness, 2*(3), 154–166. doi:10.1007/s12671-011-0054-5

Hanson, R., & Mendius, R. (2009). *Buddha's brain: The practical neuroscience of happiness, love, and wisdom.* Oakland, CA: New Harbinger Publications.

Harrington, A., & Dunne, J. D. (2015). When mindfulness is therapy: Ethical qualms, historical perspective. *American Psychologist, 70,* 621–631.

Kabat-Zinn, J. (2013). *Full catastrophe living, revised edition: How to cope with stress, pain and illness using mindfulness meditation.* New York, NY: Bantam Books.

Linehan, M. M. (1993). *Cognitive-behavioral treatment of borderline personality disorder.* New York, NY: Guilford Press.

Lutz, A., Jha, A. P., Dunne, J. D., & Saron, C. D. (2015). Investigating the phenomenological matrix of mindfulness-related practices from a neurocognitive perspective. *American Psychologist, 70,* 632–658.

McCown, D., Reibel, D., & Micozzi, M. S. (2010). *Teaching mindfulness: A practical guide for clinicians and educators.* New York, NY: Springer.

Olendzki, A. (2012). Wisdom in Buddhist psychology. In C. K. Germer & R. D. Siegel (Eds.). *Wisdom and compassion in psychotherapy: Deeping mindfulness in clinical practice.* New York, NY: Guilford Press.

Rechtschaffen, D. (2014). *The way of mindful education: Cultivating well-being in teachers and students.* New York, NY: W. W. Norton.

Rosenberg, E. L. (2004). Mindfulness and consumerism. In K. Tim & A. D. Kanner (Eds.), *Psychology and consumer culture: The struggle for a good life in a materialistic world* (pp. 107–125). Washington, DC: American Psychological Association.

Shapiro, S. L., & Carlson, L. E. (2009). *The art and science of mindfulness: Integrating mindfulness into psychology and the helping professions.* Washington, DC: American Psychological Association.

Siegel, D. (2010). *The mindful therapist: A clinician's guide to mindsight and neural integration.* New York, NY: W. W. Norton.

Sternberg, R. J. (2012). The science of wisdom: Implications for psychotherapy. In C. K. Germer & R. D. Siegel (Eds.). *Wisdom and compassion in psychotherapy: Deeping mindfulness in clinical practice.* New York, NY: Guilford Press.

Vygotsky, L. S. (1978). *Mind in society.* Cambridge, MA: Harvard University Press.

Waters, L., Barsky, A., Ridd, A., & Allen, K. (2015). Contemplative education: A systematic evidence-based review of the effect of mediation intervention in schools. *Educational Psychology Review, 27,* 103–134.

Weare, K. (2013). Developing mindfulness with children and young people: A review of the evidence and policy context. *Journal of Children's Services, 2,* 141–153.

Zenner, C., Herrleben-Kurz, S., & Walach, H. (2014). Mindfulness-based interventions in schools—A systematic review and meta-analysis. *Frontiers in Psychology, 8,* 1–20.

CHAPTER 5

THE MINDFUL CLASSROOM: CREATING SUPPORTS AND STRUCTURE FOR MINDFUL TEACHING AND LEARNING

In the end, we conserve only what we love.
We will love only what we understand.
We will understand only what we are taught.

—Bab Dioum, Senegalese Teacher and Poet
(Dioum, 1968)

The quote by Bab Dioum speaks to the importance of cultivating mindfulness in your class-room and school from the ground up. Yes, we can love things we don't understand and, yes, we understand more than we are taught. Yet, it is by teaching students how to see clearly, to appreciate subtleties and nuances in their world, and to understand the interconnected-ness of our world that we will more effectively lead them to be protectors of the world and each other. Teaching students mindfulness is essential. To do this, we must work toward building and cultivating mindfulness—giving thought to the layout of the room, the tools provided to the students, the routine and structure of the school day, and our way of being as we teach. So many educators, from elementary schools to universities, complain about the neurological states of children, how they can't pay attention, do not value each other or themselves, and seem solely driven by needs and wants. As I argue in Chapters 1 and 2, our students reflect what is practiced and presented in our culture. To shift toward a more effec-tive, thoughtful, and kind way of being in our world, in school, toward each other, and in how we approach schoolwork, we must shift what and how we teach. For students to value reflective thinking and acting, they must have a sense of what that is. For them to have an understanding, we must teach and practice it. What we do shows what we value.

The first step in preparing to implement mindfulness practices in school is to get you and your classroom ready. In this chapter, you find a brief overview of the nature of mind-fulness practices (i.e., beginner's mind, the four foundations of mindfulness, and the process of meditation), guidance for preparing your classroom, and tips for delivering mindfulness practices in school. Chapters 6 and 7 detail specific formal and informal practices for you.

BEGINNER'S MIND AND PRACTITIONER'S WISDOM

As a teacher of mindfulness you need two qualities: beginner's mind and practitioner's wisdom. First, no matter how long you have been practicing or how old you are, begin with a beginner's mind (Cook-Cottone, 2015). For you and your students, beginner's mind is a quality of awareness that allows you to see things as if you have never seen them before. As you practice, work toward noticing your experience with openness and curiosity (Cook-Cottone, 2015; Kabat-Zinn, 2013; Stahl & Goldstein, 2010). In this way, as actual beginners, your students have an advantage (Cook-Cottone, 2015; Marlatt, Bower, & Lustyk, 2012). Unlike other skills in which we intentionally develop automaticity (e.g., moving from decoding words to immediate word recognition, or thinking through the steps of driving a stick shift to skilled shifting), in mindfulness practices you want to stay with the beginner's advantage of noticing things as if you have never seen them before. With a beginner's mind, students can be present to and curious about each nuance of their internal and external worlds so that, when risk of acting without thinking or missing an opportunity to learn more about themselves is headed their way, they clearly see it (Marlatt et al., 2012).

> *What we do speaks so loudly to children*
> *that when we talk they cannot hear us.*
>
> —Gandhi

Second, no matter how many books you read, in-services or trainings you attend, or instructional videos you watch, you will not be able to share the wisdom of mindfulness unless you practice. Think about your most beloved and effective teacher. Without even knowing them, I know that you are thinking about someone who is authentic and grounded in that which they teach from a felt, experiential sense. If they taught you to read, they love reading and read every day, like my mom. If they taught you how to ride a horse, they love horses and have a deep knowledge of training and working with horses, like my Uncle Scott. The same is true for mindfulness and yoga. If they taught you mindfulness and yoga and you loved it, they practice. It is that simple. Deepen your practice and you will gain even more insight as to how to effectively and powerfully share your experience (Willard, 2016). If you come to each moment with a beginner's mind, open and curious, and bring with you the wisdom of all your hours and love of practice, you will be both competent and inspirational.

THE FOUR FOUNDATIONS OF MINDFUL PRACTICE

McCown, Reibel, and Micozzi (2010) describe four foundations of mindfulness practice: body, feelings, mind, and mind objects (Figure 5.1). For children and adolescents, begin with the first foundation (i.e., body awareness) and work your way through the foundations (i.e., feeling awareness, mind awareness, and mind-object awareness). You will want to work from the most concrete, or tangible, experience as a starting point. This is much more accessible for younger children and beginners.

First, there is mindfulness of the body, or physical self. This involves bare attention to the breath, then to the calming of the body, and finally to awareness of the body in sensation, postures, movements, and breath in both formal practice and daily living (Cook-Cottone, 2015; Kabat-Zinn, 2013; McCown et al., 2010). This can be done by guiding the students

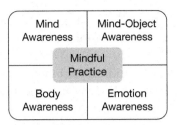

Mind Awareness	Mind-Object Awareness
Mindful Practice	
Body Awareness	Emotion Awareness

FIGURE 5.1 Four foundations of mindful practice.

verbally through an awareness of their bodies from the ground up. If they are seated in a chair, you begin with the connection of their feet on the floor, awareness of their legs and hips, and a sense of themselves sitting on the chair. You can have them notice the chair, how it feels, hard or soft. You can bring them to awareness of their spine and belly. You can guide them into their shoulders, arms, and hands. As much as possible, bring their awareness to the physical sensations that they feel. You can move through the body to the crown of the head. I am careful not to mention "private parts" (e.g., the pelvic floor) of the body in school. It can quickly distract the class without adding substantial benefit to the meditation. You can easily speak of the *sitting bones* (i.e., ischial tuberosity) and teach students where they are.

The next foundation is mindful awareness of feelings in which bare attention is focused on the feeling-tone that accompanies the experiences of each moment (Cook-Cottone, 2015; Grabovac, Lau, & Willett, 2011; McCown et al., 2010). These are the feeling-tones of unpleasant, neutral, or pleasant (McCown et al., 2010). For students, you can guide them to notice what feels good or not so good. You can teach them broad definitions of the words *pleasant* (i.e., things that feel good) and *unpleasant* (i.e., things that feel not so good) and ask them to give examples. Have them notice that there are *physical feelings* (e.g., how my feet and toes feel in my socks and shoes, pressing into the carpet on the floor), and then there are *emotional feelings* (e.g., not liking how it feels to sit still for 3 minutes [unpleasant] and wanting to wiggle and move [something that feels pleasant]). The emotional feelings tell us how we feel about what is happening (Cook-Cottone, 2015). In mindfulness practice, these feeling-tones are simply noticed as they arise and pass away. So, Joey, who feels unpleasant feelings about sitting for more than 90 seconds, notices this rather than letting himself wiggle. He can share with the class what this was like and how he stayed focused.

The third foundation is mindfulness of the mind (Cook-Cottone, 2015; McCown et al., 2010; Siegel, 2010). Note, this is a difficult concept for young children. For students who are younger than 10 or 11 years old, it may be best to move right to awareness of objects of the mind. Objects are concrete, or tangible, and therefore a little easier for children who have not entered formal operative thought to consider (i.e., the ability to think about the world in more abstract ways). In the case of mindfulness of the mind, bare attention is focused on the activity, or processing, of the mind, noticing shifts in states of awareness, concentration, and distraction (Kabat-Zinn, 2013). It can be helpful to take some time and define the different states for the students and have them give examples of how that is experienced by them. In a curriculum my research team developed for children with fetal alcohol exposure, we aligned the states of consciousness with animals or characters to increase understanding. We used terms such as "hunting dog" for alert and engaged, and "sloth" for feeling slow and lazy. It can be fun to work with the class and create these distinctions and methodologies for each of them. You want to be sure to include states of arousal, engaged attention, distraction, and sleepiness. You can include more if you'd like. It can be helpful to do an Internet search for various examples of states of consciousness (note: add "neuropsychology" to the search to keep the search results secular).

Finally, the fourth foundation of mindfulness practice is mindfulness of mind-objects. In this practice, bare attention is brought to the things the mind is thinking about. Thought objects come from within, such as your cravings (e.g., chocolate, lunch, sleep), your feelings (e.g., anger, frustration, worry, doubt), your memories, plans, and so on (McCown et al., 2010). You can add an intentional object of concentration (e.g., a word or phrase or plant or statue). I have used videos of various objects (e.g., a fireplace) in class, rather than the real thing, to ensure safety and inspire focus. The four foundations of mindful practice align with the principles of embodied learning: (1) I am worth the effort; (3) I am mindfully aware; (4) I work toward presence in my physical body; (5) I feel my emotions to grow and learn; (6) I ask questions about my feelings, thoughts, and physical experiences; (7) I choose my focus and actions; and (8) I do the work (see Chapter 3).

BEGIN WITHIN: ESTABLISHING YOUR OWN MEDITATION PRACTICE

As a mindful and yoga informed educator, you may already have an established meditation practice. As introduced in Chapter 1, it is important to develop your own practice. This is because your own practice will be your best teacher and help you be the best teacher for your students (Cook-Cottone, 2015; David, 2009; Willard, 2016). Let me tell you a story about how your own practice can teach. In 2013, I was preparing for a trip to Africa to do research on the Africa Yoga Project. With all the running around I was doing, I had everything in my truck: my briefcase, passport, yellow fever card, purse, yoga bag, a speaker for my yoga music, and more. At the same time, I was co-teaching a summer-camp yoga class on the East Side of Buffalo. This is the part of town where there are fewer jobs and resources, a higher crime rate, and absolutely no yoga studios or classes. I was excited for the neighborhood kids enrolled in the class. When I got to the classroom, I realized that I had forgotten the speaker. We needed it in order to play a song for the kids as they rested in savasana (i.e., resting pose). I had not been gone 5 minutes, but my truck window was smashed in and nearly all of my belongings were stolen, including critical things I needed for my trip to Africa. I called the police to make a report. I ran with a few of the older kids to see if we could find anything tossed aside. There was nothing. Then, I went in and taught the yoga class. It was a beautiful class. I used nearly all of the principles of embodied learning and growth (see Chapter 3). I knew my mission was worth the effort (principle 1). I used my breath as it was my most powerful tool (principle 2). I worked on presence (principle 3) and allowed my feelings to move through me (principle 4). I knew I had a choice in the present moment (principle 7), and I did the work that needed to be done (principle 8).

Fast forward. In 2015, the location of the day camp program was now the main studio for a not-for-profit I founded, Yogis in Service, Inc. (i.e., YIS; www.yogisinservice.org). Specifically, YIS was developed to create access to yoga. We had recently won a grant from Lululemon Athletica to rebuild our studio, and they were sending a film crew to interview our YIS team members who lived on the East Side about how yoga had affected their lives. One of the team members, Diane, told the crew about the day my truck was broken into. Imagine my astonishment as I listened to the story from her point of view. She described how she assumed that there would be no yoga that day. She thought for sure I would be too upset to teach. Yet, she said she saw me calm, breathing, and present for the class. She said, "If that is what yoga does,

I am going to do yoga." She said that it was my calm response and my ability to be with and for the class, despite what had just happened, that inspired her to keep doing yoga.

It is during moments like these that I know exactly why I practice. As an educator, you will model the benefits of mindfulness practice as you stay steady in the face of challenge and stress. Your successes and struggles in developing your mindfulness skills will allow you to speak authentically as a teacher about the process of learning. You will be able to use your experience to inform your mindfulness and meditation instruction to your students (Cook-Cottone, 2015; Rechtschaffen, 2014). So let's get started. This book, and others, can be wonderful guides in developing your own practice (see the references at the end of this chapter). Nevertheless, I found that some of my most powerful learnings occurred during lived experiences with a mentor. Others agree. Willard (2016) recommends finding your own mindfulness teacher, mentor, and/or center to help you get started in your practice. For many in small towns, rural areas, or in certain parts of the country, there is simply nowhere to go. In these cases, seek out professional conferences and rally for mindfulness-based speakers to be brought to your district. Consider mindfulness retreats for mini vacations. There are dozens of helpful web resources as well (e.g., search Mindfulness Practice Guidance and Mindfulness in Schools; see also The Collaborative for Academic, Social, and Emotional Learning [CASEL]; Mindful Teachers: Living, Learning, and Teaching with Mindful Awareness; The Garrison Institute; The Mindfulness Education Network; Daniel Rechtschaffen's page at www.danielrechtschaffen.com or www.mindfuleducation.com).

Making Time

There will always be roadblocks to any new behavior. First, it is new. Creating a new routine behavior or habit is a challenge for all of us. Accept that. Then, begin anyway. Willard (2016) suggests that you ask yourself when you might have a few minutes to set aside for practice. He suggests that you build your practice into an existing habit. For example, when I practice yoga or run, I meditate as a form of coming to rest after my more rigorous work. Many yoga studios and meditation centers have classes and group practices. Being part of a group with a regular schedule can be a good way to develop a practice.

Formal mindfulness practice can begin small. The key is consistency. In fact, Willard (2016) suggests that, if you have a goal of meditating an hour every day starting tomorrow, you will be less likely to have a steady practice in a year than if you began today at 3 to 5 minutes. There are several wonderful meditation apps for smartphones that offer options such as setting an interval timer and an end timer (Cook-Cottone, 2015). The Insight Timer (www.insighttimer.com) is my favorite with many scripted meditations, progress tracking tools, and bell and chime options. This app, as others, allows you to plan and track your practice, which can also help you in establishing a routine.

Setting Up Your Meditation Space at Home

First, it is important to note that you don't need a dedicated space to meditate. One of the benefits of mindfulness practice is that it requires absolutely no equipment. Most importantly, the area should be a space that is quiet, free from distractions, and cultivates a sense of peacefulness. You should be able to sit comfortably. That is all. Still, it can be a lot of fun setting up your space. At our house, we have a room dedicated to yoga and meditation with mats, meditation pillows and benches, and various artifacts that we find centering (Cook-Cottone, 2015). Try to make your mindfulness space a dedicated space that you do not use for sleep, work, or entertainment (Cook-Cottone, 2015; Wallace, 2011). Here are some things you can consider including in your meditation area/room (Cook-Cottone, 2015):

- Meditation bench or cushion (zafu, a round cushion used for seated meditation) or a good bench/chair
- One or two heavy blankets that can be folded and placed for comfort under your sitting bones or knees
- A meditation object (e.g., a photo, plant, battery-operated candle)
- Something to help you count the number of times a mantra, or affirmation, has been recited (e.g., stones and a set of bowls, a beaded necklace or bracelet)
- A timer with chimes or a pleasing sound
- A speaker or headphones for recorded meditations
- A mindfulness meditation app for your phone

Once you have set aside the time and the space (if you choose), you are ready to begin. The guidelines for helping you and your students develop your mindfulness and meditation practice (Cook-Cottone, 2015) follow.

SUPPORTING MINDFULNESS PRACTICES IN THE CLASSROOM

Supporting mindfulness practices in the classroom begins with you and your practice, extends to formal teaching of skills in the classroom, and expands to the interweaving of mindfulness throughout the school day (see Chapter 6).

Begin With What You Know

Building on your own practice, begin teaching the practices that resonate with you (Willard, 2016). When I first began teaching mindfulness practices at the university, I began with body scans and systematic relaxation (described later). As a classic type-A personality, mindful awareness and focused concentration meditation were substantial challenges for me. I did not feel authentic trying to teach them to others. It was the direct connection to and relaxation of the body that was first accessible to me. As the well-known saying goes, "It is difficult to have a stressed mind in a calm body." Accordingly, that is where I started teaching. The Advanced Graduate Certificate in Mindful Counseling, now offered at the University at Buffalo, was built from these early beginnings. It started in my counseling with children and adolescents class, with me teaching students how to teach relaxation to children with anxiety. So, find what is comfortable and what works for you, and start there.

Practices Feel and Look Different From Student to Student

Don't assume that what feels good for you feels the same for all students (Olson, 2014). Willard (2016) reminds us that, while some students love the feeling of slowing down and becoming aware of their breath and bodies, others feel very uncomfortable. Some students will come to your classroom or school with trauma, and some of the practices can be anxiety provoking (Cook-Cottone, 2015). For most of us, silence feels like a healing place, whereas for some, it is a trigger for danger, loneliness, and even abandonment (Willard, 2016). It is important to carefully assess the motives behind behaviors (Jennings, 2015). Jennings (2015) notes that many children come to the classroom with a host of unmet needs that can drive disruptive behavior. It is important to provide structure, options, and compassion, and to balance effort and rest while working with these practices (see Chapter 3, principle 7: I choose my focus and actions; principle 9; I find balance between structure and rest; and principle 10: I honor efforts to learn and grow).

Let go of your notion of what a mindfulness practice is supposed to look like (Willard, 2016). For example, in seated meditation, there are specific instructions to press your feet into the floor, sit with a straight spine, and rest your hands in your lap or on the desk. These are good recommendations. However, for some students, these positions might feel unfamiliar, mean something different in different cultures, or feel unsafe socially or interpersonally (Willard, 2016). It can be easy for a teacher to get caught up in the rigidity of specific instructions and lose the bigger picture of the mindfulness practice. For example, as Willard (2016) suggests, when I ask students to close their eyes, I give them the options of lowering their eyelids slightly or looking down in front of them, rather than insist everyone closes their eyes.

Be Mindful of How You Teach Mindfulness

When teaching mindfulness, be the presence that you want to cultivate in your students (Cook-Cottone, 2016). That is, if you are guiding the student through a relaxation exercise with the goal of helping to bring them to a calm and relaxed state, cultivate calmness and relaxation in your own body. This is where your own practice can come into play. Ground your feet. Take deep, mindful breaths, and speak from your belly.

Use your voice and words mindfully. Speak at a pace that reflects calmness and contentment. It can be a common mistake to speak too quickly (David, 2009; Willard, 2016). Notice that, when speaking too quickly, your breath does not keep up. Use your breath to pace yourself (Willard, 2016). Speak loudly enough to be heard, yet softly enough to avoid the impression of yelling. It took me quite a while to cultivate this voice. It comes from the belly and is supported by breath. Ask for feedback from your students and consider developing your voice a practice. Work toward a calm, confident, and assertive tone (Willard, 2016).

Last, use your own voice. When I travel for work, I attend a yoga class wherever I go. I have taken classes across the United States. I have noticed a tendency of some teachers to use a *yoga-teacher-voice*. This often is a singsongy voice that seems to be an attempt to be relaxing or calming. However, because it is, most often, not the teacher's authentic voice, it sounds inauthentic and distracting. I often hear the teacher speaking before and after class in a much different voice. In her own voice, she sounds grounded, confident, and authentic. That is the voice I hope to hear in class—the teacher's own voice. The same is true for words. Use words that are your words. If a word does not resonate for you or in your classroom, find a word that does (Willard, 2016). The practices will be most effectively delivered when they come directly from your practice, aligned with your breath, using your authentic voice, and resonating words.

Use Mindful Words

Rechtschaffen (2014) suggests using mindful language. In essence, this is like teaching content vocabulary in any of the core subjects. There is a specific set of words that can be very useful in teaching mindfulness. Key terms include *mindful body, anchor breaths,* and *heartfulness* (Rechtschaffen, 2014). A mindful body means that students are aware of their bodies and aware of the space around them (Rechtschaffen, 2014). It also means that students are aware of what Rechtschaffen (2014) calls the two legs of mindfulness: focus and relaxation. Another key term is "anchor breath" (Rechtschaffen, 2014). Anchor breath is a way of focusing in which students notice the way their breathing feels in their bellies (Rechtschaffen, 2014). Paying attention to anchor breath helps remind students that even when there is a lot of chaos in their lives, they can bring themselves back to feeling calm and grounded (Rechtschaffen, 2014). Another term is "heartfulness" (Rechtschaffen, 2014). Heartfulness refers to mindfulness practices that cultivate emotions such as compassion, happiness, and kindness when working with more difficult emotions such as anger and sadness (Rechtschaffen, 2014). Rechtschaffen (2014) explains that if students are struggling with one another, feeling very emotional or difficult emotions, we can guide them back to their heartfulness. This can be contrasted with hurtfulness, which would be an angry and hurtful reaction that had neither compassion nor kindness. It is the heartfulness perspective that calls forth prosocial problem solving.

Explain Mindfulness to Students

Rechtschaffen (2014) suggests that it is helpful to explain to children how their brains work. You can do this in a variety of ways. For example, I have successfully used this explanation with children as young as 6 or 7 years old, and it is part of our curriculum, *Girls Growing in Wellness and Balance: Yoga and Life Skills to Empower* (Cook-Cottone, Kane, Keddie, & Haugli, 2013). I explain that the thinking brain and the feeling brain need to work together to make the best choices. When we use our breath, body, and focus to help the two parts of the brain to work together, we are being mindful. When the thinking brain works alone, sometimes all the important feelings, including how much you love and care about others and things that are important to you, are not included. On the other hand, when we use only our feeling brain, especially when we are upset or really mad, we can make poor choices. The two parts of our brain work best together (Cook-Cottone et al., 2013). I explain that the brain is like hot soup. The soup is wonderful, but when you are upset, it is too hot. I ask, "What do you do when your soup is too hot?" The students always say, "You blow on it," and "You wait." I agree. When things are too hot, they need time and air. The same is true for your brain. Once you take time to stop and breathe, the thinking and the feeling parts have a chance to work together, and you will be more likely to make the best decision (Cook-Cottone et al., 2013).

Overall, I find it helpful for students to have a bigger understanding of what we are doing and why. For older students, this can include an explanation of any of the key mechanisms of mindfulness, reading and discussing review articles, or showing them models of mindfulness. Having a larger sense of the *why* of mindfulness can help them with the *how* and the motivation.

Use Imagination, Metaphor, and Story

We are all captivated by imagination, metaphor, and story. You can create a fun and accepting context for mindfulness practice by integrating the students' imagination and sense of story (Olson, 2014; Willard, 2016). Willard (2016) tells a story of Lev Vygotsky, the child development expert, who asked two little boys to stand as long as they could. He explains that the children lost focus and were off doing the next thing within a few minutes. However, when he asked the boys to first imagine they were factory guards, the boys were able to stand still for nearly four times as long (Willard, 2016). I recall being in swim team practice, putting in the thousands of yards required for competitive swimming. I imagined swimming to Alcatraz with fish and turtles swimming under me. The hours would pass by as I imagined the press interview and photographs that would be taken once I finished my historic swim. When teaching poses, you can ask students to sit like a mountain, breathe like a bellow, and lengthen their necks like a giraffe (Willard, 2016). While mindfully walking, you can take them through the journey of a great explorer noticing the stones, leaves, and wildlife along the path. As great explorers who need to document their observations for the university when they return, their mindful awareness flourishes. Harnessing the power of the imagination is a powerful way to invite students into the world of mindfulness.

Connect to the Senses

Connecting to your sensory experiences is a shortcut to the present moment (Willard, 2016). Often, our thinking minds are engaged in reflections about the past or worries about and plans for the future (Willard, 2016). The senses are connected to right here and now. Consistent with principle 4, in Chapter 3, "I work toward presence in my physical body," mindfulness and mindful awareness often integrate a connection to sensory experiences. No matter what the experience or mindfulness activity, take time to bring students' awareness to the present sounds, smells, touch sensations, sights, and tastes.

Create a Mindful Space in Your Classroom

Create a space that enhances the practice (Willard, 2016). You might have a whole room or dedicated space, as they do in some schools, or a corner of your classroom. You can add secular posters on mindfulness, and photos, drawings, and artifacts that are calming and peaceful. In the yoga studio of Yogis in Service, we have small sculptures of frogs doing yoga poses (a secular choice) and have decorated the studio in the basic elements of nature (i.e., wood, plants, natural light). In your space, have sitting pillows or small benches. Provide headphones, recordings of guided meditations, meditation jars (described later), and stones in bowls for counting affirmations, breaths, or calming phrases. If there is no space, students can keep a small meditation jar or set of stones in their desks. In this way, they are available any time throughout the day.

Rechtschaffen (2014) describes the peace corner concept. This concept was pioneered by Linda Lantieri and is said to be used in schools across the globe (Rechtschaffen, 2014). The peace corner is a dedicated space, collaboratively created by students for students to find peacefulness. There is calming music playing, pillows, coloring materials, and various tactile objects for soothing. Students are not sent to the peace corner; rather, they self-refer (Rechtschaffen, 2014). Students go to the peace corner when they feel dysregulated. Once they feel centered and calm, they return ready for learning (Rechtschaffen, 2014).

I acknowledge that this might not be possible in some schools. For 10 years, I implemented and researched a yoga program for middle schools girls. We taught yoga in the music room, in the library (with students studying at tables around us), in the middle of the cafeteria, and even on the school stage. Some semesters, the space rotated each week. Some weeks, the custodial staff did not get to mopping the cafeteria floor in time for us to put down the mats. We did the best with what we had, always working to make it better. I have also been able to run mindful groups in some very beautiful spaces, such as a church loft and outside on an Adirondack deck. In these beautiful spaces, it seemed easier to settle into mindfulness. I am reminded that this is internal work. The goal is to connect to your own mind, body, and breath while attuned and connected to your world. In this way, our space can become a tool for our practice—either to give us the opportunity to let go and not react, or to see the peacefulness and beauty that is possible.

Plan and Schedule Mindful Practices

Mindfulness can be infused every day (Rechtschaffen, 2014). Cultivating a daily commitment to practice helps students cultivate mindfulness habits. Formal mindfulness practices in the classroom can be completed in a few moments or in an hour-long block. In fact, you could have a day of mindfulness or a week or even a month-long mindful retreat (Cook-Cottone, 2015). Over many years of researching school-based yoga and mindfulness programs, I have learned that when you look at what can happen during the school day, it does not matter how wonderful and effective the program is. If a teacher can't fit it into her school day, or a school district can't find a way to practically implement the program, it will have no effect. This is why the National Institutes of Health has implemented funding programs for feasibility and acceptability studies. They agree: If it can't feasibly be done and the population, in this case school personnel and students, doesn't accept it, the program will have a very hard time finding effects.

Schedule your mindfulness activities into your day. I have a guiding principle I use often when I teach yoga; "After great effort, take great rest." Mindfulness practices are wonderful ways to bring a sense of equanimity into the school day. Begin the day with 3 to 8 minutes of mindfulness activity. Engage in cycles of teaching curriculum, student academic skills work, and then 3 to 5 minutes of mindfulness and mindfulness movement practices. With a short practice in the morning and an additional three to four mindful breaks throughout the day, you can build up to 30 minutes or more of mindfulness in the classroom each day.

There are also district- and school-wide options. Some schools have a mindfulness and yoga teacher and schedule social-emotional learning time into the students' academic day (Cook-Cottone, Lemish, & Guyker, 2016). Classes are sometimes called wellness or wellness and health classes. In high school, mindfulness is sometimes woven into the health curriculum. Mindfulness and yoga can be integrated into the three-tier systems as universal intervention for all students or a targeted intervention for students who struggle (see Chapter 2). Finally, mindfulness and yoga can be part of before-and-after school programs.

Teach to the Developmental Level and Age

Be mindful of the developmental capabilities of the students with whom you are working. The manner in which tools are taught must match the developmental level of the students for mindfulness programming to be effective, see Table 5.1.

To illustrate, Mrs. Jones, a second-grade teacher, began her mindfulness practice 2 years ago. After an in-service session on mindful schools, she feels ready to begin teaching mindfulness to her second graders. She uses her own experience with meditation to inform her mindfulness teaching; however, she does not stop to consider the developmental level of her students and their neurological ability to pay attention. She begins with a 10-minute guided meditation she has downloaded from a well-known mindfulness resource page. It does not go well. She stops several times to redirect students who are talking or fidgeting, and a student who gets out of his seat is given a time out. After the 10 minutes, Mrs. Jones is exhausted, has yelled twice, which always feels bad, and isn't sure if mindfulness is a good idea. She rationalizes that her class this year feels immature, and perhaps she will try this again next year with hopes of a more attentive

TABLE 5.1 Mindfulness Practice by Age

Age	Developmental Notes	Mindfulness Practice Tips
Grades K–2	• In preoperational/operational thought (need concrete examples and lived experiences) • Use mindfulness practices to learn focus, self-regulation, and self-care • Live in the present moment • Reactive • Unfiltered bare awareness • Few self-limiting beliefs • Eager, curious, and ready to learn	• Mindfulness lessons 10–30 minutes • Present concept with a short practice (2–5 minutes) • Use props (breathing buddies) • Establish rituals and routines • Make it fun, safe, and warm • Don't explain everything; let them experience • Help them see cause and effect • Keep practices embodied and filled with movement
Grades 3–5	• In operational thought (still need concrete examples and lived experiences, can learn some abstractions, can think about their thinking) • Use mindfulness practices to learn focus, self-regulation, and self-care • Learn in a step-by-step fashion • Rational minds developing rapidly • Emerging self-awareness • Increased ability to describe emotions and physical states • Beginning to wonder why they are learning things • Eager to please • Emerging impulse control • High need for positive reflection • Peers becoming very important	• Mindfulness lessons 10–30 minutes • Can spend up to 10 minutes in silent practice • Can begin to include dialogues and reflection time • Use mindfulness journals • Embodied games and practices are still important; engage through play • Routine still important • Stress related to testing and other pressures real for them • Allow them to learn through experience, rather than telling them • Give them the rational reason for learning a lesson

(continued)

TABLE 5.1 Mindfulness Practice by Age (*continued*)

AGE	DEVELOPMENTAL NOTES	MINDFULNESS PRACTICE TIPS
Grades 6–8	• In formal operative thought (still benefit from concrete examples and lived experiences, can learn some abstractions, can think about their thinking) • Mindfulness practices are used to defuse stressors, support reliance on inner value systems, and further develop impulse control • Bodies, minds, and social roles are changing rapidly • Aware of violence and trauma in the community and culture • Increased risk for self-harm, substance use, risky sexual decision making, and school failure • Self-doubt, sexual orientation, and gender identity issues begin to emerge • Bullying experiences peak in middle school • Benefit from an honoring of independence and connectedness to others	• Mindfulness lessons 30–60 minutes • Silent practice can extend to 20 minutes • Teach lessons along with explanations of their benefits • Teach how lessons can be integrated into lives out of school • Rotating class schedules create implementation challenges and necessitate team work • After-school mindfulness clubs, mindfulness-based interventions, and mindfulness/yoga integrated into wellness and physical education classes create accessibility • Lessons learned in mindfulness/ yoga training can be used in service requirements (e.g., teaching younger students mindfulness)
Grades 9–12	• In formal operative thought (still benefit from concrete examples and lived experiences, can learn some abstractions, can think about their thinking) • Mindfulness practices are used to defuse stressors, support reliance on inner value systems, and further develop impulse control • Getting pulled in many directions—family, friends, media, school pressures, and larger life decisions • Questioning who they are with tensions between fitting in and personal authenticity • Peer-centered • Body issues and body image problems can be central • Long to be self-determined	• Mindfulness lessons 30–90 minutes • Present new concept, practice tool, and allow for dialogue and reactions • Practices can be used before tests, athletic events, and other potential stressful experiences • Rotating class schedules create implementation challenges and necessitate team work • After-school mindfulness clubs, mindfulness-based interventions, and mindfulness/yoga integrated into wellness and physical education classes create accessibility • Lessons learned in mindfulness/ yoga training can be used in service requirements (e.g., teaching younger students mindfulness) • Journals can be useful tools of self-reflection and growth • Use body-positive talk • Integrate sharing and partner work • Support self-determination • Encourage mindfulness-based school projects

Source: Cook-Cottone (2004), Cook-Cottone, Tribole, and Tylka (2013), David (2009), and Rechtschaffen (2014).

and mature class. Things take a turn for Mrs. Jones and her class. In a second in-service on mindful schools, she realizes in a small group discussion that beginning with a short 2 to 3 minutes of breath exercises and working up to a 10-minute guided meditation could take up to half the school year. This gave her a new perspective. Excited, she took her new viewpoint back to the classroom and experienced a more positive and energizing interaction with her students.

THE MINDFUL LESSON

Mindfulness can be integrated into the school day (i.e., informal mindfulness practices; see Chapter 7) or formally taught as skills in a more structured and extended lesson or practice (i.e., formal mindfulness practices; see Chapter 6). When skills are being taught or reinforced, it is good to allow for an extended mindfulness lesson (Rechtschaffen, 2014). For elementary school students this can take 15 to 20 minutes, and for middle and high school students this can take up to an hour (Rechtschaffen, 2014). You will want time to introduce a new concept and skill, practice, and have time for reflecting, dialoguing, and integrating (Rechtschaffen, 2014). A typical lesson looks like this (Rechtschaffen, 2014, p. 145):

• Opening mindfulness moment (a short centering practice)
• Time for checking in and reporting back
• Introduction of new mindfulness skill or concept
• Practice time for new mindfulness skill or concept
• Sharing through discussion and dialogue
• Journaling
• Sharing ideas for generalizing use of skills to school and life
• Closing mindfulness moment

Opening and Checking-in

Begin mindful lessons with a short 2 to 5 minute mindful lesson (Rechtschaffen, 2014). Begin with something familiar. Breath work, a guided meditation, or mindful listening are all good choices (Rechtschaffen, 2014). Then, transition to the checking-in component of the lesson. Here, students share how they are using their mindfulness lessons in their everyday life (Rechtschaffen, 2014). I usually help to stimulate the sharing by calling up specific life domains: schoolwork, school, family, friends, thinking, emotions, decision making, challenges, and possibilities. It can be helpful to recall a specific homework or skill that the students have been working on (Rechtschaffen, 2014). Allow a few minutes here for discussion and sharing.

New Lesson, Practice, and Dialogue

Following the opening and check in, introduce the new lesson. Depending on the age of the class, you may explain the concept or therapeutic underpinning of the practice. Rechtschaffen (2014) warns not to tell the students what the practice should or will be like.

Rather, set them up with the specific skills. You may model the practice or simply walk the students through the experience. Take about 3 to 5 minutes to do this, depending on the age of the students. Next, the students will practice what they have learned. This can be done individually, in pairs, or in small groups. Another 2 to 5 minutes here. At this point, the lesson should be at about the 12 to 20 minute mark, depending on the age of the students. Students can share with the whole group the discoveries made in pairs or small group work (Rechtschaffen, 2014).

Journaling, Generalizing, and Closing

Journaling is often reserved for older students (Rechtschaffen, 2014). However, I have found that elementary students enjoy drawing and writing about their experience in a similar, yet less formal, way. This allows younger students to reflect on their mindfulness lesson in a personal and creative way and cultivate a practice of processing experiences through writing. For older students, ask them to draw or write about their mindfulness lesson practice. Ask them to make connections that bridge the lesson that was taught and the meaning that is experienced within the lesson. Ask, "How did it feel to learn this practice? What does this type of practice mean to you and offer you?" Ask them to be as descriptive as possible. Next, at the end of each lesson, Rechtschaffen (2014) suggests the group explore ways in which the theme, concept, or practice of the mindfulness lesson can be used in the students' daily lives. The goal is for the students to become investigators into how mindfulness can play a role in their lives (Rechtschaffen, 2014). Invite them to practice at home and in school so that they can share. Finally, close the session with a short mindfulness lesson (see Rechtschaffen, 2014 for a more detailed breakdown of the mindfulness lesson).

CONCLUSION

Mindfulness practice in the classroom offers students an opportunity to practice valuing the reflective and intentional process. As we seek to graduate self-motivated and skilled problem solvers, we must also seek to develop reflective thinking. These processes go hand-in-hand. By building the mindful classroom from the ground up and from the inside out (i.e., from your own practice to your teaching), you will model the work that is needed to build a mindful and reflective life.

REFERENCES

Cook-Cottone, C. (2004). Childhood posttraumatic stress disorder: Diagnosis, treatment, and school reintegration. *School Psychology Review, 33,* 127.

Cook-Cottone, C. P. (2015). *Mindfulness and yoga for self-regulation: A primer for mental health professionals.* New York, NY: Springer Publishing.

Cook-Cottone, C. P. (2016). Yoga for the re-embodied self: The therapeutic journey home. *Yoga Therapy Today, Winter,* 40–42.

Cook-Cottone, C. P., Kane, L., Keddie, E., & Haugli, S. (2013). *Girls growing in wellness and balance: Yoga and life skills to empower.* Onalaska, WI: Schoolhouse Educational Services.

Cook-Cottone, C. P., Lemish, E., & Guyker, W. (2016). *Secular yoga in schools: A qualitative study of the Encinitas Union School District lawsuit*. Presented at the Yoga in the Schools Symposium, April 2015, Kripalu, Lenox, MA.

Cook-Cottone, C. P., Tribole, E., & Tylka, T. L. (2013). *Healthy eating in schools: Evidence-based interventions to help kids thrive*. Washington, DC: American Psychological Association.

David, D. S. (2009). *Mindful teachers and teaching mindfulness: A guide for anyone who teaches anything*. Somerville, MA: Wisdom Publications.

Dioum, B. (1968). *Paper presented at the General Assembly of the International Union for the Conservation of Nature and Natural Resources*, New Delhi, India. Seattle Public Library Archive.

Grabovac, A. D., Lau, M. A., & Willet, B. R. (2011). Mechanisms of mindfulness: A Buddihist psychological model. *Mindfulness, 2*(3), 154–166. doi:10.1007/s12671-011-0054-5

Jennings, P. A. (2015). *Mindfulness for teachers: Simple skills for peace and productivity in the classroom*. New York, NY: W. W. Norton.

Kabat-Zinn, J. (2013). *Full catastrophe living, revised edition: How to cope with stress, pain and illness using mindfulness meditation*. New York, NY: Bantam Books.

Marlatt, G. A., Bower, S., & Lustyk, M. K. B. (2012). Substance abuse and relapse prevention. In C. K. Germer & R. D. Siegel (Eds.). *Wisdom and compassion in psychotherapy: Deepening mindfulness in clinical practice*. New York, NY: The Guilford Press.

McCown, D., Reibel, D., & Micozzi, M. S. (2010). *Teaching mindfulness: A practical guide for clinicians and educators*. New York, NY: Springer.

Olson, K. (2014). *The invisible classroom: Relationships, neuroscience, and mindfulness in schools*. New York, NY: W. W. Norton.

Rechtschaffen, D. (2014). *The way of mindful education: Cultivating well-being in teachers and students*. New York, NY: W. W. Norton.

Siegel, D. J. (2010). *The mindful therapist: A clinician's guide to mindsight and neural integration*. New York, NY: W. W. Norton.

Stahl, B., & Goldstein, E. (2010). *A mindfulness-based stress reduction workbook*. Oakland, CA: New Harbinger Press.

Wallace, B. A. (2011). *Minding closely: The four applications of mindfulness*. Ithaca, NY: Snow Lion Publications.

Willard, C. (2016). *Growing up mindful: Essential practices to help children, teems, and families find balance, calm, and resilience*. Boulder, CO: Sounds True.

CHAPTER 6

MINDFULNESS ON THE CUSHION: FORMAL MINDFULNESS PRACTICES IN EDUCATING FOR SELF-REGULATION AND ENGAGEMENT

[T]he faculty of voluntarily bringing back a wandering attention,
over and over again,
is the very root
of judgment, character, and will.

No one is [a master of oneself] if he have it not.

An education which should improve this faculty
would be the education par excellence.

William James, *Principles of Psychology* (1890)

MINDFUL TOOLS FOR SELF-REGULATION AND INTENTIONAL, REFLECTIVE ENGAGEMENT

Mindfulness practices are the skills that students can effectively learn (Jennings, 2015). We have spent a lot of time talking about the big ideas of mindfulness and yoga in education in the first section of this book. We now move on to the practical applications of mindfulness in the classroom. The mindfulness practices described here are the specific tools that will help your students manage stress, self-regulate, and engage intentionally in their school day. This chapter offers a review of specific *formal mindfulness-based practices* that can help you and your students embody self-regulation, self-care, and intentional, reflective engagement (see the Mindful and Yogic Self as Effective Learner [MY-SEL] model in Chapter 1).

Willard (2016), in his book, *Growing up Mindful: Essential Practices to Help Children, Teens, and Families Find Balance, Calm and Resilience*, defines mindfulness practices as having these three components: paying attention on purpose, present moment connection, and nonjudgmental acceptance (Willard, 2016, p. 28). Mindful practice cultivates an effective sense of self that can negotiate both internal and external challenges (see Figure 6.1). Mindfulness practices empower students to be more intentional in their schoolwork, in relationships, and with themselves. As students learn to *notice* and *allow* internal and external experiences,

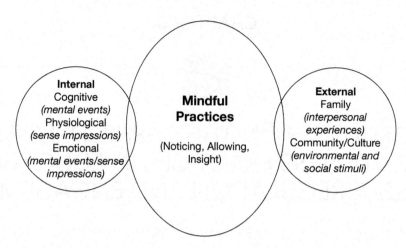

FIGURE 6.1 Mindful practices.
Source: Cook-Cottone (2015).

they will gain valuable *insights* and the ability to be more intentional and effective in their behavioral choices (see Figure 6.1; Cook-Cottone, 2015; Waters, Barsky, Ridd, & Allen, 2015).

This chapter details structured practices that can be used with your students as well as support the development of your own mindful path. Thereafter, the practices are presented in terms of developmental accessibility. The first set can be used with all ages. The later practices are best used with adolescents and adults. Each of the practices is linked to the associated principle of embodied growth and learning (see Chapter 3). Examples are provided to illustrate the utility of these practices with specific struggles, in-class challenges, and disorders.

FORMAL MINDFULNESS PRACTICES

The term *formal* refers to the *on-the-cushion* nature of the practices. A formal mindful practice is a systematic meditation practice with the specific aim of cultivating the cognitive process of mindfulness (Lutz, Jha, Dunne, & Saron, 2015; Shapiro & Carlson, 2009; Stahl & Goldstein, 2010). In other words, formal refers to the specific setting-aside of time to practice (e.g., 5–60 minutes; Cook-Cottone, 2015; Shapiro & Carlson, 2009; Willard, 2016). Formal practices also have a structure or format for practice (Cook-Cottone, 2015). It is important to make a distinction between formal and informal practices. Specifically, informal practices involve the intentional weaving in of the elements of mindfulness into typical daily classroom and at-home activities (Willard, 2016). Here, we learn about the formal practices.

What Is Meditation?

Meditation is one of the formal mindfulness practices. There are many different popular meditation practices, all with the underlying premise of attending deliberately to external and/or internal phenomena (Cook-Cottone, 2015; Waters et al., 2015; Willard, 2016). It is the intentional act of regulating attention through the observation of thoughts (i.e., mental events), physiological experiences (i.e., sense impressions), and emotions (i.e., mental events/sense impressions; Cook-Cottone, 2015; Waters et al., 2015). Also essential, meditation includes an acceptance and knowing that it is the nature of the mind to become distracted (Willard, 2016). What happens next is one of the many different ways one type of meditation is different from another. Broadly speaking, there are at least two broad forms of meditation: meditation with simple awareness of the present moment and focused concentration meditation (Cook-Cottone, 2015; Stahl & Goldstein, 2010; Waters et al., 2015).

Mindful awareness meditation is practiced in a manner that brings full attention and awareness to the present moment and to the internal and external phenomena that are present (Cook-Cottone, 2015; Stahl & Goldstein, 2010). Awareness meditation involves a simple noticing of these experiences (Cook-Cottone, 2015). In some forms of this type of meditation, there is no effort to change anything that the meditator is noticing (Hanh, 1975; Kabat-Zinn, 2013; Waters et al., 2015). The practice is to observe dispassionately without volition, distraction, grasping, or aversion (Wallace, 2011; Waters et al., 2015). You may notice sense impressions such as sight, sounds, tastes, and sensations of the skin. You may notice cognitive processes via the working of your mind, such as thoughts, memories, and cognitive reactions (Cook-Cottone, 2015). You will also notice emotions that present in both body and mind (Cook-Cottone, 2015; Kabat-Zinn, 2013). *Acem meditation* is an example of awareness meditation. In this form of meditation, thoughts, memories, feelings, and sensations arise and pass through the meditator's objective awareness without any intentional attempt to control the content (Waters et al., 2015).

Mindful awareness meditation also includes forms of meditation that involve awareness of internal and external experiences, along with an intention to keep focus on the present moment and to turn attention away from mental distractions (e.g., memories or planning; Cook-Cottone 2015; Waters et al., 2015). Willard (2016) explains that mindfulness meditation practices can be summed up using the four Rs that he learned from Vancouver-based mindfulness instructors Brian Callahan and Margaret Jones Callahan: *Rest, Recognize, Return,* and *Repeat* (Willard, 2016). According to Willard (2016), the process is quite simple (Figure 6.2).

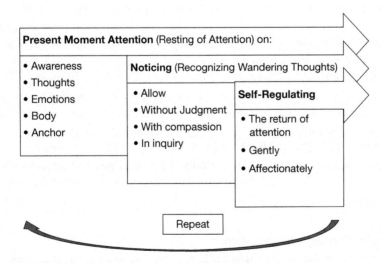

FIGURE 6.2 The process of meditation.
Source: Cook-Cottone (2015) and Willard (2016).

First, find present moment attention as you *rest* your awareness on an anchor (e.g., the breath or a series of words). Second, without judgment and with compassion, simply notice, or *recognize*, when your mind wanders and where it goes when it wanders. That is, as you meditate, your allowing and noticing the patterns of the mind include the process of inquiry: "What are my patterns," and "Where are the thoughts, feelings, sensations that draw my attention time after time?" It is this process that is an access point for knowing ourselves. Third, when your mind wanders, perhaps when you are drawn into a line of thinking, or you are trying to avoid a feeling or thought, all you need to do is notice that this has happened, self-regulate, and *return* awareness gently and affectionately back to the anchor. Fourth, *repeat* the process as necessary (Willard, 2016). To illustrate, imagine you are meditating. You are resting your focus on your breath as it moves in and out of your body. You suddenly become aware that you are beginning to think about your plans for the rest of the day. At this point, you might say to yourself, "I am thinking." You simply recognize what you are doing without judgment. Next, you compassionately bring your awareness back to the present moment and breath, away from thinking and recognizing that you are thinking. Yoga Nidra is an example of this type of meditation. Specifically, in Yoga Nidra, neutral attention is withdrawn from desiring to act (e.g., get up and move) and turned toward the senses or imagination (Waters et al., 2015).

Concentration meditation involves a focus on an object of meditation (Cook-Cottone, 2015; Hanh, 1975; Kabat-Zinn, 2013; Stahl & Goldstein, 2010; Waters et al., 2015; Willard, 2016). Awareness is brought to a single point, an anchor (i.e., one-pointedness; Stahl & Goldstein, 2010). Willard (2016) explains that use of an anchor for meditation strengthens the skill of concentration. This anchor could be a mantra (i.e., a centering statement), a concept, an object, or the picture of a calming place or loved one (Willard, 2016). There are many examples of this type of meditation. For example, in Transcendental Meditation (TM), the meditator silently repeats a word or mantra as he or she works toward a meditative state (Waters et al., 2015). In TM, when a distracting thought arises, the meditator brings his or her awareness directly back to the mantra (Waters et al., 2015). Another example is the metta meditation, or loving-kindness meditation. This involves the deliberate focus of attention on positive feelings of love, kindness, and compassion for self and others (Waters et al., 2015). Shamatha meditation practice, yet another form of meditation, involves placing attention on a mental image or attending to a visual object as the meditator works toward stability of attention, vividness in seeing, and introspection (Waters et al., 2015). In Zen meditation, the meditator focuses attention on a word puzzle or the breath in an effort to exclude mental distractions and work toward a heightened state of consciousness (Waters et al., 2015). Last, Kabat-Zinn's (2013) mindfulness-based stress reduction (MBSR) program utilizes a few different types of concentration meditation. These include a technique-specific mindfulness meditation in which attention is focused in a nonjudgmental manner on an object without distraction (Waters et al., 2015). Also, within the 8-week MBSR program, meditators engage in breath awareness, body scan exercises, walking meditations, and mindful eating (Kabat-Zinn, 2013; Waters et al., 2015). More on this and other specific mindfulness programs are detailed in Chapter 8.

Finding Insight Through Meditation

Insight is the capacity to know your inner self. It is inward looking. Insight comes from what you notice as you practice the level of awareness found in meditation (Cook-Cottone, 2015). As a person practices meditation, cycling through the process of focusing, wandering, and returning to the anchor, the capacity for concentration is further developed (Willard, 2016). Every time the meditator focuses on the anchor and disengages from the ongoing stream of thoughts, there is an increase in the capacity to let go of distraction (Willard, 2016). Perhaps one of the most misunderstood aspects of meditation is the exact process through which there is the greatest opportunity for growth and insight. Specifically, each time the meditator notices his or her mind wandering, this is "a moment of mindfulness—not a moment of failure" (Willard, 2016, p. 33). In this way, formal meditation cultivates the space between stimulus, or being distracted, and response (i.e., training back to focus, going with the stimulus, or reacting; Wallace, 2011). It is in the moment within which the mind wanders, as well as in the direction of the wandering (i.e., the where of the wandering), that the meditator has an opportunity to see his or her own habits and patterns (Willard, 2016). This is the source of what some call wisdom, self-understanding, or insight (see Figure 6.3; Cook-Cottone, 2015; Willard, 2016).

Here is a more detailed breakdown for you. As you sit in meditation, you will notice stimuli (Grabovac, Lau, & Willett, 2011). It may be a mental event or a thought (as Hanh [1975] describes), or it may be a sense impression, information coming from one of your senses or your body. You simply notice. Because you are human, each stimulus is automatically and immediately tagged by the brain with a feeling-tone: pleasant, neutral, or unpleasant (Cook-Cottone, 2015; Grabovac et al., 2011; Hanson & Mendius, 2009). Research suggests that there is an added challenge. That is, owing to biological mechanisms of self-protection, "negative trumps positive" (Hanson & Mendius, 2009). According to neuropsychologists and neurologists, these things we cannot control (Cook-Cottone, 2015). However, it is at exactly this point in the process that you have a choice (Chapter 3, principle 7: I choose my focus and actions).

In meditation we dig into this space, the space right after the stimulus and feeling-tone (Cook-Cottone, 2015). This is the space of insight, in which lives can be changed (Cook-Cottone, 2015). As you sit in meditation, you notice stimuli and feeling-tones, then you choose to attach, avoid, or allow. This is not an easy practice as the natural tendency is to attach and build on the feeling-tone cultivating concepts, emotions, and maybe even a line of thinking or ruminating (Grabovac et al., 2011). More insight is available here. Many times,

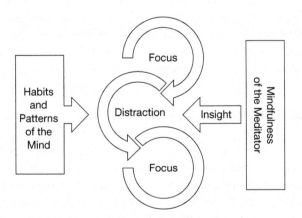

FIGURE 6.3 Meditation insights.
Source: Cook-Cottone (2015) and Willard (2016).

we have a default script we fall into in which we are the victim; everything is out of control; or we have no power. Often these stories are activated when we attach to the unpleasant feeling-tone. This is identification. We experience things as if these experiences are, in fact, who we are (Cook-Cottone, 2015; Wallace, 2011). Other times, the feeling-tone is so unpleasant that we move into aversion. We want to avoid this feeling. By staying present, moving your awareness to your breath or object of concentration (e.g., plant, object, word, concept), you bring yourself to allowing the stimulus to run its course. Any behavior you choose after this can be unencumbered, full of freedom, and full of your intentions.

Grabovac et al. (2011), Bien (2008), and Hanh (1998) distill the essence of what is to be learned in meditation practice to these three ideas (i.e., impermanence, suffering, and not self):

1. Sense impressions and mental events arise and pass away (i.e., *impermanence*).
2. Habitual reactions (i.e., attachment and aversion) to the feeling-tones accompanying sense impressions or mental events are the source of *suffering*.
3. Sense impressions and mental events are *not self*.

Siegel (2010) suggests that, over time, meditation practices can help us neurologically enhance the ability to notice and discriminate various incoming sensations and mental events from our narrative-based sense of self. Students can begin to realize that just because they think or feel something, that is not who they are (Cook-Cottone, 2015). They are their choices (Chapter 3, principle 7: I choose my focus and actions).

As you practice, minute after minute, session after session, you come to know your habits. As you come to know the habits of your mind, you learn to see them for what they are—habits—rather than the truth. For example, David, a sixth-grade boy, has a tendency to say, "I can't," when anything gets outside of his comfort zone. When he begins to read a long story, he says aloud, "I can't. It's too hard." If he attempts new math problems, he says, "I can't." Not surprisingly, this was the same approach he took to mindfulness practice. When the class was asked to sit in stillness and focus on their breath, David said, "I can't." His teacher asked him to shift "I can't" to "I'll try." She asked him to try for 30 seconds. She asked him to notice his body, breath, and how he was feeling. Then, she counted aloud as David focused and breathed. She celebrated with him when he finished and asked him to check back in. He felt calmer and happier. Trying became his practice. With small accomplishable steps in his mindfulness and classwork, he slowly moved to an "I'll try," or growth, mindset. David gained insight into what was possible for him (Chapter 3, principle 12: I work toward the possibility of effectiveness and growth in my life).

SPECIFIC MEDITATION PRACTICES FOR SCHOOLS

I have divided the formal practices into two sections: (a) formal meditation practices for all ages (i.e., elementary to adult), and (b) formal meditation practices for older students to adult (i.e., later middle school and high school). It is important to remember that there can be wide variation in students' ability to attend, concentrate, reflect, and have insight. Children with cognitive and/or attention difficulties will routinely need more support, concrete guidance, and tangible objects of focus (i.e., guided meditations) no matter what their age.

Formal Mindfulness Practices for All Students

This first set of practices is a set of basic tools for students and educators of all ages. The second smaller set is more complex and more appropriate for children with better developed cognitive skills. The practices are presented in an intentional order, from the most basic guidance for sitting in meditation, moving toward increasingly more complex practices.

Getting Seated

Finding a good seat is important for meditation practice (Cook-Cottone, 2015). If you are not comfortable, how you are seated becomes an obstacle to your practice (Wallace, 2011). Traditionally, meditators such as Hanh (1975) suggest sitting in the lotus position (i.e., left foot placed on the right thigh and right foot placed on the left thigh); half lotus (i.e., only one foot on one thigh); knees bent resting on your two legs or a small bench; or sitting on a cushion (Zabutan). The photos show a student sitting with legs crossed in easy pose with two options; (a) one hand on the heart and one hand on the belly, and (b) hands resting on thighs, face up (Instructional Photograph 6.1).

Wallace (2011) notes that many people simply do not feel comfortable sitting on the floor. Further, depending on your classroom or space, sitting on the floor may not be an option. Thus, in a firm supportive chair, keep your back straight (Cook-Cottone, 2015; Hanh, 1975). The head and neck should be aligned with the spine (Hanh, 1975). Sit with your knees hip-distance apart and feet on the floor (Davis, Eshelman, & McKay, 2008)

INSTRUCTIONAL PHOTOGRAPH 6.1: SEATED MEDITATION

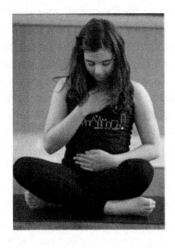 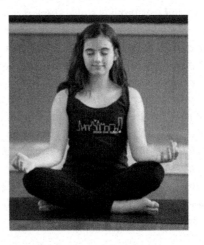

Photographer: Madison Weber; model, Kayla Tiedemann.

Eyes can be open, partially closed, or closed (Stahl & Goldstein, 2010; Willard, 2016). If open, eyes should be focused a yard or two in front of you (Hanh, 1975). If sleepiness is present, it can be helpful to keep the eyes open or slightly open (Cook-Cottone, 2015; Stahl & Goldstein, 2010). Maintain a soft smile (Hanh, 1975). A soft smile helps you relax the "worry-tightening" muscles in your face (Hanh, 1975, p. 34). If you'd like, place the left hand, palm side up, in your right palm (Hanh, 1975). You can also place your hands on your thighs or at your heart and belly (Cook-Cottone, 2015; Stahl & Goldstein, 2010). The position that is ultimately selected should allow for alertness and comfort (Stahl & Goldstein, 2010).

The practice script that follows should be read for each of the seated meditations. It helps students get settled and prepared for the meditation or mindfulness practices. Accordingly, each meditation scripted here begins with the words, "Start with the Getting Seated for Meditation Script."

Visualizations

Visualizations are a powerful way to help students develop meditation skills without a need to fully understand the meditation process. Willard (2016) offers an entire chapter on visualization for children in his text, *Growing Up Mindful*. In visualization, you provide metaphors for the elements of meditation. In the following visualization, the student's mindful awareness and beginner's mind is represented by the little boy. The meditation anchor is the moon. The passing thoughts and feelings are reflected by the clouds (Instructional Story 6.1).

PRACTICE SCRIPT 6.1: GETTING SEATED FOR MEDITATION

Approximate timing: 2 minutes for practice

Sit comfortably. Be sure that you are well grounded (e.g., your feet are touching the floor if in a chair, or your body and legs provide stable support if you are seated on the floor). Roll your shoulders back, draw your belly in, and extend and straighten your spine as you reach the very top of your head toward the ceiling. If you would like, close your eyes. If you decide to leave your eyes open, choose a focal point a few feet in front of you and rest your eyes there. Place your left hand, palm facing up, within the palm of your right hand, and rest your hands on your lap or legs. Let a gentle half smile come to your face. Take a few moments to bring your awareness to your body becoming present from the soles of your feet to the crown of your head. [Read slowly here, taking a pause as you move through the body.] Notice your feet, legs, body, arms, hands, chest, heart beating, lungs breathing, and the very top of your head reaching to the ceiling. How do you feel? Notice your heart beating and any tense places in the body. These are places in which it feels like your muscles are holding on tight. Breathe into any tense places you may feel and exhale to release them. With each exhalation, release tense places and soften through your whole body. Let go of everything. Hold on to nothing but your breathing and your half smile.

Source: Cook-Cottone (2015), Hanh (1975), Kabat-Zinn (2013), McCown, Reibel, and Micozzi (2010); Wallace (2011), and Willard (2016).

INSTRUCTIONAL STORY 6.1: THE BOY, THE MOON, AND THE CLOUDS

Approximate timing: 2 minutes for introduction; 5 minutes for practice

Find your comfortable seat [use Getting Seated for Meditation Script]. *Once upon a time, there was a little boy who loved the moon. His favorite part of the month was the day the moon was full, a giant, big round circle in the sky. He loved the moon so much that his mom and dad cut a hole in the roof and put in a window so he could watch the moon every night as he fell asleep. The little boy loved the moon so much that they became friends. They supported each other. Every night the moon would move up to its place in the sky and look down for the boy. As much as the moon inspired the boy to rest, the boy inspired the moon to shine. And so it went. They helped each other every night.*

Earlier today, the little boy and his family went to visit his grandmother. The little boy is not going to be able to take care of the moon. I told him that you would help him take care of the moon. He was so happy. He said that it was easy to take care of the moon. You simply have to relax, breathe, and watch the moon. The moon loves to be seen. He said that if clouds pass by, you simply notice them and keep your eyes right on the moon. He said to remember that the clouds will come and go, and your job is to breathe and watch the moon so that it knows you are there, and it is inspired to shine. It is your turn now to watch the moon.

You are resting comfortably right under the sky window. You are relaxed and feeling calm. Looking up through your special window to the sky, you are breathing slowly: in—one, two, three, and four, and out—one, two, three, four. You notice your breath is steady and calm as you look up through your window at the moon. As you look at the moon, you notice how round it is, and how it is white and gray with shaded areas and brighter areas across its surface. You look carefully at its coloring and wonder if it is slightly blue, red, or yellow. What is the color of the moon you see? It seems as if the moon feels you watching and brightens just a bit. As you carefully look at the moon, you breathe steadily in—one, two, three, and four, and out—one, two, three, four.

As you watch the moon, you notice some clouds coming in from one side of the sky and moving toward the other side. You know it is your job to watch the moon, so you let the clouds float by. Some of the clouds are big, and some are small. Some of the clouds move slowly, and some move quickly. You keep watching the moon, and the moon is so happy. The clouds keep moving by. As you watch the moon, you might see that a cloud or two gets stuck in front of the moon. You can breathe in deeply for one, two, three, and four, then use your exhale to move the cloud out of the way of the moon, one, two, three, and four. The moon can feel how hard you are working to take care of its shining and is thankful. You notice that the clouds are coming by less often. You notice that eventually there are no more clouds and all that you see is the beautiful moon. You breathe in—one, two, three, and four, and out—one, two, three, and four. You are so happy you could help the little boy. He is on his way home and will watch the moon tonight. He wants you to know that you can watch the moon with him any time you want. All you need to do is close your eyes, imagine his moon window, and breathe.

Source: Informed by Willard (2016).

The Basic Meditation Practice

Hanh (1975) says that, as you begin practice, you should "Hold onto nothing but your breath and the half smile" (p. 35). Hanh (1975) describes it as achieving total rest. He states that in order to achieve total rest you must do two things: (a) watch your breath, and (b) let go of everything else. It is a continual watching and letting go, watching, letting go, and watching and letting go (Cook-Cottone, 2015). During this process, allow yourself to release every muscle in your body (Hanh, 1975). According to Hanh (1975), relaxation is a necessary point to commence meditation. The story that follows was inspired by Hanh (1975) and originally created for Cook-Cottone (2015).

To introduce this in class, it can be fun to give each student a small pebble and a permanent marker. Have them create their own meditating pebble with a gentle half smile (Instructional Photograph 6.2). They can place the pebble on their desk or hold it in their hands while they breathe softly and listen to the story.

INSTRUCTIONAL PHOTOGRAPH 6.2: THE MEDITATING PEBBLE

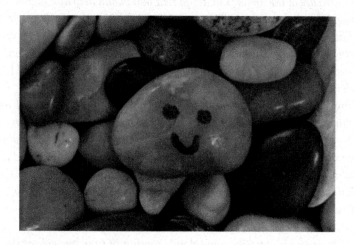

Photographer: Catherine Cook-Cottone.

Note: When telling the story, it is good to explain to the younger children that the Meditating Pebble is like the cartoon characters that live underwater: It too can breathe.

INSTRUCTIONAL STORY 6.2: THE MEDITATING PEBBLE

Approximate timing: 2 minutes for introduction; 5 minutes for practice

Imagine that you are a little pebble. You have been gently tossed into a river. You are a little pebble in the water, and pebbles like water. The water is just the right temperature. You feel calm and happy. You safely sink down through the water without effort. As a pebble, you are free from everything (no homework, no tests, no practice); you can just watch and let go and gently float down to the bottom of the riverbed. You are at the point of complete relaxation there on the bed of the river. It does not matter how long it took you to fall or how far you fell to get there on the riverbed. Once you reach the riverbed, you have found your own special place to relax. Here, you are no longer pushed or pulled by the water or anything else. You can just watch as the river and all that is in it—fish, leaves, and water bugs—float by.

At the bottom of the river, you are at the point of perfect relaxation. It feels cozy and soft. You can let go of everything. Being a special kind of pebble, you can breathe under the water. At the very center of you is your breath. You gently breathe in and out, noticing how comfortable and calm you feel. You breathe in and out slowly and softly, feeling and watching the water drift by and letting go of everything else.

(continued)

INSTRUCTIONAL STORY 6.2 (continued)

In this special spot you, feel happiness, peace, and calm right now. Things are so calm and peaceful right now that you settle in even more and breathe, watch, and let go. You notice that, if you turn to look at the water and the things coming your way (i.e., the future), you miss this really great moment of being and watching right now. So you let go of looking to what is coming. You also notice that, if you look to the water or the things that have floated by (i.e., the past), again you miss this wonderful moment right now. So you let go of looking to what has passed. You notice that the best place to find peace, joy, and calm is right here in your current spot and in the current moment. You settle in even more, breathe, watch, and let go. Whenever you find yourself thinking about anything else, you notice. Then, you come right back to your spot, your breathing, watching, and letting go. Cuddle into your spot on the riverbed and breathe in and out slowly and deeply.

Take a few more breaths knowing that it is time to bring your attention back to the classroom. Breathing in—one, two, three, four, and breathing out—one, two, three, four. Breathing in—one, two, three, four, and breathing out—one, two, three, four. Breathing in—one, two, three, four and breathing out—one, two, three, four. Breathing in—one, two, three, four and breathing out—one, two, three, four. Now, slowly bring your hands up to your eyes. Slowly open your eyes and allow light through your fingers. Slowly bring your hands down to your desk or lap. Check in with how you are feeling.

Source: Inspired by Hanh (1975), Cook-Cottone (2015), and Greenland (2010).

As in this instructional story, the breath is used as an anchor, or tool, to help your mind focus. Attention to breath and breathing is not meant to be used to chase thoughts and feelings away (Cook-Cottone, 2015; Greenland, 2010; Hanh, 1975; Kabat-Zinn, 2013). Breath is the methodology for uniting the mind and the body and bringing them together in one spot, like the pebble in the riverbed (Cook-Cottone, 2015; Hanh, 1975; Kabat-Zinn, 2013). Explain to the students that when they feel a thought or feeling arise, do not follow it with their attention. Invite them to notice the presence of the thought or feeling and bring their attention back to their breath, just like the pebble in the riverbed (Hanh, 1975). Greenland (2010) suggests writing a focus word on the back of a pebble or stone (e.g., calm, peaceful, happy, joy, focus, health, or safe). She calls these "focus rocks" (Greenland, 2010, p. 96). Students can bring to awareness the concept written on their pebbles as they breathe and watch the water, thoughts, and other distractions float by.

Breath Awareness

Breath awareness and breath control are critical aspects of the physiological components of self-regulation (Cook-Cottone, 2015). As well explicated by Davis et al. (2008) and Willard (2016), breathing exercises have been found to be effective in the relief of many triggering symptoms, such as anxiety and mood symptoms, irritability, muscle tension, headaches, and fatigue. Breath awareness is a wonderful place to begin a meditation practice. Hanh (1975) begins his instruction on meditation with instruction on the breath. This ancient proverb on breath is powerful; I frequently use it when teaching mindfulness and yoga (Cook-Cottone, 2015):

He who half breathes, half lives.

—Author Unknown

There are several ways to utilize the breath in meditation. You can follow the length of the breath (Hanh, 1975). You can notice the role the body, specifically the diaphragm, stomach, and rib cage, plays in the extension of breath (Hanh, 1975). Hanh (1975) suggests that beginners lie down. Unless you are in physical education class or have yoga mats on hand, this might not be feasible. Notice in Instructional Photograph 6.1, students can place one hand on their hearts (chest area) and one hand on their bellies. Adding the external points of contact with the hands helps students become very aware of the depth of their breathing. In deep breathing, the chest fills and then the belly. Next, the belly empties and then the chest. They will be able to notice this as their chests rise and fall. Extension of the length of the breath can help anchor awareness of breathing. Begin with a few breath cycles—a four-count inhalation and exhalation (i.e., *breathing in—one, two, three, four, and breathing out—one, two, three, four*). Eventually, have them move to a five-, six-, or seven- count breath (Hanh, 1975). Hanh (1975) suggests that 20 breath cycles are a sufficient practice of noticing and lengthening the breath.

In Yogis in Service, Inc. and in my yoga-based eating disorders prevention program, Girls Growing in Wellness and Balance: Life Skills to Empower (Cook-Cottone, Kane, Keddie, & Haugli, 2013), we use breathing buddies (see Instructional Photograph 6.3). Breathing buddies are stuffed, beanbag-based animals or handmade beanbags crafted to look like animals (i.e., with glued-on googly eyes, felt ears, and a permanent-marker smile). You want your breathing buddy to have some weight to it so that it provides external sensory feedback to the student. The breathing buddy rests on the student's belly as the student takes deep breaths. The student knows he or she is breathing deeply enough when

INSTRUCTIONAL PHOTOGRAPH 6.3: BREATHING BUDDY

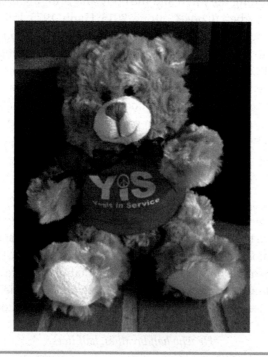

Photographer: Catherine Cook-Cottone.

the breathing buddy moves up and down on his or her belly (Cook-Cottone et al., 2013; Greenland, 2010).

Fiona, a second grader, found breathing buddies to be really helpful as she worked through her separation anxiety. Over the summer, Fiona's grandmother passed away suddenly in a car accident. Her mother was also in the car. Although Fiona's mother suffered only mild physical injuries, she was struck with grief and loss. Fiona's father and older sister did their best all summer to cope and take care of Fiona during this time. Still, it was a very difficult summer for everyone. After the accident, Fiona struggled when she was away from her mother. She became overwhelmingly anxious every time they had to be apart. When Fiona's mom eventually returned to work, Fiona texted and called her many times throughout the day. When Fiona began school in the fall, she was not able to focus in class, broke phone and texting rules in the classroom (hourly), and was beginning to fall far behind. She was referred to the school psychologist for a brief assessment and prereferral intervention. The school psychologist quickly assessed her separation anxiety and set up a behavior plan with the teacher to address time-on-task and phone use behaviors. She also set up regular counseling sessions during which she worked with Fiona to help her manage her anxiety. As part of the intervention, Fiona and the school psychologist made breathing buddies together from felt and dried beans. Fiona loved the way the deep breathing lowered her anxiety. She showed her breathing buddy and how it worked to her mom. They practiced Fiona's breathing work together before bed. Her mom stitched a heart onto her breathing buddy so Fiona would be able to feel how much her mom loved her while she was in class. After 3 weeks with her behavioral plan and regular sessions addressing anxiety, as well as using her breathing buddy, Fiona returned to her typical functioning in the classroom, with her breathing buddy right in her desk.

Breath work is one of the most effective mindfulness tools you can use. Awareness-of-breath practice integrates the following principles of embodied learning and growth (see Chapter 3): principle 2, my breath is my most powerful tool; principle 3, I am mindfully aware; principle 4, I work toward presence in my physical body; principle 6, I ask questions about my physical experience, feelings, and thoughts; principle 7, I choose my focus and actions; and principle 8, I do the work. Provided here is a script that you can use with your whole class and in your own practice.

PRACTICE SCRIPT 6.2: BREATH AWARENESS

Approximate timing: 2 minutes for introduction; 20 minutes for practice

Start with the Getting Seated for Meditation Script. Bring your awareness, your focus, to your body. Now, just breathe, letting your breath move in and out and in and out. Really pay attention to your breath. If possible, try closing your mouth and breathing through your nose. Do not try to change your breathing. Just let it happen. Notice the qualities of your breath. (Speak slowly here, allowing time for students to really process each question.) …. Is it smooth? …. Is your inhalation the same length as your exhalation? …. Can you feel your heart beat as you breathe? …. What is the pace of your breathing? Is it fast, slow, moderate? …. Do not do anything. Do not change your breathing. Simply notice. As you are aware of your breathing, you may notice that other

(continued)

PRACTICE SCRIPT 6.2 (continued)

thoughts, feelings, memories, or ideas enter your awareness. Simply notice that they are there, then bring your attention directly back to your breath. Do this as often as needed as you practice breath awareness.

Bring your awareness to the muscles of the face. Notice your jaw, cheeks, lips, eyes, and forehead. Breathe into these muscles. As you breathe out, release any tension. You want your face to feel as soft and relaxed as the face of a sleeping baby or puppy. Bring your awareness to the very tip of your nose. Notice the air as it passes just underneath the tip of your nose. Breathe while you notice the tip of your nose. Now, bring your awareness to your nostrils. Notice the quality of the air, the warmth as the air leaves your body and the coolness of the air as it enters. Notice if the air is dry or moist as it enters and leaves your body. As you breathe, remain aware of your focus. Continuously bring your attention back to your breath, your nose and your nostrils, the quality of the air, the pace of your breath. There is so much to notice right here in your present moment.

Begin to notice how the air feels as it enters your nose. See if you can feel it enter your body, move from your nose to your throat and into each of your lungs. Can you feel the breath divide as half enters one lung and half enters the other? Notice how your rib cage rises and falls as you inhale and exhale. You may begin to notice that your rib cage expands from front to back and from side to side as you inhale. You may notice that the ribs and the side of your body gently soften as you exhale. Continue breathing here. As before, notice your focus. If you need to, bring your focus back to your breath.

Now, bring your awareness to the qualities of your breath. Notice the length of the breath going in and the breath going out. Bring awareness to the fullness of your breath. Is it shallow and in your chest? Does it go deep into your body, expanding both your chest and your belly?

Slowly begin to deepen your breath. Count to four as you inhale—one, two, three, four—then count to four as you exhale—one, two, three, four. Continue this for four breaths. (Note, pause here and allow time for breath.) Now, continuing with deep breath, notice the transition from inhalation to exhalation. Once you feel as if you cannot inhale any further, allow your body to move, without effort, to letting the air go. As you feel you cannot exhale any further, allow your body to shift to taking the air in. Continue this for four breaths. (Note, pause here and allow time for four breaths.) Think to yourself as you breathe, "I breathe in a long breath," and "I breathe out a long breath."

Now, allow your breath to return to your normal breathing. When breathing your own normal breaths, pay attention. Are your breaths shorter? Think to yourself, "I breathe in a shorter breath," and "I breathe out a shorter breath." Notice the qualities of your normal breathing. Describe them to yourself as you breathe. You might think, "My breathing is smooth and even," or you might think, "My breathing is deep and strong." Breathe and notice the qualities of your breath.

Now, expand your awareness from your breath to your chest and head and then to your entire body, all the way from your feet to the very top of your head. Breathe as if you could breathe into your entire body. Inhale, a big, whole body inhale and exhale a big, whole body exhale. Notice your body again. Notice any changes in how your body feels. Slowly bring your palms together and rub them together, palm to palm, generating a little warmth. Then, take the palms of your hands to your eyes, softly cupping them. Slowly open your eyes into the palms of your hands and spread

(continued)

PRACTICE SCRIPT 6.2 (*continued*)

your fingers slightly to allow light in. Slowly withdraw your hands from your eyes, breathing normally.

Source: Bien (2008), Cook-Cottone (2015), Davis et al. (2008), Greenland (2010), Kabat-Zinn (2013), Stahl and Goldstein (2010), and Wallace (2011).

Body Scan

The body scan is a good practice for integrating mind and body (Davis et al., 2008; Jennings, 2015; McCown et al., 2010; Stahl & Goldstein, 2010). The body scan meditation has traditionally been done lying down (Jennings, 2015). Again, this is fine if you have yoga mats in your room or can do this during physical education or wellness class. However, in the classroom, you can ask your students to lean back into their chairs. You want them to feel grounded and comfortable in the position that they select (Cook-Cottone, 2015; Jennings, 2015). If the meditation is done in a yoga room with supports, blankets, and pillows, a rolled blanket can be placed under the knees and a small pillow under the head (Cook-Cottone, 2015). Read through the scan a few times before you work with it in class. It may be helpful to do some basic anatomy with the class so that they know the names and location of the body parts to which you will be referring. Use a figure drawing as in Figure 6.4. Have students draw a line to each body part and then draw in heart and lungs. For older children, this is a good time to show a video on the action of the diaphragm (e.g., see the 3D View of the Diaphragm, www.youtube.com/watch?v=hp-gCvW8PRY).

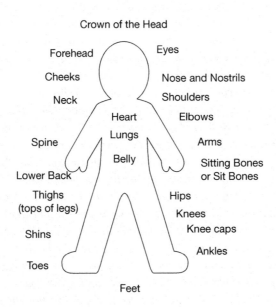

FIGURE 6.4 Basic body parts.

It can also be helpful to have students explore a felt-sense of what tension and relaxation feel like. Have them grip their hands into fists and hold, then have them soften and relax their fists. Do this for various parts of their bodies so that they have a sense of what it feels like to hold tension in their bodies. You will be referring to tension and softness within the script that follows. Note, the body scan practice integrates these principles of embodied learning and growth (see Chapter 3): principle 2, my breath is my most powerful tool; principle 3, I am mindfully aware; principle 4, I work toward presence in my physical body; principle 6, I ask questions about my physical experience, feelings, and thoughts; principle 7, I choose my focus and actions; and principle 8, I do the work.

PRACTICE SCRIPT 6.3: BODY SCAN
Approximate timing: 1 minute for introduction; 20 minutes for practice

Once you are in a comfortable position, close your eyes and bring your awareness to your breathing. Notice the rise and fall of your chest and belly as you breathe. Slowly begin to extend your breath, lengthening each inhalation and exhalation, pausing slightly at the turn of the breath. Inhale. Hold. Exhale. Hold. Do this for five complete breath cycles. (For young students or students who struggle with attention or self-regulation, count this out for them.)

Now, bring your awareness all the way down to your feet. Notice your toes, your big toes, second toes, third, fourth, and baby toes. Breathe as if you can breathe down into your toes. Notice any tension or holding you might feel in your toes. Let them settle. Notice where your toes connect to your feet, the balls of your feet, and move your awareness to the arches of your feet. If your feet are bare, notice the feeling of the air on your skin, the muscles beneath this skin. Notice your heels, the skin, the muscle and bone. Feel your heels resting on the floor, in shoes, or on the mat. Let them settle on the mat. Notice the tops of your feet. Breathe as if you can breathe into your feet, noticing any sensations you may feel.

Move your awareness to your ankles. Feel the connection of your ankles to your feet. Feel the space in your ankle joints. Next, notice the muscles and the skin. Can you feel the air or socks around your ankles? Are your ankles warm or cold? Breathe as if you can breathe right into your ankles.

Next, move your awareness into your lower legs. Move your attention from your heels through your Achilles tendons and into your calf muscles. Notice the feeling of your calf muscles touching the floor or the chair. Let them settle. Feel any tension or relaxation that is there. Just notice and breathe into your calves. Now, move your awareness to your shins. Focus on the area where the top of your feet meet your shins, then let your awareness move up your shin bones to your knees. Breathe as if you can breathe into your shins, noticing the bones, the muscles, and skin. Let them settle and soften.

Move your awareness, your attention, to the tops of your knees. Notice your knee caps as they cover the knee joints. Bring your awareness to all the muscles and tendons that meet the joint of your knees, some under the knee caps, some at the sides of the knee. Feel what you feel. Feel the space within the joint and the air or clothes around your knee. Move your awareness up your thighs. Feel the tops of your upper legs. Notice if they are holding tension or relaxed. Have a sense of the skin, the muscles, and the bones. Breathe as if you can breathe into your legs. Next, move your awareness to the undersides of your knees and up the backs of your upper legs. Feel your legs as they rest on the floor or chair. Breathe as if you can breathe into your legs. Let your legs settle and relax.

(continued)

PRACTICE SCRIPT 6.3 (continued)

Next, move your awareness up into your sitting bones. Feel the connection of your sitting bones with the chair or the floor as you rest, gently supported. Bring your awareness to the connection of your legs to your hips and body. Notice if you feel tension or softness. Breathe as if you can breathe into your hips and body. Slowly, bring your awareness into your belly. Notice your belly rise and fall as you breathe. Does your belly rise and fall easily with your breath? Breathe as if you can breathe directly into your belly.

Now, bring your awareness to the very bottom of your spine. Notice your low back. Does your low back feel supported or is there tension? Notice the connection of the low back to your whole back, the sides of your body, and the upper sections of your spine. Breathe as if you can breathe into your lower back and up into your entire spine. Let your awareness travel up your spine to the upper middle section of your back, the space between your shoulder blades. Notice if you feel supported by the floor or the chair. Is your back soft or tense? Bring your awareness across your upper back, spanning your focus of attention wide to reach the backs of your shoulders, the shoulder blades, and the very base of the neck. Notice any tension or softness. Breathe as if you can breathe across your whole upper back. Feel the support of the back as it meets the chair or the floor. Let your spine settle, soften, and relax.

Move your awareness to the area between the shoulder blades just under your heart. Bring your awareness to your lungs, noticing them fill with air as you breathe in and empty as you breathe out. Become very aware of your heart, your heartbeat, and the rhythm with your breath. Notice how your heart is supported by your mid back, your shoulder blades, and your lungs. Your heart is held by your body. Notice your breath and breathe as if you could breathe directly into your heart. Keep your attention here and breathe.

Bring your attention to your chest. Notice the muscles on top of the rib cage and those that span to the tops of your shoulders. Bring your attention to your shoulders, to the tops of your arms. Notice the upper arms as they are supported by the chair or the floor. What do you feel? Breathe as if you can breathe into your upper arms. Next, move your awareness to your elbows. Notice the muscles that come from the upper arms and the lower arms to your elbow joints. Breathe into the center of the elbows. Next, let your awareness travel down your forearms. Notice the skin, the muscles, and the bone. What sensations do you feel? Notice your wrists and the connections to your hands. Do you feel space here? Do you feel tension or softness? Notice what you are feeling here. Breathe as if you can breathe into your wrists. Now, notice your hands. Notice your thumbs, your first, second, third, and pinky fingers on each hand. Notice how your fingers feel. Are they straight, bent, slightly curled? Do you feel lightness or tension in your fingers? Just notice. Move your attention to the palms of your hands. What sensations do you feel? Breathe as if you can breathe into the palms of your hands, and notice what you notice. Keep your focus here and breathe.

Bring your awareness back to your chest. Notice your chest as you breathe in and out. Become aware of any movements in your chest as you breathe. Let your awareness travel to your throat. Can you feel the air pass through your throat as you breathe? Let your awareness move to the back of your neck and then to the base of the skull. Notice the connection of the neck to your head. Notice any tension or softness. Keep your awareness here and breathe.

Move your attention around to the front of your neck and up into your jaw. Feel your jaw. Are you clenching or relaxed in your holding of your jaw? Breathe as if you can breathe into your jaw. Next, allow your awareness to flow around to the back of your head. Notice your head resting on the chair or on your mat. Notice any support offered to your head by the floor or your chair. Breathe here.

(continued)

PRACTICE SCRIPT 6.3 (*continued*)

Bring your awareness to your cheeks, your mouth, your lips. Notice any sensations here. Notice your nose. Feel the air as it moves past your nostrils as you breathe. Breathe here and notice. Next, bring your awareness to your eyes. Do they feel soft, tense? Breathe as if you can breathe into your eyes. Keep your awareness here and breathe.

Slowly, move your awareness to your eyebrows and your forehead. Notice the skin, the muscles underneath the skin, and the bone. Breathe as if you can breathe into your forehead and notice what you feel. Now, bring your awareness to the very center of your forehead. Notice the skin, the muscles, the bone. Bring your awareness to the center of your forehead to the area that some call the mind's eye. Breathe here. With your eyes closed and your awareness at the very center of your forehead, what do you see? What do you feel? Notice and breathe as if you can breathe into the very center of your forehead. Hold your awareness here and breathe (long pause of at least 60 seconds).

Now, bring your awareness to your whole body. Extend your awareness to the soles of your feet, the palms of your hands, and the crown of your head. Breathe as if you can breathe into your whole body, the soles of your feet, the palms of your hands, and the crown of your head. Take a big inhale—one, two, three, four, five, and a big exhale—one, two, three, four, five. Take another big inhale—one, two, three, four, five, and another big exhale—one, two, three, four, five. Slowly allow your breath to return to normal.

When you are ready, begin to wiggle your fingers and your toes. If you are lying down, bend your elbows and your knees and slowly roll to your right side. Gently come to a seated position, ankles crossed, hands on your thighs. Bring your hands together and rub them together gently, bringing warmth into your hands. Place your hands over your eyes, and open your eyes into the palms of your hands. Open your fingers slowly to let in light and gently withdraw your hands from your face.

Note: To modify for younger students, you can do a shorter body scan focusing only on the feet, legs, belly, hands, arms, and head. Do two deep breaths in each spot.

Source: Adapted from Cook-Cottone (2015), informed by Davis et al. (2008), Jennings (2015), Kabat-Zinn (2013), McCown et al. (2010), Shapiro and Carlson (2009), Stahl and Goldstein (2010), Wallace (2011), and Willard (2016).

The Calming Mind Jar (or Meditation Jar)

If you want to give students an object of focus, there are lots of secular and fun options. For example, a creative colleague of mine, Kellie Love, a teacher in a Bronx elementary school, uses *calming mind jars* to help kids focus (see Instructional Tool 6.1: Calming Mind Jar). The mind jar is used as an anchor for attention. Students shake their calming mind jar, set it on the desk, and breathe as they watch the glitter settle as a metaphor for their minds settling. Willard (2016) recommends using different sizes or colors of glitter to represent thoughts, feelings, and urges to do things (i.e., engage in behaviors). If you would like to see what the use of a mind jar looks like in a classroom, you can watch the video, "Aliza and the Mind Jar," which illustrates the utility of this tool (vimeo.com/119439978). Aliza is one of Kellie Love's students. The calming-mind-jar practice integrates the following principles of embodied learning and growth (see Chapter 3): principle 2, my breath is my most powerful tool; principle 3, I am mindfully aware; principle 4, I work toward presence in my physical body; principle 7, I choose my focus and actions; and principle 8, I do the work.

INSTRUCTIONAL TOOL 6.1: CALMING MIND JAR

- Get materials together:
  - Empty water bottle (no glass jars)
  - Clear glitter glue (gives the liquid a viscosity that allows the glitter to more slowly settle in the water. You can also use clear glue and extra glitter. Be sure not to use white glue.)
  - Glitter of all sizes
  - Sequins of all sizes
  - Funnel
  - Water
  - Duct tape
- Create the calming mind jar:
  - Fill three fourths of the bottle with water.
  - Add glue or glitter glue and shake the bottle. Add more water as needed.
  - Add glitter and sequins using the funnel and shake the bottle. Start with a little of each size and add until you find it to your pleasing.
  - Cut duct tape to size and seal the bottle closed.
- Use the calming mind jar:
  - Ask the students to notice how they are feeling. Have them check in with their bodies, thoughts, and feelings.
  - Ask the students to shake their calming mind jars and then set them on their desks or in front of them if they are seated on the floor to practice.
  - Ask them to watch (i.e., rest their attention on) the glitter slowly fall to the bottom of their calming mind jars as they breathe deeply and closely.
  - If they notice that they are paying attention to something other than the glitter as it settles, they simply bring their focus back to the glitter.
  - After everyone's jar has settled, ask the students to notice how they are feeling. Have them check in with their bodies, thoughts, and feelings.
  - Ask the students to share their experiences with the class.

The Sensory Sloth

Connecting to the here and now can be difficult. Students are often lost in their thoughts, distractions, or feelings. Getting connected to sensory experiences can bring students back to the here and now (Greenland, 2010; Rechtschaffen, 2014). The sensory sloth activity provides an opportunity for kids to slow down, connect to the present moment, and engage each of their senses. It is fun to do this activity along with mindful eating (see Mindful Eating, this chapter). You can set up a series of sensory stations. At each station, students observe the artifacts with each of their senses (saving taste for mindful eating) moving slowly in a walking meditation from station to station. The main objective is awareness of what is observed through the senses as they work to stay present to each step and breath as they move as slowly as a sloth. Stations can include a scent tray for the sense of smell, with items such as bay leaves, whole nutmeg, cinnamon sticks, dried flowers, and peppercorn. For the sense of sound, set up a music station with headphones and songs from which they can pick out one or two instruments and describe their sounds and how they blend, or do not blend with other instruments in the piece. For mindfulness of the sensation of touch, students can explore a bin of textures with tree bark, granite, cotton balls, feathers, and so on. For the sense of sight, there are many options, from artwork to a microscope to prisms and crystals. As they move through each station, guide them to check into their sensations and out of their thinking. Guide them to describe what they observe without evaluating or judging. Remind them that their only job is to describe. As they finish, have them check in on how they experienced their thoughts, the need to judge, distractions, and being present. Ask them which sensations brought them most effectively to the here and now and which sensations were not as effective. The sensory sloth practice integrates the following principles of embodied learning and growth (see Chapter 3): principle 2, my breath is my most powerful tool; principle 3, I am mindfully aware; principle 4, I work toward presence in my physical body; principle 6, I ask questions about my physical experiences, feelings, and thoughts; and principle 7, I choose my focus and actions.

Mindful Eating

Mindful eating can be both a formal and informal practice (Cook-Cottone, 2015). As a formal mindfulness practice, the food is the object of attention in a focused-concentration meditation (Cook-Cottone, 2015; David, 2009; Davis et al., 2008; Greenland, 2010; Kabat-Zinn, 2013; Rechtschaffen, 2014). Mindful eating is a long-standing mindfulness practice. It is often done at the beginning of MBSR classes (see Chapter 12 for a full description of MBSR; Kabat-Zinn, 2013; Stahl & Goldstein, 2010). I use this as the first introduction to mindfulness in my course at the University at Buffalo, *The Mindful Therapist*. Typically, this activity is done with raisins. I offer a choice between a raisin and a dark chocolate chip (Cook-Cottone, 2015). Mindful eating practice integrates the following principles of embodied learning and growth (see Chapter 3): principle 3, I am mindfully aware; principle 4, I work toward presence in my physical body; principle 7, I choose my focus and actions; and principle 8, I do the work.

PRACTICE SCRIPT 6.4: MINDFUL EATING

Approximate timing: 1 minute for introduction; 10 minutes for practice

Preparation: *Bowl of raisins, bowl of dark chocolate chips, and napkins—enough for your class*

Find a comfortable seat. Be sure your feet can rest on the floor or a stable surface. Hand out napkins then place either raisins or chocolate chips on each napkin. Be sure to make accommodations for students with allergies.

Now, settle into a steady even breath and relax. Breathe slowly in for one, two, three, and four. Breathe slowly out for one, two, three, and four. Begin by simply looking at your raisin or chip. Pretend that you are from another planet, and you have never seen a raisin or a chocolate chip before. This is your first time here on Earth and your first time with this food. Notice the color, the texture, the shape, ridges, contours, and how it is resting on your napkin. Pretend that you have to tell the people on your planet what this raisin or chip is like. You must look at every detail. See the raisin or chip exactly as it is right there on your napkin. Shift the raisin or chip on your napkin. As a good investigator on this new planet, you must look at every detail. What do you see now? Does the light fall in new ways on your raisin or chip? Do you see new contours or shades

(continued)

PRACTICE SCRIPT 6.4 (continued)

of color? As you practice concentration on your object, you will also notice your mind and body as feelings and thoughts come and go. Try to simply notice any thoughts, judgments, cravings, and bodily sensations, then bring your awareness back to your object. Maybe you really want to eat the raisin or chip. See if you can just notice that urge to eat and keep looking at your raisin or chip.

Next, pick up your raisin or chip with your fingers. Lift it closer to your eyes so you can see it in yet another new way. Bring your attention to what your object feels like. Is it soft or hard; smooth or rough; does it melt or get softer; is it cold? As you explore the touch sensation of your raisin or chip, you will also notice the sense impressions coming from your body in other areas. Maybe the room is cold or your chair is hard. Maybe your legs are tingling as you sit very still. Work on just noticing the feelings, the sensations from your body, and the thoughts that come to mind. Simply notice and bring your attention back to your raisin or chip.

Bring your raisin or chip to your nose. Smell. What do you smell? Do you smell the earthy fruitiness of the raisin, the essence of grapes? Do you smell chocolate? What if you had never smelled these smells before? How would you describe the smell you are smelling right now? Remember, you can't say, "I smell chocolate," or "I smell raisins." People from your planet do not know what those are. Without these words, how would you describe what you are smelling right now? As before, notice any other sense impressions or mental events as they arise and fall way.

Now, bring the raisin or chip to your mouth. Let it touch your lips so that you can feel the texture and smell the essence. Slowly place the object in your mouth without chewing. Let the object rest on your tongue. What do you taste? Find the words to describe the taste without using the words raisin or chocolate. What comes up for you? Slowly move the raisin or chocolate around in your mouth. Experience the taste and sensations. When you are ready, chew your raisin or chocolate. Has the taste changed? Did the texture change? Be aware of how your body, your mouth, and your saliva respond to the raisin or chocolate in your mouth. Once you are ready to swallow, notice any shifts in awareness in your presence. With intention, swallow your raisin or chip. Notice your mouth, your nose, your hands now. What do you notice?

Take a moment to offer gratitude for the raisin or chip, for your awareness, and for the opportunity to explore mindful eating. Now, write a few notes as a report to the people of your planet. Describe what you saw, smelled, felt, and tasted. Be very specific.

Source: Adapted from Cook-Cottone (2015), Informed by David (2009), Davis et al., (2008), Greenland (2010), Kabat-Zinn (2013), Rechtschaffen (2014), Stahl and Goldstein (2010), and Willard (2015).

Walking Meditation

Walking meditation involves a moment-by-moment presence with each step (Cook-Cottone, 2015; David, 2009; Davis et al., 2008; Hanson & Mendius, 2009; Jennings, 2015; Stahl & Goldstein, 2010). Walking meditations are nice for younger students and students who have difficulty sitting or paying attention. Walking meditation involves noticing each foot as you lift it and move it forward and place it down on the ground (Cook-Cottone, 2015; David, 2009; Kabat-Zinn, 2013; Jennings, 2015; Stahl & Goldstein, 2010). Walking meditation is not about getting somewhere. It is bare awareness of each aspect of the act of walking. Mindful walking can be done indoors or outdoors (Cook-Cottone, 2015; David, 2009; Davis et al., 2008). You need a space about 10 to 20 feet in length (Shapiro & Carlson, 2009). To complete a walking meditation, you and your students should choose a quiet and pleasant space, although this is not entirely necessary.

To illustrate, when I teach walking meditation at the University at Buffalo, we meet late in the evening. The building is quiet, and the class walks together throughout the building. I lead, and the students simply need to follow the person in front of them. We walk past classrooms with instruction ongoing, up and down stairs, through the quiet hallways, and across more crowded meeting places. The focus is on the walking and the noticing. Students find it compelling to explore what they noticed as they walked the same hallways they walk every day. The shift is substantial. When we share what was observed, the students describe the humming of the building, the moving of the water in the walls, and the echoing of our steps in the hallway. There is an expansion of awareness that comes with tuning in and slowing down.

You can adapt walking meditations for younger children by adding a simple narration as you walk (Willard, 2016). This is much like the verbal tracking done by a play therapist. You simply track what is happening while you walk. For example, you might say the following:

> I am watching each step as I walk carefully and mindfully. I notice my heel as it connects to the floor and the ball of my foot as it connects to the ground just before my toes feel the ground. I am noticing my breath moving in and out as it moves along with my footsteps. I see the path as we walk and notice the gravel beneath my feet. I hear the sounds as my feet crunch into the gravel with each step. I see the grass along the path and its green blades—some bending into the path and some reaching to the sky. I see my friends walk in front of me and hear my friends walking behind me. I feel the sun on my cheeks as I move.

Other ideas include walking with pennies on your shoes and trying not to drop one (Willard, 2016). Where should you walk? The choice is yours and your students'. Gardens and labyrinths can be beautiful places for walking meditation. It can be a fun class project to create a walking-meditation labyrinth. Rechtschaffen (2014) recommends nature walks and getting outside to bring awareness to the elements of nature. Walking meditation incorporates the following principles of embodied learning and growth (see Chapter 3): principle 3, I am mindfully aware; principle 4, I work toward presence in my physical body; principle 6, I ask questions about my physical experience, feelings, and thoughts; principle 7, I choose my focus and actions; and principle 8, I do the work.

PRACTICE SCRIPT 6.5: WALKING MEDITATION

Approximate timing: 1 minute for introduction; 20+ minutes for practice

Begin your walking meditation by standing with your feet hip distance apart, hands at your sides, shoulders soft, and tailbone neutral. Eyes open, chin neutral, look around. See what you see. Take in the external. Do you see people? Are there trees or grass? Are you inside; do you see the floor and furniture? Take it all in. Check in on what you are experiencing inside as well. How do your feet feel on the ground? Is the surface hard or soft? Do you feel supported? Scan your body from your feet to the crown of your head, across your shoulders and down your arms to your fingertips. Do you feel tension? Are you relaxed? Can you breathe into any tension you are feeling and let

(continued)

PRACTICE SCRIPT 6.5 (*continued*)

it go? Take a big breath in and hold for a count of four, then release your breath slowly returning to regular breath.

Take your gaze about 5 feet in front of you. You will feel as if you have a gentle downward gaze. From grounded feet, lift your right foot off the ground, bending at the knee, then move your foot forward. Notice how your leg feels when you lift your foot. Notice how your foot lands on the ground. Do all four corners of your foot connect to the ground at once, or does the heel meet the ground followed by the ball of the foot and then the toes? Place your weight on your right foot and lift your left foot. Now that you are in motion, how does the action of lifting your left foot differ from the action of initiating movement with the lifting of your right foot? How does lifting your left foot feel in your leg, your core? Place your left foot on the ground and notice the nature of the contact of your foot on the ground.

Commence a slow and steady pace that allows you to notice each and every step as you lift, propel, and place each foot. For a period of time, keep your awareness on the stepping aspects of walking. Be very curious about any changes in your steps. Perhaps you turn a corner or avoid a small rock. What does that feel like in your body? Does your pace change? Does your breath stop? Notice your feet in your shoes and the sensation of the foot to shoe, to ground. How does the wearing of shoes feel as you walk? Do you notice qualities of the shoe?

As you walk, bring your awareness to your breath. Your body is a system. Your breath fuels your walking as oxygen is sent to the muscles in your body to propel you. Notice the rhythm of your steps, your breath, your heartbeat. Notice the synchrony of your body as it moves step by step. Expand your awareness to your whole body. Feel your body move through space as you breathe and take step after step. Feel the air on your skin as you move forward.

Be mindfully aware of any thoughts or feelings that may be arising as mental events. Simply notice them and bring your awareness back to your feet and the aspects of each step, the lifting, the moving the foot forward, and the placing of your foot on the ground.

Once you have reached your allotted time for walking meditation, return to your point of origin. Place your feet hip distance apart, your hands at your sides; soften your shoulders and neutralize your chin. Take a moment to offer gratitude for your feet, your body, your breath, and your heart. Offer gratitude for your awareness during your walking meditation and the insight brought to you by your practice.

Source: Adapted from Cook-Cottone (2015), informed by David (2009), Davis et al. (2008), Hanson and Mendius (2009), Jennings (2015), Kabat-Zinn (2013), Shapiro and Carlson (2009), and Stahl and Goldstein (2010).

Loving-Kindness Meditation

The Loving-Kindness Meditation, or Metta, brings a focus to loving-kindness, helps reduce resistance, and enhances compassion and presence, especially with difficult people in our lives and in the lives of our students. A process of acceptance, slowing, and letting go, practicing this meditation helps us dissolve barriers that can build up in our minds, such as self-centeredness, resentment, bitterness, and anger (Cook-Cottone, 2015; David, 2009; Greenland, 2010; Rechtschaffen, 2014; Stahl & Goldstein, 2010). According to Siegel (2010), practicing the Loving-Kindness Meditation can help students make a neurological shift. It is believed that this practice can activate students' social and self-engagement system, bringing a valance of compassion and kindness toward self and others into our choices and actions (David, 2009; Greenland, 2010; Rechtschaffen, 2014; Siegel, 2010). Much time and energy can be ineffectively spent in reaction to people in our lives who don't behave as we would like them to (Cook-Cottone, 2015; David, 2009; Greenland, 2010; Rechtschaffen, 2014; Wallace, 2011). The Loving-Kindness Meditation helps to shift the focus away from the unproductive, or triggering, feeling states and allows a return to present moment awareness and connectedness (Cook-Cottone, 2015; Rechtschaffen, 2014; Wallace, 2011). Hutcherson, Seppala, and Gross (2008) found that a brief practice of the Loving-Kindness Meditation, compared with a closely matched control task, significantly increased feelings of social connection and positivity toward novel individuals on both explicit and implicit levels. The Loving-Kindness Meditation incorporates the following principles of embodied learning and growth (see Chapter 3): principle 3, I am mindfully aware; principle 5, I feel my emotions in order to grow and learn; principle 6, I ask questions about my physical experience, feelings, and thoughts; principle 7, I choose my focus and actions; principle 8, I do the work; principle 10, I honor efforts to grow and learn; and principle 11, I am kind to myself and others.

PRACTICE SCRIPT 6.6: LOVING-KINDNESS MEDITATION
Approximate timing: 2 minutes for introduction; 20 minutes for practice

---

Start with the Getting Seated for Meditation Script. Cultivate the qualities of relaxation, stillness, and presence. Grounded in your seat, bring your awareness to your breath. Breathe deeply, inhaling and exhaling. Focus on your breath and allow a sense of calm in your shoulders, arms, and legs. Begin to expand your awareness to encompass your whole body. Imagine that you are surrounded by a large circle of loving-kindness, and you are at the very center. Imagine that the circle of loving-kindness is like a child holding a sleeping puppy or kitten with care, warmth, and love. This is the nature of the sphere that is around you now. As you sit within the sphere of loving-kindness, say these words:

May I be happy.
May I be well.
May I be safe.
May I be peaceful and at ease.

Once you have finished, bring your awareness back to your breath, to your whole body, then out the circle of loving-kindness. Breathe easily.

Now, bring to mind a good friend or someone who has shown you great kindness. Imagine that the circle of loving-kindness that surrounds you is expanding to include your friend. Breathe and visualize, you, your loved one, and the circle of loving-kindness. Repeat these words:

May you be happy.
May you be well.
May you be safe.
May you be peaceful and at ease.

(continued)

PRACTICE SCRIPT 6.6 (continued)

Now, bring to mind a friend or neighbor, somebody for whom you feel a warmth and kindness toward. This can be someone from your daily travels, the person who lives next door to you, or your teacher. It can be anyone you choose. Breathe and visualize, you, your loved one, and your friend or neighbor within the circle of loving-kindness. Repeat these words:

May you be happy.
May you be well.
May you be safe.
May you be peaceful and at ease.

Now, think about someone about whom you feel neutral. You don't feel good about them, and you don't feel bad about them. Think about someone in your life with whom you interact, yet have no feelings, good or bad, associated with this person. Maybe it is the person who drives the bus, checks you in at dance class, or lives a few doors down from you. Maybe it is another student at the bus stop some mornings or in a class with you. Hold this person in your awareness. Breathe and visualize, you, your loved one, your friend or neighbor, and the neutral person within the circle of loving-kindness. Repeat these words:

May you be happy.
May you be well.
May you be safe.
May you be peaceful and at ease.

Now, bring to mind someone with whom you struggle or gets on your nerves. Thinking of this person brings up feelings of frustration. Perhaps it is someone close to you, in your family, or someone right here at school. Bring that person to mind. Breathe and visualize, you, your loved one, your friend or neighbor, the neutral person, and the difficult person within the circle of loving-kindness. Repeat these words:

May you be happy.
May you be well.
May you be safe.
May you be peaceful and at ease.

Now, it is time to expand your loving-kindness circle to include all beings everywhere. Bring to mind those who are hungry, cold, tired, and poor, as well as those who have great wealth and abundance. Bring to mind beings that are sick and those who have great health. Bring to mind all beings in your town, city, state, and nation. Bring to mind all people across the world. Bring to mind all people everywhere. Breathe and think about you, your loved one, your friend or neighbor, the neutral person, the difficult person, and all beings everywhere within the circle of loving-kindness. Repeat these words:

May all beings be happy.
May all beings be well.

(continued)

PRACTICE SCRIPT 6.6 (continued)

May all beings be safe.
May all beings be peaceful and at ease.

Feel the expanding love-and-kindness circle as you breathe. Feel the expansiveness of your sphere and the possible connections with all beings. Slowly, bring your awareness back to your breath and your body. When you are ready, rub your hands together, warming them gently. Raise your hands to your eyes and slowly open your eyes into the palms of your hands. When you are ready, rest your hands on your thighs, eyes open, breath steady.

Note: To be trauma-sensitive, do not follow classic instructions that bring to mind someone who hurt you or makes you angry. Asking students to think about someone who gets on their nerves is less triggering replacement.

Source: Adapted from Cook-Cottone (2015), informed by David (2009), Greenland (2010), Hanson and Mendius (2009), Shapiro and Carlson (2009), Rechtschaffen (2014), Siegel (2010), Stahl and Goldstein (2010), and Wallace (2011); www.mettainstitute.org/mettameditation.html.

FORMAL MINDFULNESS PRACTICES FOR OLDER STUDENTS

A substantial proportion of all our students are struggling (Rechtschaffen, 2014). A review of the extant research on mental disorders among youth found that approximately one fourth of youth had experienced a mental disorder during the past year, and about one third at some other time in their lives (Merikangas, Nakamura, & Kessler, 2009). Many students are at risk. As students reach later middle school and high school, their ability to understand concepts changes, as do their stressors and the complexity of their decisions. Risk increases for eating disorders, depression, suicide, substance use, sexual decision making, sexual activity, pregnancy, and self-harm. Faced with the more complex challenges of adolescent social networks, academic pressures, and the developmental task of individuation, students can benefit from basic mindfulness skills—as well as more sophisticated mindfulness skills that help them cognitively negotiate their experiences and stressors.

Further, older students are more aware of the violence present every day in culture. As we are all too well aware, in recent years, violence has made its way into nearly every aspect of daily life (Olson, 2014; Rechtschaffen, 2014; Wiest-Stevenson & Lee, 2016). Wiest-Stevenson and Lee's (2016) review of the literature suggests that up to 60% of students have been exposed to some form of trauma, either in or out of school. A recent report in the *Communiqué*, a publication of the National Association of School Psychologists, details a lawsuit filed in Compton, California (*Peter P. et al. v. Compton Unified School District, 2015*). The article and the lawsuit highlight the prevalence of trauma exposure among all youth, emphasizing the higher rates of exposure among underserved youth (Ahlers, Stanick, & Machek, 2016). The authors cite research detailing the effect of trauma on youth mental health, learning, and relationships (Ahlers et al., 2016). Highlighted by the lawsuit was the fact that the schools were not apprised of trauma-informed approaches to students, and students were not receiving adequate support or intervention (Ahlers et al., 2016).

How does this look in practice? I will illustrate using the case of Jennifer, a student in the ninth grade. I share it because it is a good illustration of how, for some students, mindfulness can be a self-care practice that helps them replace dysfunctional and self-destructive approaches to their stress, trauma, and emotions. It is also timely as schools move toward trauma-informed practice in the classroom (Ahlers et al., 2016; Olson, 2014; Rechtschaffen, 2014).

Jennifer is currently 15 years old. Jennifer's experiences can be described as complex trauma (Ahlers et al., 2016). Her parents divorced when she was 3 years old. Jennifer readily explains to anyone who asks that her parents never should have been together. Her mom has not secured a long-term relationship since her divorce from Jennifer's father 9 years ago. Jennifer lives in an impoverished, underserved community. The neighborhood averages one fatal shooting every 6 weeks. One of her mother's previous boyfriends sexually abused Jennifer from age six to age eight. Jennifer was afraid to tell her mom what was happening because the boyfriend had told her it was her fault. He also told her that, if her mom found out, she would be mad at Jennifer for trying to steal him and would kick her out of the house. Jennifer told a school counselor who informed her mom. The situation was investigated. Jennifer went to live with her grandmother until the boyfriend was removed from the house. There was a trial and Jennifer testified. Her mom did not show for court. With all the stress, Jennifer's mom was diagnosed with depression and began drinking heavily in a misdirected effort to cope. When Jennifer was 11, she was removed from her mother's care. Although Jennifer doesn't tell many people, her mom still drinks every day.

At her grandmother's, Jennifer lives with 2 cousins, an 11-month-old and a 3-year-old. Jennifer's life can feel very chaotic. When she was going through the trial, she experimented with cutting her arm. She had heard about it at school and thought that it was what kids did who were from families like hers. She heard it helped them cope. She never thought it would become a problem (Cook-Cottone, 2015). Now at 14, she thinks about cutting herself all the time. If her grandmother and uncle start fighting, her mom gets drunk and texts her all night, or things get chaotic with the kids, Jennifer sneaks off to her room and takes a pair of scissors to her forearm. In summer, when her arms show, she takes the scissors to her thighs, so that her shorts will conceal the cuts. Jennifer says that she feels like she has no other options. She explains that cutting feels like something she can control when the rest of her life feels very out of control.

For students who struggle like Jennifer, emotional experiences, even mildly uncomfortable situations, feel very distressing and intolerable (Cook-Cottone, 2015; Wupperman, Fickling, Klemanski, Berking, & Whitman, 2013). Without other tools, students may rely on self-destructive behaviors to cope (Cook-Cottone, 2015). By relying on self-destructive behaviors, they are looking for self-regulation and calm in the wrong place. Epstein (2001) tells an old story of a seeker looking in the wrong places. The story told here was inspired by his story.

INSTRUCTIONAL STORY 6.3: SEEKING IN THE WRONG PLACES

A long, long time ago, a group of raccoons was walking after dinner. Raccoons like to be up at night. It was a dark night, and they kept to the lighted path to find their way. Ahead of them on the walkway, they noticed another raccoon, Rocky, digging in the ground underneath a lamppost. Rocky was digging and sniffing, his face close to the walkway. He continued to dig and sniff as his friends approached.

(continued)

INSTRUCTIONAL STORY 6.3 (continued)

They saw that Rocky seemed to be looking for something. Stepping forward, one of the raccoons asked, "What are you looking for? Can we help?"

"I am looking for my snack. I have lost it," Rocky explained to them.

The other raccoons began to help. They looked on the pathway. They looked in the plants that lined the walkway. Some of the raccoons searched the street, while the other night animals shuffled by. They looked for quite a while with no success. Tired from work, full from dinner, still quite a ways to walk, they were becoming very weary.

Looking for a better strategy, one of the raccoons asked, "Hey Rocky, where do you think you first lost your snack? We can focus our search there."

"I lost it in my house," Rocky said. "Over there," and he pointed down the street to his raccoon den.

Confused, one of the raccoons asked, "Then why, for goodness sake, are you searching here, under the lamppost?"

"Because the light is better here," Rocky replied.

Source: Inspired by Epstein (2001).

Epstein (2001) explains that this story is not quite as dismaying as it may seem. In the same way, neither is Jennifer's behavior (Cook-Cottone, 2015). The seekers' activity may not have been completely in vain after all. You see, "*Looking* is the key" (p. 20). Jennifer and Rocky most certainly are not going to find satisfaction cutting for emotional regulation and stress reduction (i.e., self-harming) or looking for a snack far from where it was lost. Still, their efforts to heal and make things right are there. They are just off course. For Jennifer and Rocky, looking in the "right" place does not seem accessible.

Jennifer has a sense that she needs tools to negotiate her stressors and her own sensitivity (Cook-Cottone, 2015). She is seeking. I honor this seeking in students. I validate their awareness of the painful experiences in their lives and their efforts to address them. Things that have happened to and challenged us and our challenges are important (Cook-Cottone, 2015). Yet, it is also critical to learn how to be with these memories and challenges and secure empowering, effective skills that can be utilized as needed (Cook-Cottone, 2015; McCown, Reibel, & Micozzi, 2010). Jennifer was referred to a psychologist who specialized in mindfulness interventions.

Research corresponds to this logic: Mindfulness may help Jennifer. In 2013, Wupperman et al. offered that mindfulness can reduce reported acts of self-injury and overall harmful dysregulated behaviors. Difficulties in the ability to be aware, manifest attention, and accept ongoing experiences appear to play a role in relation to harmful dysregulated behaviors (Cook-Cottone, 2015). Wupperman et al. (2013) hypothesize that mindfulness may disrupt and prevent the cycles of trauma, distress, and self-harm. Mindfulness helps create a space between triggers (e.g., emotional and interpersonal) and the behavioral response (Cook-Cottone, 2015). That is, mindfulness may help develop decentering, or the ability to step back from automatic reactions and judgments, to create a space for a better and safer choice (Wupperman et al., 2013). With this space, Jennifer can become aware of her urges to engage in dysregulated behaviors (Cook-Cottone, 2015). She can choose a healthier response rather than injuring herself. With these tools, Jennifer may also learn to prevent these cycles from occurring in the first place (Cook-Cottone, 2015). As she becomes increasingly aware of the processes in her mind and her body, she can be more effective at noticing when negative affect is arising and address it before it evolves into a distressful or seemingly unmanageable feeling (Cook-Cottone, 2015; Wupperman et al., 2013). In fact, Wupperman et al. (2013) cite research that suggests that continued mindfulness practices may help develop more functional neural pathways that enhance affect and behavioral regulation (Figure 6.5).

As a student practices, he or she notices the space, the choice, and the competence that comes from allowing and being present with what is (Cook-Cottone, 2015). This can change the way a student experiences his or her struggles. For example, before Jennifer began her meditation practice, her thinking process looked like this: stimuli (i.e., family fighting and feeling overwhelmed), feeling-tone (i.e., unpleasant), choice (i.e., aversion), and response (i.e., cutting; see Figure 6.6).

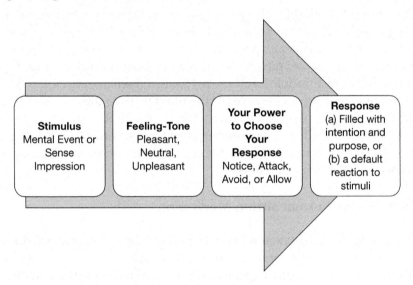

FIGURE 6.5 The space between in meditation.
Source: Cook-Cottone (2015).

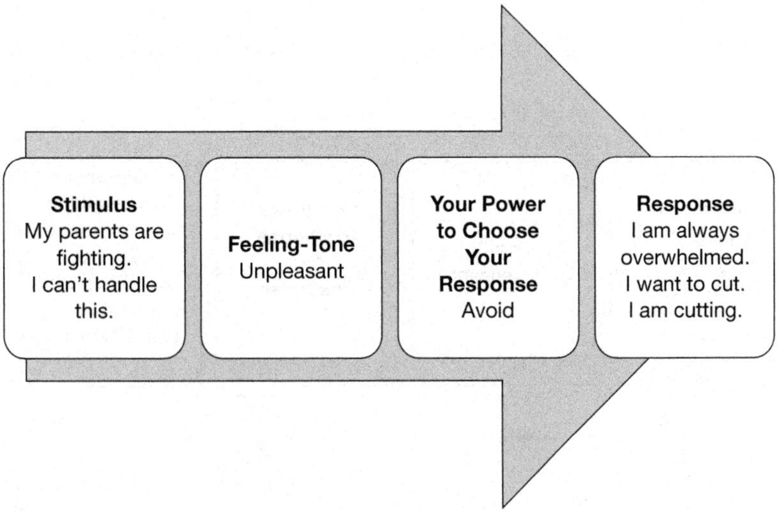

FIGURE 6.6 Jennifer's default reaction to stimuli.
Source: Cook-Cottone (2015).

Jennifer focused her meditation on the noticing of the arising and passing away of her awareness of mental events and sensations, and on the way her brain tagged mental events and sense impressions as pleasant, unpleasant, and neutral (Cook-Cottone, 2015). She watches the nearly automatic tendency to attach to the feeling-tone, the mental event, or the sense impression. She noticed how simply sitting for meditation could trigger her personal narrative, or belief system, "I am overwhelmed, and I can't handle this." Before she began to work on mindfulness, she had no awareness of mental events or sense impressions arising and passing away. She did not know that they were attached to a feeling tone. Most troublesome, Jennifer believed her story that she was always overwhelmed and that she could not handle anything. She thought that maybe she was just like her mom. Her meditation practices and work with her psychologist gave her insight to this path of events, and she began to question her old narrative. She began to find space, choice, and power (see Figure 6.7). See principles of embodies learning and growth (see Chapter 3); principle 1, I am worth the effort; principle 3, I am fully aware; principle 4, I work toward presence in my physical body; principle 5, I feel my emotions in order to grow and learn; principle 7, I choose my focus and actions; principle 8, I do the work.

The following practices provide several structured ways to dig into the space between stimulus and response (Cook-Cottone, 2015). These include the sitting meditation script unique to this text, designed to bring awareness and competence to cultivating the space between stimulus and response. As you and your students practice, use Figure 6.8 to record your experience and growing awareness.

The Space Between: Formal Sitting Meditation

The *Space Between* formal meditation is intended to bring awareness and insight. This script will help you and your students bring awareness to stimuli that include sense impressions and mental events, the accompanying feeling-tones, the choice to notice and then attach or allow, and, finally, the active choice of a response (Grabovac et al., 2011; Wallace, 2011).

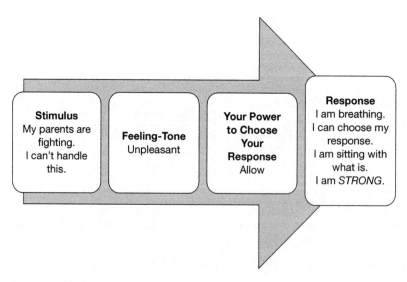

FIGURE 6.7 Jennifer's new choices.
Source: Cook-Cottone (2015).

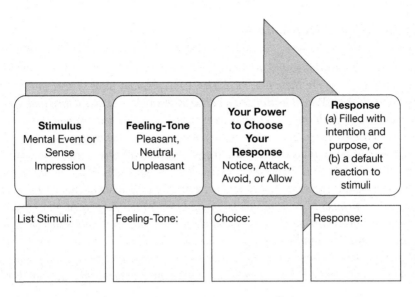

FIGURE 6.8 Cultivating growing awareness and change.

PRACTICE SCRIPT 6.7: THE SPACE BETWEEN
Approximate timing: 2 minutes for introduction; 20 minutes for practice

Start with the Getting Seated for Meditation Script. Take a few moments to bring your awareness to your body. How do you feel? Pause and be present here in this moment. Take a deep breath in and exhale.

Bring your awareness to your breath. Take a few breaths and observe. Notice if it is even, regular, and smooth. Your breath will be your object of concentration for this meditation. You will continually bring yourself back to your breath as an anchor. Do not try to change your breath. Simply be present to it. Notice it.

As you breathe, you will become aware of sense impressions. These can be things that you see, smell, taste, hear, or feel on your skin or inside your body. You may hear children outside, birds chirping, a lawn mower or snow blower going. You may have a candle lit and notice a flicker in the flame and feel a slight breeze on your skin. Your stomach may grumble or your muscles tighten. These are sense impressions. Notice them as they arise. As they arise into your awareness, say to yourself, "I am hearing the chirping of the birds," or "I am feeling the grumbling of my stomach." Notice that these sense impressions arise and pass away and that your breath is a constant. Notice this and bring your awareness back to your breath.

As your sense impressions arise, you will also notice that they feel pleasant, neutral, or unpleasant. Notice this. Notice how your brain tends to automatically label your sense impressions. Perhaps you hear the birds chirping and you feel a feeling-tone, a pleasant feeling-tone. Or maybe you hear a lawn mower, and you feel an unpleasant feeling-tone. Notice this. Notice that the feeling tones arise and pass away as well. The feeling-tone comes to your awareness; it peaks; then it softens and passes away. As you notice the sense impressions and the feeling-tones, allow them to be and bring your awareness back to your breath.

(continued)

PRACTICE SCRIPT 6.7 (continued)

As you are sitting, breathing, and attending to the nature and quality of your breath, you may notice mental events. These are thoughts, memories, concepts, and ideas. These can also be feelings tied to ideas and memories. When mental events arise as feelings, you will notice that there are sense impressions that may go with them. You might feel sadness in your belly as you think about the dog you loved when you were little. You notice these mental events—memories, ideas, stories—as they arise. As you notice, bring your awareness back to your breath. Your breath is your anchor. Notice that the mental events arise in your consciousness, gain a stronger presence, then pass away, getting softer as they move out of your awareness. Notice this pattern. Notice that, as mental events arise and pass away, your breath is a constant cycle of inhalation and exhalation. As you sit and breathe, you may notice that your mental events also have associated feeling-tones. You notice that your brain labels them as pleasant, neutral or unpleasant. Notice that you think and the feeling-tone is right with the thought. As you see these feeling-tones, you notice that they arise and pass away, just as your sense impressions and mental events arise and pass away. Notice this and bring your awareness back to your breath.

As you practice, sitting and breathing, you may notice that some sense impressions and feeling-tones pull for your attention. They snag, like Velcro, on your thinking self. As you sit, you hear the lawn mower (sense impression), and you notice that the feeling-tone that goes with that sense impression is unpleasant. "It is early," you think. "It is too early for mowing," you think. You start to become angry as the whole story of your neighbor's thoughtlessness comes to mind. You think about her dog that barks late into the night; how she fails to weed her garden, making the neighborhood look bad; how someone who never mows her lawn is highly inconsiderate to do it before 9 a.m. when you are trying to meditate. You notice that, as your mind works and works, your breath and your choice are lost.

Your power is in your anchor, your breath. The moment that you notice that you have left your breath, go back to it. It does not matter if you brought your awareness back at your first sense impression or mental event, or if you were well into a long story. Bring yourself back to your breath. The growth is in your noticing. As you sit, you will see the habits of the mind. You will get to know them. As you see them, notice them. "Ah, there it is. I notice my 'neighbor story.' I notice it, and I will bring myself to my breath." Perhaps it is different, pleasant. "Ah, there are the birds chirping. I notice them. I notice the pleasant feeling-tone. I bring myself back to breathing." Breathe.

As you are sitting, bring your awareness wholly to your breath. Notice the qualities of your breath. Is it even, smooth; does it move in and out without pause? Breathe and notice. (Pause here for 60 seconds.) *When it is your time to finish, cultivate gratitude for your practice, your ability to sit and notice, and for your insights gained during your practice today.*

Source: Cook-Cottone (2015), inspired by Grabovac et al. (2011) and Wallace (2011).

Soften, Soothe, Allow

The Soften, Soothe, Allow Meditation is one of my favorite meditations for working with difficult emotions (Germer & Neff, 2013). It was written by Dr. Kristen Neff, the leading expert in self-compassion research. The full version of the meditation can be found at www.centerformsc.org/sites/default/files/Soften-Soothe-Allow.pdf. Also, the Insight Timer www.insighttimer.com) has a guided meditation titled, "Soften, Soothe, Allow," read by Dr. Neff. I recommend it to nearly all my patients who struggle with emotion regulation. The Soften, Soothe, Allow Meditation begins with labeling the emotion (Germer & Neff, 2013). Dr. Neff asks you to recall a mild to moderately difficult situation that you are experiencing right now and to visualize the emotion. Next, she asks if you can name the strongest emotion associated with the situation (e.g., longing, grief, anger, betrayal). She then asks you to work toward mindfulness of the emotion in the body. This process begins with an awareness of the body as a whole and then the location of the spot in the body where the emotion is expressing itself most strongly.

Once the emotion is located, Dr. Neff asks you to soften into the location of the emotion in your body. She asks you to let your body be soft without demanding that it become soft. She asks you to gently let go of any gripping or holding around the edges of the emotions. Next, she requests that you soften your body around the edges of the emotion and use a loving awareness of how the emotion feels in your body. Once you have softened the edges, she asks you to soothe yourself by placing a hand on your heart and acknowledging to yourself how painful the feeling is and to repeat the word, "soothe .... soothe .... soothe."

Last, Dr. Neff asks you to allow discomfort to be in the spot of the emotion. She asks you to notice discomfort and to let it come and go as it may. As you do this, she asks you to repeat, "allow .... allow .... allow." Next, Dr. Neff suggests that you use all three words as a mantra, "soften .... soothe .... allow." And remember: If you feel too much discomfort, stay with your breath until you feel better. Ultimately, the goal is not to get rid of the emotion. Rather, the goal is to be with the emotion with a sense of ease. This meditation is especially useful with adolescents and young adults who often experience intense and sometimes painful emotions. This meditation is the essence of principle 5 (see Chapter 3), I feel my emotions in order to grow and learn.

TIPS FOR PRACTICE AT HOME FOR STUDENTS

Mindfulness practices are a set of tools for self-regulation and stress management. To create access to these tools, there are a few things you can do as an educator: Offer tips for home as you practice in class, use broad and general recommendations, and be secular (Rechtschaffen, 2014).

First, what you model in school and in the classroom will give students a good sense of how to practice at home. Each time you engage in a classroom, or school-based, practice, it can be helpful to add, "And when you do this at home you can. ..." An open suggestion—that is, consider trying this at home—serves as a friendly invitation rather than a requirement. In this way, a home practice can evolve organically from intrinsic interest.

Next, keeping it broad and general is important (Cook-Cottone et al., 2013). Because families have varied resources and family routines and rules, it is important to keep home practice tips general enough to be assimilated into each student's home life. To illustrate, Shana, a second grade student, lives in a small apartment with her three siblings and her mom. There is no place that she can set up a meditation room, or even a meditation space. She does have her favorite quiet spot at the foot of her bed where she sometimes does homework or plays board games with friends. For her, a more general suggestion to find your favorite spot works. Essentially, students can practice meditation anywhere. It can be helpful to guide them to find a quiet place (e.g., at their study desk or table) or a favorite place (e.g., under a tree in the backyard). That is really all they need.

It is very important to be transparent and culturally sensitive regarding what you recommend for at-home practice (Cook-Cottone, Lemish, & Gyker, 2016; Rechtschaffen, 2014). Some families do not feel comfortable with practices that appear to be connected to the historical roots of mindfulness (Cook-Cottone et al., 2016). For some parents, it can feel as if the practices are in conflict with their own religious practices. For example, when I was in elementary school, I was learning to use the rosary and preparing for my first communion. I believe it would have been uncomfortable for my mother, who taught Sunday school, to have me come home from school with mala beads and a Sanskrit mantra. She would have found it interesting, as she did the cardboard pyramid I brought home or the sign language alphabet I learned. Still, in the absence of context and an explanation from the teacher, me coming home with mala beads may have been concerning for her. In this way, being transparent and informative, and keeping mindfulness practices secular and free of artifacts that resonate with historical roots, ensure access to practices for kids.

Rechtschaffen (2014), author of *The Way of Mindful Education*, explained it this way. Coffee originated in Ethiopia, where it was used as a stimulant beverage for a millennia before it was exported to places like Egypt and the Middle East. Coffee is now a ubiquitous beverage and key menu item in coffee shops and restaurants all over the world. Coffee is loved by people of all ethnicities, races, and religions. While coffee has been used to wake us up, mindfulness practices are used to tune us in and create focus. Drinking coffee to wake up will not make you Ethiopian any more than using mindfulness practices to tune in and engage will make you Buddhist (Rechtschaffen, 2014).

In discussions about secular practices for schools, I have heard educators argue that there are central tools that have historical roots, that have been used effectively for centuries, and that there is no need to change something that works (e.g., mala beads, singing bowls). The main motivation to engage in secular practices is that it increases access. For some parents, the perceived link to religious practices creates unnecessary tensions especially when alternative, secular forms of the tools are available. It can be helpful to think about the function of the tools that you are using and make substitutions that allow access for all. For example, if you were using mala beads to help students concentrate, substitute cups of pebbles or dried beans for counting breaths or affirmations.

Writing and Recording Your Own Mindful Meditation Script for Home

A foundation of constructivism is this: When students create their own meaning, they learn. Teaching students formal meditation practices can help them create a set of tools to use to handle stress, self-regulation, and practice intentionally engaging in the world around them. Recall, our next goal is to help them become architects of their own learning. Students can write their own meditation scripts for use at home (Willard, 2016). When students create their own meditation scripts, they become architects of their own learning. To create a script, students need to include breath, physical presence, and sensations, an object for focus, perhaps a story about the object, a section to bring awareness back to breath, and a closing bringing them back to current moment awareness (see Table 6.1). Once they have written out their scripts, have them trade scripts so that a peer can read it to them. They should

TABLE 6.1 Creating Your Meditation Script

Describe the process of getting seated for your meditation. Include details that are relevant to your home (e.g., the type of chair or pillow)	Getting Seated:
Provide instruction on breath. Write about how you would like to bring your awareness to your breath. Would you like to count breaths? Watch inhalations shift to exhalations? Provide the details here.	Breath Awareness:
Provide guidance as to how you would like to attend to the physical body and sensations. Here, you can detail awareness of your body parts (as in the body scan), or you can bring your awareness to your senses, asking yourself to notice smells, feelings, and sounds. Be descriptive and specific.	Physical Presence:
Next, you may choose to explore your emotions. You can add a section that asks you to notice your feelings. You may want to locate the feelings in your body and breathe into the feelings (see Soften, Soothe, Allow Meditation).	Emotion Awareness:
Many meditations ask you to bring your focus to an object. You can choose your breath, your feelings, a statement (e.g., I can be present in the moment), a color, a favorite place, or an imaginary place. Whatever you choose, give yourself detailed guidance. If it is a place, describe the place in detail, including what it looks like, sounds, smells, the wind, etc. As this is your focus object, also remember to tell yourself to notice other thoughts as they arise and pass away and to bring your focus back to the object.	Focus Object and Thoughts:
Once you have spent time with the focus object, you want to bring your awareness back to your body and your breath. Slowly guide yourself to the present moment, the sensations of the body and the breathing that you described during the early part of your meditation. Once you have brought yourself back to the present moment, guide yourself to slowly moving back to engagement in your current world (e.g., sitting up, slowly opening your eye and checking in). This should be the closing of your meditation.	Centering and Closing:

make any corrections they feel are needed. Last, record the script digitally on their phone or other electronic device so that they can e-mail it or text it to themselves. Now, they will have a customized meditation script that they can use at any time. Note, students may want to make several versions of the script at various lengths, 3, 5, 10, and 20 minutes.

CONCLUSION

Mindfulness practices on the cushion offer a formal, structured way to cultivate insight. Both internal and external experiences affect us. The awareness of sense impressions, mental events, and the associated feeling-tones provides an opportunity to shift *out* of habitual ways of thinking and acting *into* active choice in our daily lives. That is, as your students notice the ways in which they are triggered, and practice allowing these sensations and mental events to arise and pass away without attaching to or avoiding them, they are empowered to choose a response that serves their emotional and relational health, athletic performance, and academic mastery.

REFERENCES

Ahlers, K., Stanick, C., & Machek, G. R. (2016). Trauma-informed schools: Issues and possible benefits from a recent California lawsuit. *Communiqué, 44*, 1–25.

Bien, T. (2008). *Mindful therapy: A guide for therapists and helping professionals.* Boston, MA: Wisdom Productions.

Cook-Cottone, C. P. (2015). *Mindfulness and yoga for self-regulation: A primer for mental health professionals.* New York, NY: Springer Publishing.

Cook-Cottone, C. P., Kane, L., Keddie, E., & Haugli, S. (2013). *Girls growing in wellness and balance: Yoga and life skills to empower.* Onalaska, WI: Schoolhouse Educational Services.

Cook-Cottone, C. P., Lemish, E., & Guyker, W. (2016, February). Plenary session: Secular yoga in schools: A qualitative study of the Encinitas Union School District lawsuit. In *Yoga in the Schools symposium*, Kipalu Center for Yoga and Health. Stockbridge, MA.

David, D. S. (2009). *Mindful teachers and teaching mindfulness: A guide for anyone who teaches anything.* Somerville, MA: Wisdom.

Davis, M., Eshelman, E. R., & McKay, M. (2008). *The relaxation and stress reduction workbook* (6th ed.). Oakland, CA: Harbinger.

Epstein, M. (2001). *Going on being-buddhism and the way of change: A positive psychology for the west.* New York, NY: Harmony/Crown.

Germer, C. K., & Neff, K. D. (2013). Self-compassion in clinical practice. *Journal of Clinical Psychology, 69*, 856–867.

Grabovac, A. D., Lau, M. A., & Willett, B. R. (2011). Mechanisms of mindfulness: A Buddhist psychological model. *Mindfulness, 2*(3), 154–166. doi:10.1007/s12671-011-0054-5

Hanh, T. N. (1975). *The miracle of mindfulness: An introduction to the practice of meditation.* Boston, MA: Beacon Press.

Hanh, T. N. (1998). *The heart of Buddha's teaching: Transforming suffering into peace, joy, and liberation.* New York, NY: Broadway Books.

Hanson, R., & Mendius, R. (2009). *Buddha's brain: The practical neuroscience of happiness, love, and wisdom.* Oakland, CA: New Harbinger.

Hutcherson, C. A., Seppala, E. M., & Gross, J. J. (2008). Loving-kindness meditation increases social connectedness. *Emotion, 8*, 720–724.

Greenland, S. K. (2010). *The mindful child: How to help your kids manage stress and become happier, kinder, and more compassionate.* New York, NY: Simon & Schuster.

James, W. (1890). *The Principles of Psychology* (vol. 2). New York, NY: Holt.

Jennings, P. A. (2015). *Mindfulness for teachers: Simple skills for peace and productivity in the classroom.* New York, NY: W. W. Norton.

Kabat-Zinn, J. (2013). *Full catastrophe living, revised edition: How to cope with stress, pain and illness using mindfulness meditation.* New York, NY: Bantam Books.

Lutz, A., Jha, A. P., Dunne, J. D., & Saron, C. D. (2015). Investigating the phenomenological matrix of mindfulness-related practices from a neurocognitive perspective. *American Psychologist, 70*, 632–658.

McCown, D., Reibel, D., & Micozzi, M. S. (2010). *Teaching mindfulness: A practical guide for clinicians and educators.* New York, NY: Springer.

Merikangas, K. R., Nakamura, E. F., & Kessler, R. C. (2009). Epidemiology of mental disorders in children and adolescents. *Dialogues in Clinical Neuroscience, 11*(1), 7–20.

Olson, K. (2014). *The invisible classroom: Relationships, neuroscience, and mindfulness in schools.* New York, NY: W. W. Norton.

Rechtschaffen, D. (2014). *The way of mindful education: Cultivating well-being in teachers and students.* New York, NY: W. W. Norton.

Shapiro, S. L., & Carlson, L. E. (2009). *The art and science of mindfulness: Integrating mindfulness into psychology and the helping professions.* Washington, DC: American Psychological Association.

Siegel, D. J. (2010). *The mindful therapist: A clinician's guide to mindsight and neural integration.* New York, NY: W. W. Norton.

Stahl, B., & Goldstein, E. (2010). *A mindfulness-based stress reduction workbook.* Oakland, CA: New Harbinger Press.

Wallace, B. A. (2011). *Minding closely: The four applications of mindfulness.* Ithaca, NY: Snow Lion.

Waters, L., Barsky, A., Ridd, A., & Allen, K. (2015). Contemplative education: A systemic, evidence-based review of the effect of meditation interventions in schools. *Educational Psychology Review, 27,* 103–134.

Wiest-Stevenson, C., & Lee, C. (2016). Trauma-informed schools. *Journal of Evidence-Informed Social Work,* 1–6. doi:10.1080/23761407.2016.1166855

Willard, C. (2016). *Growing up mindful: Essential practices to help children, teems, and families find balance, calm, and resilience.* Boulder, CO: Sounds True.

Wupperman, P., Fickling, M., Klemanski, D. H., Berking, M., & Whitman, J. B. (2013). Borderline personality features and harmful dysregulated behavior: The mediation effect of mindfulness. *Journal of Clinical Psychology, 69,* 903–911.

CHAPTER 7

OFF THE CUSHION: INFORMAL MINDFUL PRACTICES

You can't stop the waves, but you can learn how to surf.

Rechtschaffen (2014, p. 147)

INFORMAL MINDFULNESS PRACTICES

During a recent trip to San Diego, California, I took surfing lessons. I was joined by my husband, Jerry; my two daughters, Chloe and Maya; and my brother, Stephen, who is an adult with Down syndrome. During the lessons, the wind was gusting, and the waves were rough and hard to predict. It was a perfect week for learning. When you are surfing, you watch the rise and fall of the water and the patterns of the waves as they roll in. If you turn your back or look away, the waves can hit you, take your breath away, and even knock you off your feet. If you try to fight the waves, you tire quickly. On a rough day, you can get a bit beat up. I speak from experience. After a day like that, you could leave convinced that you did not like surfing.

There is another way to be with the waves. If you stay present, line up your board, and align your actions with the direction of the incoming waves, things shift. Instead of impact, you are on top, moving and flowing, gliding toward shore. It can be beautiful. There are no promises that you won't fall or that you will have a soft landing. I have a felt sense of this, too. Still, the difference between the fight or the ride is one moment. It is a moment when you can either miss it all and get hit from behind, battle the wave head-on suffering inevitable impact and fatigue, or you can ride. To do this well requires a certain level of letting go.

I was paired with my brother Stephen. He lives in the moment as a way of being. As much as I try to understand and think to manage my world, Stephen is present and open to what is next. While surfing, Stephen tried and crashed and tried and crashed over and over, all with the same eagerness. Because of this, he, more than me, was able to ride the wave. It was his ability to let go, be present, allow the wind and the waves, and do it all with an attitude of happiness that made his surfing even more effective and fun than mine. Stephen's surfing, like everything else he does, is a constant reminder to me that we cannot cognitively mediate the world. He reminds me that understanding, seeking control, and solving problems is not always the best approach. Surfing the waves of life's ups and downs with joy and gratitude can, at times, be the best option.

Informal mindful practices are like bringing the *surfer mind* to everyday activities. They are defined as the daily cultivation of mindful awareness, inquiry, a half smile (i.e., an inclination toward happiness), gratitude, and a sense of nonattachment to daily activities and challenges (Cook-Cottone, 2015; Kabat-Zinn, 2013; Rechtschaffen, 2014; Stahl & Goldstein, 2010). This chapter provides an overview of the methodology for informal mindfulness techniques. The first section of the chapter addresses the cultivation of thought processes and attitudes, such as being in inquiry and cultivating thoughts, feelings, and actions that serve you. The second section provides instruction for and examples of informal practices.

THOUGHTS AND ATTITUDES THAT CULTIVATE AND SUPPORT MINDFUL AWARENESS

Informal mindful practices are the cultivating of a mindful way of being throughout the day. The thoughts and attitudes that support mindful awareness throughout the day include inquiry, happiness, and gratitude (Rechtschaffen, 2014).

Inquiry

Sustaining presence and mindfulness within the context of intra- and interpersonal challenges can be difficult (Brach, 2012). Recall the Mindful and Yogic Self as Effective Learner Model (MY-SEL, see Chapter 2) and the ongoing tensions and attunements that move through the internal and external aspects of self. It can be a challenge to be in active self-care and reflective, intentional engagement without effective, daily tools. Brach (2012) describes RAIN (i.e., Recognize, Allow, Investigate, and Nonidentification), a methodology for cultivating mindful awareness and engagement in difficult weather or rough seas. Figure 7.1 illustrates the experience of self as learner through the perspective of informal practice (i.e., RAIN) in the embodied expression of self.

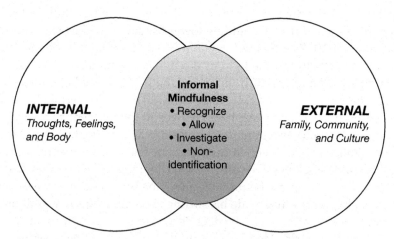

FIGURE 7.1 Informal practice as the embodied expression of self.
Source: Brach (2012) and Cook-Cottone (2015).

The RAIN mindfulness tool of inquiry provides support for working with challenging states of mind (Brach, 2012). It is an acronym to help trigger mindful presence and inquiry during your current situation, whatever it may be. According to Brach (2012), RAIN stands for: "Recognize what is happening, Allow life to be just as it is, Investigate inner experience with kindness, Non-identification [and] rest in Natural awareness" (p. 40; see Figure 7.2). Steps one and two (i.e., recognizing and allowing) are considered the basic components of mindfulness (Brach, 2012). The last two components are opportunities for deeper insight (Brach, 2012).

Informal mindful practice can be viewed using these four steps: recognize (e.g., A wave is coming or the water is calm), allow (e.g., I accept and allow the wave or the stillness as present in my life), investigate (e.g., What is the nature of the wave? How am I experiencing the wave?), and nonidentification (e.g., I am not the wave). To follow the metaphor, the waves can arise from within us via body sensations, emotions, or thoughts and memories. The waves can also arise from our external world as events and challenges for our close friends and family, our communities, or our culture (see Figure 7.1).

Recognizing What Is Happening

Recognizing involves mindful awareness, presence, and attention to what is happening right now in your internal experience (i.e., mental events, sense impressions, thoughts, or emotions). It involves a noticing of what is arising. This presence can be awakened by asking yourself, "What is happening inside me right now?" (Brach, 2012, p. 40). This is done without judgment and with an attitude of inquiry and curiosity (Cook-Cottone, 2015).

Allowing Life to Be Just as It Is

Once you have checked and asked yourself what is going on intrapersonally, the next task is to allow what is to simply be (Brach, 2012). This includes mental events, sense impressions, emotions, and thoughts (Cook-Cottone, 2015). You ask yourself, "Can I let this be just as it is?" (Brach, 2012, p. 40). You will notice the feeling-tone and any natural sense of attachment

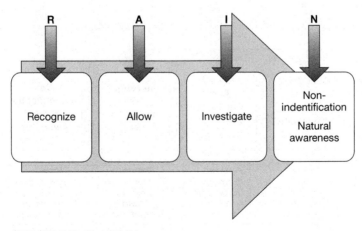

FIGURE 7.2 The RAIN process.
Source: Cook-Cottone (2015); used with permission.

or aversion to what you are allowing to let be (Grabovac, Lau, & Willett, 2011). Development of this skill, the mindful competency, to allow what is with nonjudgment, facilitates freedom of choice and the ability to stay in your intention no matter the circumstances (Brach, 2012; principle 7: I choose my focus and actions).

Investigating With Kindness

After recognition and allowing comes the opportunity to investigate what is happening (Cook-Cottone, 2015). Brach (2012) suggests that this step is especially suited for the therapeutic relationship. It involves asking deeper questions: "How am I experiencing this in my body?," "What does this feeling want from me?," "What am I believing about myself?," or "What does this mean for me?" (Brach, 2012, p. 42). This line of inquiry goes beyond a noticing and allowing and digs into our personal narrative, the truths or untruths that we hold about others and ourselves. Through this step, we can get ourselves and our students closer to the truth and the authentic experience of self.

Realize Nonidentification: Rest in Awareness

Brach (2012) explains that nonidentification means that your "self-sense is not fused with, or defined by, any limited set of emotions, sensations, or stories about who you are" (p. 44). Nonidentification leads to an awareness of simply being. Nina is a seventh-grade student who experiences a lot of anxiety. She has been working on her anxiety with the school's social worker, Miss Lolly, and they have partnered with her classroom teacher to help her bring her anxiety remediating skills into the classroom. Her teacher, Mrs. Curry, has been cultivating a mindful classroom for a few years now. This is the perfect setting for Nina, who gets overwhelmed when she thinks about her mother. Her mother is fine now, after treatment and recovery from breast cancer when Nina was in second and third grade. Since her mom's illness, Nina's anxiety gets in the way of her ability to attend to and engage in schoolwork. She is using the RAIN method to explore her experiences with anxiety (see Figure 7.3). Nina is able to deconstruct her worries when she breaks them down

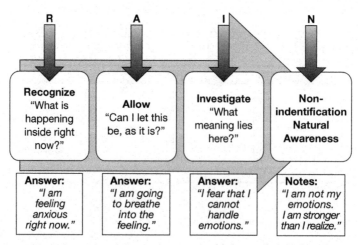

FIGURE 7.3 Nina's RAIN example.
Source: Cook-Cottone (2015); used with permission.

using RAIN. First, she recognizes and identifies her anxiety (principle 3, I am mindfully aware). Next, Nina asks herself to allow the feelings then uses her breath (principle 5, I feel my emotions in order to grow and learn; principle 2, my breath is my most powerful tool). In inquiry, with the help of Miss Lolly, the social worker, Nina asks, "What meaning lies here?" She has come to understand that she has a belief that she cannot handle her emotions. Both Miss Lolly and Mrs. Curry are working with Nina as she gains the skills she needs to know that she can, in fact, handle her emotions (principle 12, I work toward the possibility of effectiveness and growth in my life). Next, Nina reminds herself that she is not her emotions and that she is stronger than she realizes (see Figure 7.3).

Half Smile (An Inclination Toward Happiness)

It is believed that the human brain has an inclination toward negative perceptions, moods, and states (Hanson & Mendius, 2009). Theory holds that our brains scan the environment for potential threats in order to protect us. It is believed that this is our default mode. If we do not intentionally cultivate happiness, our brain simply defaults to scanning for threat (Hanson & Mendius, 2009).

The half smile is the second of the overarching mindfulness qualities that can change the tone of your day in a positive and helpful way (Cook-Cottone, 2015). The half smile is an informal practice that activates the body (i.e., the muscles of the face into a smile; Cook-Cottone, 2015). This activation triggers a positive approach mode in the mind. The half smile is an embodiment practice (Cook-Cottone, 2015). Specifically, embodiment in psychological research and theory refers to the idea that the body plays an essential role in emotional, motivational, and cognitive processes (Cook-Cottone, 2015; Price, Peterson, & Harmon-Jones, 2012). Price et al.'s (2012) review suggests that there is growing evidence that supports the notion that manipulated facial expressions, among other embodied practices, can influence physiological activity related to approach motivation and may play a role in the cultivation of positive affect. This means that turning the corners of your mouth up into a smile may actually help you feel more positive.

What can this look like as a daily informal practice? Hanh (1975) suggests that you bring a half smile to your face when you first wake up. He encourages the use of a sign, a cue, to remind you to bring a half smile to your face. I have a reminder note set in my phone alarm that I see when I go to turn it off. Upon waking, before getting out of bed, take a half smile and three gentle breaths (Cook-Cottone, 2015). Hanh (1975) suggests that—when you are sitting, standing, looking at someone you care about, noticing a flower—cultivate a half smile.

Gratitude

Gratitude is the third overarching quality that can change the tone or tenor of your day in a positive and helpful way (Cook-Cottone, 2015; Rechtschaffen, 2014). According to Wood, Froh, and Geraghty (2010), gratitude involves noticing and appreciating the good things in the world. Bringing a sense of gratitude to your daily living can help sustain presence and cultivate a positive attitude toward challenges (Cook-Cottone, 2015; Rechtschaffen, 2014). Reviews by Emmons and Stern (2013) and Wood et al. (2010) suggest that gratitude has a unique and causal relationship with well-being. Gratitude practices cultivate both happiness and a positive mindset (Rechtschaffen, 2014). Here is an easy one: Throughout the day, pause and notice what you are grateful for in the moment (Cook-Cottone, 2015; Rechtschaffen, 2014). Similarly, gratitude practice can include daily journaling in which, at the end of each school day, you or your students record three things for which you are grateful.

Following their review of the literature, Wood et al. (2010) identified several mechanisms that may be involved in the relation between gratitude and well-being. These include: schematic biases, coping, positive affect, and broaden-and-build principles. Of note, broaden-and-build emotions (e.g., gratitude, joy, interest, contentment, pride, and love) broaden people's momentary thought-action repertoires and help build enduring resources (e.g., physical, social, and interpersonal resources; Fredrickson, 2001). The associated principles of embodied growth and learning are 1, I am worth the effort, and 3, I am mindfully aware.

Cultivating Thoughts, Feelings, and Actions That Serve You

Several years ago, I ran across a very simple and effective technique for being intentional in everyday thinking. This works best for students who are in late middle school and high school, who are of typical or higher cognitive functioning. If a student is not able to think reflectively, this technique may not be a good fit. The technique is called the *Morita Table*. Astrachan-Fletcher and Maslar (2009) describe Morita Therapy (see Morita, Morita, Kondo, & LeVine, 1998) in which you are guided to act with purpose regardless of the automatic thoughts, feelings, and sensations that arise. The concept is similar to Brach's description of nonidentification. That is, you are not your thoughts, feelings, or impulses. Who you are is what you choose to cultivate, extend, and do. The first step in determining which thoughts and feelings to cultivate is to work from a sense of purpose or intention (Astrachan-Fletcher & Maslar, 2009). I like to use the purpose, or intention, "to have a life that I want to be present in." For older adolescents, it can be fun to explore various guiding intentions for them to use. Some students have said things like, "to enjoy valuable friendships," "to make a difference in the field of medicine," or "to be kind to myself and others" (see David [2009] for more guidance on setting intentions). Once you have the purpose set, you are ready to create a Morita Table. The table divides experiences into two types: controllable experiences and uncontrollable experiences (see Table 7.1).

Experiences that are considered uncontrollable include automatic thoughts, feelings, sensations, and events (Cook-Cottone, 2015). Consistent with mindfulness teachings, students are asked to accept their automatic thoughts, feelings, and sensations, along with the notion that these are not within their control. I add that automatic thoughts, feelings, and sensations are not permanent. They arise and pass away. We can experience them then let them go. There is no need or reason to keep them (Cook-Cottone, 2015). Controllable experiences, on the other hand, include conscious and deliberate thoughts (e.g., intentions and plans) and actions. The next step is to have students consider acting in a manner that aligns with their purpose (Cook-Cottone, 2015). In this clear and simple way, those things we can control, those we cannot, and those we keep and cultivate are made distinct by this simple rule of thumb: Does this serve my intention or life purpose (Astrachan-Fletcher & Maslar, 2009)? You can use Table 7.1 with your students as a tool to reflect on their experiences and choices.

TABLE 7.1 Mindful Morita Table Template

Intention/Purpose: _____

(e.g., *To create a life I want to be present in*)

Present Moment Choices

Things I Cannot Control	Things I Can Control
(Immediate Thoughts, Feelings, Events)	(Awareness, Breath, Focus, Behaviors)

Source: Adapted from Astrachan-Fletcher and Maslar (2009); Cook-Cottone (2015); David (2009).

I use a simple story to help students understand the Morita Table. I believe it is the simplicity of the story that helps students see the silliness in cultivating thoughts that don't serve them (Cook-Cottone, 2015). See Instructional Story 7.1.

INSTRUCTIONAL STORY 7.1: THE ICE CREAM SANDWICH WRAPPER

Imagine that you are standing in a park on a hot summer day. There is a cart near you selling ice cream sandwiches. People have been eating ice cream sandwiches all day and the garbage can is full. Some of the wrappers have fallen out and are now blowing in the wind. One of the wrappers blows onto your leg and sticks to your skin. Do you stand there and think, "Oh well, this is the way it is going to be. I now have an ice cream sandwich wrapper stuck to my leg for the rest of my life"? No, of course not. That would be silly. You look down. You see clearly that the ice cream sandwich wrapper is garbage and not part of what you want on your leg. Knowing this, you peel it off your leg and throw it away. Done.

Your automatic thoughts, feelings, and sensations are this way. There are things people have told you during your life, messages you have heard in the media, perhaps even things you have told yourself that do not serve your life purpose. There are feelings and sensations that don't serve you to cultivate. How do you know which ones are which? You ask yourself, "Does this thought, feeling, or sensation help me to create a life in which I want to be present?" If your answer is "No," see it for what it is then let it go. Shift your energy to cultivating thoughts and actions that serve you, that work toward your life purpose.

Source: Cook-Cottone (2015, pp. 152–153); used with permission.

For younger students, it can be helpful to use a gardening metaphor—for instance, pulling weeds and planting flowers (Hanson & Mendius, 2009). Students can gradually supplant a negative, implicit memory encoding process (i.e., remembering only the bad things that happen). This can be done by consciously making the positive aspect of your experience prominent in your awareness (Cook-Cottone, 2015). Simultaneously, the negative aspect of memory or experience is placed in the background and given less attention and energy (Cook-Cottone, 2015; Hanson & Mendius, 2009). Hanson and Mendius (2009) suggest that, by planting flowers (i.e., tending to the positive aspects of memory and experience) and pulling weeds (i.e., reducing focus on or cultivating an anecdote for), you can help shift how your brain neurologically processes information. Importantly, the authors emphasize that active effort is required as the brain has a negative bias for reasons such as self-protection. You and your students must actively work to heal negative experiences and to internalize positive ones (Hanson & Mendius, 2009). When guiding students through short meditations, you can have them garden their thoughts, carefully looking for kindness, beauty, gratitude, and curiosity, and watering those thoughts so that they grow. Ask them to notice negative thoughts like judging, worrying, and complaining, then weed them out and place them in the recycle bin. If there is time for reflection after the meditation, they can reinforce the process by drawing on paper the watering and weeding they imagined. Sometimes, we can weed and water the wrong plants. Students can share and give each other feedback.

These overarching informal processes of inquiry, happiness, gratitude, and active intention address many principles of embodied growth and learning (see Chapter 3), including 1, I am worth the effort; 3, I am mindfully aware; 4, I work toward presence in my physical body; 5, I feel my emotions in order to grow and learn; 6, I ask questions about my physical experience, feelings, and thoughts; 7, I choose my focus and actions; 8, I do the work; 11, I am kind to myself and others; and 12, I work toward the possibility of effectiveness and growth in my life.

INFORMAL PRACTICES

Opportunities for informal practice of mindfulness can be found everywhere and at any time. In a busy classroom and bustling school, there are endless opportunities. Informal practices can be taught during a structured mindful lesson (see Chapter 5 and Rechtschaffen, 2014). A posted listing on a classroom wall, gentle reminders, and mindful mini sessions can help create an atmosphere of ongoing mindfulness in the classroom. Here are a few informal practices that illustrate the opportunity to practice mindfulness anywhere and at any time.

Single Tasking and Mindful Engagement

Willard (2016) suggests that single tasking is a simple way to bring mindfulness into our daily lives. It can be very powerful to intentionally bring an accepting, open, and discerning awareness to whatever you are doing (Kabat-Zinn, 2013; Shapiro & Carlson, 2009). One of the many potential stressors children experience is multitasking (Chadha, 2015). According to Grabovac et al. (2011), attention is a sequential process during which we pay attention to one thing after another after another. When we feel as if we are multitasking, we are really just paying attention to several different things in a rapid sequence (Willard, 2016). It is not an effective or healthy way to process information. Courage, Bakhtiar, Fitzpatrick, Kenny, and Brandeau (2015) suggest that today's work, play, and learning environments require multitasking activities from children and adolescents. Specifically, advances in web-enabled and multifunction devices may create a perception among children that they must stay connected (Courage et al., 2015). According to Courage et al. (2015), young children with less mature attention systems and executive functions may be especially *at risk*. According to a review of the literature, multitasking is almost always less efficient in terms of time and accuracy. Further, multitasking can result in more superficial learning than single-task performance (Courage et al., 2015). Single tasking is an ongoing effort to do one thing at a time and do it mindfully, integrating all the senses, deep presence, and awareness. Essentially, to be mindfully aware, you must be single tasking.

Hanh (1975) describes his work doing dishes at the monastery many years ago. There were over one hundred monks, cold water, no dish soap, and only ashes, rice, and coconut husks to use for scrubbing. The practice was "while washing dishes, one should only be washing dishes" (Hanh, 1975, p. 3). Hahn (1975) speaks of one-mindedness, bare awareness, being in breath, and presence while washing dishes. It may seem silly to worry about being mindful when doing such tasks, especially for children and adolescents. However, shifting your relationship with these more mundane tasks can affect the quality of your life (Kabat-Zinn, 2013; Rechtschaffen, 2014). You gain the ability to be peacefully present during the simplest of tasks. The associated principles of embodied growth and learning are 3, I am mindfully aware; 4, I work toward presence in my physical body; and 7, I choose my focus and actions.

Your Body Doesn't Speak English (Or Any Other Language), It Speaks Breath

I like to explain to the children and adolescents with whom I work that the body does not speak English. You can tell it to calm down, stop getting all worked up, and so on. That might work a little, so long as you use the right tone of voice. Imagine talking to someone who does not speak English. If you use a calm voice, they will have a sense from your tone that things are okay. Still, they won't really know what you mean. The language that speaks most clearly to your body, especially in times of stress, anger, or other challenging emotions, is breathing. Your body understands breath. As a way of modeling, you can ask your students to help you. Ask, "I am so upset and afraid about the test coming up. Tell me what kind of breath I could use to tell my body it is going to be okay." The students can take turns offering suggestions. You might tell them you are very angry, sad, overwhelmed, or too excited. Together you problem solve. Are you scared? Maybe a hand on your heart and one on your belly will help. If you are sad, maybe belly breathing with your breathing buddy. There are lots of choices. Your students will learn a lot by helping you speak to your body with breath. The associated principles of embodied growth and learning are 2, my breath is my most powerful tool; 3, I am mindfully aware; 4, I work toward presence in my physical body; 7, I choose my focus and actions; and 8, I do the work.

Your Breath in Footsteps, Numbers, and Soup

There are many ways to notice the breath as an informal practice. I offer a few here to get you started. First, following the breath is a body settling, informal mindful practice that you can do anywhere, anytime (Cook-Cottone, 2015). As with the other informal practices, you can teach these during a structured mindful lesson giving students opportunities for guided practice. You begin by inhaling and exhaling normally. Notice the qualities of the breath. On your next inhalation, inhale gently and normally, being aware and saying to yourself, "I am inhaling normally" (Hanh, 1975, p. 83). Teachers can model this thinking as a think-aloud for the students. As you exhale mindfully, say to yourself (or aloud), "I am exhaling normally" (Hanh, 1975, p. 83). Continue this process for three to four breaths (Cook-Cottone, 2015; Hanh, 1975). On the next breath, extend the inhalation. Do this with awareness and intention. Say to yourself (or aloud), "I am breathing in a long inhalation" (Hanh, 1975, p. 83). Exhale a long and mindful exhale and say to yourself (or aloud), "I am breathing out a long exhalation" (Hanh, 1975, p. 83). Again, continue this process for three or four breaths (Cook-Cottone, 2015; Hanh, 1975). Next, follow your breath from inhalation to exhalation and move toward body awareness. Be present to the movement of your body as you breathe. Notice the rib cage, the lungs, the stomach, and the passage of the air through your nostrils moving in and out (Cook-Cottone, 2015; Hanh, 1975). Say to yourself (or aloud), "I am inhaling and following the inhalation from its beginning to its end. I am exhaling, following the exhalation from its beginning to its end" (Hanh, 1975, p. 83). Continue this for at least 20 breaths.

Second, measuring your breathing by your footsteps is similar to a more traditional walking meditation and a great way to practice single tasking (Cook-Cottone, 2015; Hanh, 1975; Kabat-Zinn, 2013; Shapiro & Carlson, 2009). This informal practice can be done anytime you, or your students, are walking. Hanh (1975) suggests taking a nice garden walk; however, you can do this walking to class or on your way to the office. Walk slowly and breathe normally. Calculate the length of your breath by counting the number of steps it takes for you to inhale completely (Cook-Cottone, 2015). Then, count the number of steps it takes for you to exhale completely. As you do this, do not force or manipulate your breath (Cook-Cottone, 2015; Hanh, 1975). Rather, allow the breath. Next, try lengthening your exhalation by one breath. Note, do not force your inhalation to change, just observe it (Cook-Cottone, 2015; Hanh, 1975). Notice if it feels as if there is a desire to lengthen it. Ask your students if they notice this. Continue this way for 10 breaths (Hanh, 1975). Try lengthening the breath even more. After 20 breaths return to normal breathing and walking (Cook-Cottone, 2015; Hanh, 1975). Teachers can model this practice for younger students. It can be helpful for students to do this while counting aloud to help them cultivate their inner observer.

Third, soup breathing involves breathing as if you are cooling soup (Willard, 2016). To do this, hold your hands as you would hold a bowl of soup (Willard, 2016). Inhale as if you are smelling the soup, thoughtfully and fully. At the end of the inhale, exhale as if you are cooling the soup (Willard, 2016). Your exhale must be done slowly and carefully as to not spill the soup by blowing too hard. Note, if you extend the exhale longer than the inhale (i.e., inhale for a count of four and exhale for a count of five), it is a message to your nervous system that everything is okay. It can help initiate a calming response. Willard (2016) suggests that you can do this with pretend tea, hot chocolate, and even pizza. It can be fun to practice when you have the actual food or drink. According to Willard (2016), evidence suggests that these types of visualizations can warm your hands and calm your nervous system. The associated principles of embodied growth and learning are 2, my breath is my most powerful tool; 3, I am mindfully aware; 4, I work toward presence in my physical body; 7, I choose my focus and actions; and 8, I do the work.

Addressing Struggles With Distraction

Within the mindfulness tradition, mindful awareness is the primary intention for practice and for daily living. Mindful awareness includes taking the perspective of the inner observer and coach. For younger students (e.g., grades K through 3), attentional and meta-cognitive systems are still developing. Children have shorter attention spans and little capacity for self-awareness. Skills can be developed through modeling and verbal coaching. For example, an older student is capable of being consciously aware: "I am walking," "I am sitting," or "I am working on math." In this manner, the older student is aware of his or her experience (Cook-Cottone, 2015). For younger students, they are simply walking, sitting, or doing math with little meta-awareness (i.e., awareness of being aware) that they are doing these things. To support the development of the inner observer, teachers can model while walking, "Students, I am noticing that I am walking, you are walking, we are walking" (note, this method is sometimes called a *think-aloud*). Through modeling, the teacher is calling to mind the notion of the inner observer. The inner observer and inner coach are key to addressing struggles with distraction.

Coming from a mindfulness perspective, Gunaratana (2001) suggests that there are several steps you can take to address distraction: notice, ignore, observe, reflect, and push through. The teacher can model these steps through think-alouds. First, once you notice that you are distracted, attempt to ignore the obstacle or distraction. The inner observer says, "I notice that I am distracted. I will ignore the distraction." When ignoring does not work, move to the next step, diverting the mind by actively engaging. Observe more deeply the intentional object of attention (i.e., math homework; Gunaratana, 2001). This can be difficult, especially regarding topics or tasks at which a student does not feel successful. Nevertheless, an intentional mindful observation of the work can be the key to active engagement: "I am working through this math problem. I notice the shapes of the numbers, the layout of the equation, and the patterns in the formula. I am breathing. I am present to my homework." Stop here and breathe.

If shifting your attention more deeply toward the object of attention does not work, Gunaratana (2001) suggests that you try reflecting on the fact that distractions arise from many causes and places both inside and outside, and these hindrances are in flux. That is, rather than thinking that there is something wrong with us or the math homework, rather than judging and reacting, we simply reflect on how obstacles, hindrances, and distractions come and go. We reflect on the notion that they always have and they always will. Still, for some, this option does not work. Using this mindful approach to attending and engaging, Gunaratana (2001) offers one last step if all others fail—to push through. I use this quote often in yoga class and when working with patients, "The way out is through." He suggests that you clench your teeth, press your tongue against your upper palate, and apply all your energy toward overcoming the obstacle. This method can be practiced during structured mindful lessons attending to simple objects. Students can share which step in the process of actively attending worked best for them and what it feels like to push through. The associated principles of embodied growth and learning inclue 1, I am worth the effort; 2, my breath is my most powerful tool; 3, I am mindfully aware; 4, I work toward presence in my physical body; 5, I feel so that I can heal; 7, I choose my focus and actions; 8, I do the work; and 12, I work toward the possibility of effectiveness and growth in my life.

Mind-O-Meter

The mind-o-meter is a tool for self-awareness and self-regulation (see Figure 7.4). The mind-o-meter provides a fun way for students to pay close attention to what is happening in their inner and outer worlds (Greenland, 2010). Print out the likeness of the meter in Figure 7.4 and have your students color in the labels as indicated. Greenland (2010) suggests using the tool as a way to check in with the class. For example, you might instruct your students, "I am going to ask you a question, and I want you to point to your answer on the mind-o-meter. Do your best to show exactly how you feel you are doing right now. Ready? How strong is your attention to this lesson right now? Go! Point to your answer" (Greenland, 2010). This way, as the teacher, you can easily get a quick read on how your students are doing. If much of the class is checked out, you can bring them back with mindful movement or breath work. In this way, the tool helps you create student-teacher attunement in the class. The mind-o-meter also promotes awareness and using think-alouds: "Wow, I see a lot of you are really struggling to pay attention right now. Let's do some mindfulness movement to settle our bodies and some breathing to get our attention focused." Greenland (2010) suggests checking on a variety of processes including: attention, patience, frustration, interconnectedness, wakefulness, relaxation, and excitement. The associated principles of embodied growth and learning are 3, I am mindfully aware; 4, I work toward presence in my physical body; and 7, I choose my focus and actions.

The Sense Doors

In Eastern tradition, the elements of our sensory systems are referred to as the sense windows. These include taste, smell, touch, sight, hearing, the vestibular systems (i.e., balance and spatial orientation), and the proprioceptive system (i.e., the body's awareness of itself—the position of its joints, how it is moving, and how much effort it needs to exert; Greenland, 2010).

In the classroom, students can work with their sense windows toward noticing, allowing, nonreaction, and presence. Willard (2016) describes an informal practice termed counting to five sensations, which offers the possibility of a neutral, calming response. You can do this with sounds, things you see, and sensations in the body (Willard, 2016). To illustrate,

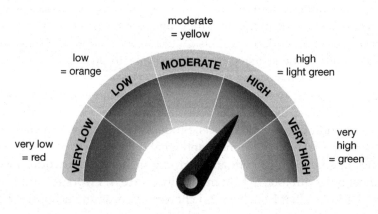

Mind-O-Meter

FIGURE 7.4 Mind-O-Meter.
Source: Adapted from Greenland (2010).

teachers can guide students in a group, or one-on-one, to notice the first five sounds they hear (e.g., the teacher in the adjacent room, a bird on a tree outside, the clock ticking, a car driving by, and the breathing of the person next to them). A focus on sensations can help downregulate the nervous system, helping students move from their reactive, stress-responding mental set to a more open, curious, and engaged mental set. Sensate focus is often used for individuals with emotion regulation difficulties for this reason.

Also in the classroom, the sense windows can be explored in informal mindful ways. For instance, you can set up sensory stations and have students fill out response sheets that ask the following (Greenland, 2010):

- Describe the sensory experience (e.g., taste, touch, smell).
- Categorize the experience (i.e., pleasant, unpleasant, neutral).
- Report your physical reaction (i.e., how did that feel in your body?).
- Describe your behavioral reaction (i.e., what did you do?).
- Report your emotional reaction (i.e., how did you feel?).
- Describe mental associations (i.e., what did you think?).

Students can review their sheets and notice any patterns. Observations can be written down in their journals, shared in pairs, or shared with the class. Students can also notice their patterns over time. Do things change if they breathe, work toward a positive or growth mindset, or attempt bare awareness?

Time In, Not Time Out

David (2009) suggests giving students a *time in*. A time in involves taking time to check in with yourself and refocus your awareness and intention. David (2009) calls practices like this *mindfulness boosters*, because they take very little time and build on the more formal mindfulness practices you are already building in class. Examples of time in include (David, 2009):

- Taking 30 seconds to stop, drop, and breathe in the middle of a working session
- Focusing students on the process of opening and closing their hands, then giving themselves a brief hand massage
- Inviting students to listen to the sounds in the room for 30 seconds
- Asking students to stand up and rock forward and backward on their feet, coming to tippy toes as they roll forward
- Guiding students through 30 seconds of breath work

Interconnectedness

Interconnectedness is the notion that all things are connected. Informal mindful awareness involves an awareness of the interconnection of all things (Rechtschaffen, 2014; Willard, 2016). According to Hanh (2002), when we are totally mindful and in direct contact with reality (not the images or ideas of reality), we realize that all phenomena are interdependent and endlessly interwoven. When aware, we come to realize that there is no such thing as a separate thing, event, or experience. We realize that no part of the world can exist apart from others. Hanh calls it the principle of *interbeing* (Hanh, 2002), which he demonstrates using a sheet of paper.

Hanh (2002) explains that if you look deeply into a sheet of paper you can see the cloud. Without the cloud, there would be no rain. Without the rain, there would be no trees. You see the sunshine in the paper, too. Without the sunshine, the forest cannot grow. With no forest, there is no wood. He explains how the logger who cut the tree is also in the paper. The logger must eat and so we see the wheat that becomes the bread that the logger eats. As with the wheat, we see the logger's parents. And so it goes. There are clouds in every paper. Hanh's (2002) beautiful description can also be found at www.awakin.org/read/view.php?tid=222 at Awakin.org. Associated principles of embodied growth and learning include 3, I am mindfully aware; 6, I ask questions about my physical experiences, feelings, and thoughts; 7, I choose my focus and actions; and 8, I do the work.

Journaling

Journaling creates an experience of reflection (Rechtschaffen, 2014). When writing about one's experiences, the student becomes one step removed from the experience. He or she is the observer. Traditional journaling about the events of the day, stressful events, and emotions can be helpful (e.g., Ullrich & Lutgendorf, 2002). Mindful journals are distinct from typical journals in that they are a writing of what students have become present to, rather than a running narrative (David, 2009). They might also take a specific *tone* such as mindful awareness, compassion, gratitude, or interconnectedness. Some suggestions:

• Take the present tense documenting what you see, smell, feel, and notice (David, 2009).
• Write three things for which you are grateful and make you happy.
• Document reflections upon mindfulness activities.
• Detail your feelings, where they show up in your body, how they are affected by breath, and so on.
• Document your daily intentions in the morning, before you start your day (David, 2009).

The associated principles of embodied growth and learning are 3, I am mindfully aware; 4, I work toward presence in my physical body; 6, I ask questions about my physical experiences, feelings, and thoughts; 7, I choose my focus and actions; 8, I do the work; and 11, I am kind to myself and others.

Mindful Communication

Mindful communication can build from English and language arts coursework (David, 2009). You can begin with students reading to each other and listening to tone, pace, content, distractions, and mindfulness (David, 2009). Next, move to mindfulness conversations. Mindfulness conversation involves awareness of how students speak, what they really say and mean, the reciprocation of communication, eye contact, and reflective listening (David, 2009). In reflective listening, students listen carefully and reflect back the content, intention, or feeling to the person who spoke (Cook-Cottone, Kane, & Anderson, 2014). For beginners, a reflective statement can begin with, "It sounds like you …," or "I hear you saying that…," followed by a summary statement of what was heard (Cook-Cottone et al., 2014). Students can provide feedback for each other. There is much to learn from both the listener and the person talking.

Rechtschaffen (2014) suggests that mindful communication is a way to de-script old and potentially harmful communication patterns. He offers an exercise in which mindful communication is used within the context of an argument. This is a wonderful tool to offer students during a mediation session, walking them through the steps of mindful communication as they work through their conflict. Here are the steps (Cook-Cottone et al., 2014; Rechtschaffen, 2014):

- Take some time to feel how your body is responding to the conflict (Rechtschaffen, 2014).
- Feel the bottom of your feet, press into the earth, and relax (Rechtschaffen, 2014).
- Notice your breathing, inhalations and exhalations, and intentionally extend your exhalations (Cook-Cottone, 2015; Rechtschaffen, 2014).
- Become aware of any sense of self-righteousness and accept that it is part of being human (Rechtschaffen, 2014).
- Work toward letting go of your perspective for a moment (Rechtschaffen, 2014).
- Orient your awareness to what the other person is saying, listen, and receive their words (Rechtschaffen, 2014).
- Do not plan what you are going to say next (Cook-Cottone et al., 2014; Rechtschaffen, 2014).
- Notice how your heart is affected by the person's words (Rechtschaffen, 2014).
- When the person is finished, refrain from giving advice or making judgments (Rechtschaffen, 2014).
- Use reflective statements to show them that you heard what they had to say: "It sounds like…" (Cook-Cottone et al., 2014), or "What I heard you feel…"
- Speak to them using "I" statements and share directly from your heart (Rechtschaffen, 2014).

The associated principles of embodied growth and learning include: 1, I am worth the effort; 2, My breath is my most powerful tool; 3, I am mindfully aware; 4, I work toward presence in my physical body; 5, I feel my emotions in order to grow and learn; 6, I ask questions about my physical experiences, feelings, and thoughts; 7, I choose my focus and actions; 8, I do the work; 10, I honor efforts to grow and learn; and 11, I am kind to myself and others.

WWW: What Went Well

Olson (2014) offers a simple tool for bringing the class together at the beginning and at the end of the day. At the beginning of the day you can ask, "What went well (WWW) for you since our last class?" (Olson, 2014, p. 156). At the end of the day, you can ask such questions as: "What went well in your mindfulness practice today?," "What went well for you in your kindness work?," or "What went well for you today in finding things for which you are grateful?" Olson (2014) notes that, when you first begin this practice in the classroom, the typical negative bias will arise as students will think it important to list the things that went wrong. With practice, you can work into a routine of reflecting happiness, gratitude, mindful problem solving, and their successful informal practices.

CONCLUSION

The focus of this chapter was learning how to surf the up-and-down waves of daily life experiences in school and at home. The chapter provided a review of informal mindfulness practices as a key support for sustained presence in a mindful classroom and school. Inquiry, gratitude practice, and setting positive intentions were reviewed as ways of cultivating an overall positive attitude, an approach mental set, and broaden-and-build emotions to challenges and daily events (Cook-Cottone, 2015). Supportive thought processes such as RAIN and the Morita method were reviewed as ways to work through daily cognitive and mental challenges and cultivate a mindset oriented to engagement and growth. Finally, several specific informal mindful practices were reviewed that can help you and your students practice informal mindfulness daily. See David (2009), Greenland (2010), Olson (2014), Rechtschaffen (2014), and Willard (2016) for even more ideas for informal mindful practice with children and adolescents.

REFERENCES

Astrachan-Fletcher, E., & Maslar, M. (2009). *The dialectic behavior therapy skills workbook for bulimia: Using DBT to break the cycle and regain control of your life.* Oakland, CA: New Harbinger Publications.

Brach, T. (2012). Mindful presence: A foundation for compassion and wisdom. In C. K. Germer & R. D. Siegel (Eds.), *Wisdom and compassion: Deepening mindfulness in clinical practice.* New York, NY: The Guilford Press.

Chadha, N. (2015). Strategies to manage stress among youngsters. *Indian Journal of Health and Wellbeing, 6,* 644.

Cook-Cottone, C. P. (2015). *Mindfulness and yoga for self-regulation: A primer for mental health professionals.* New York, NY: Springer Publishing.

Cook-Cottone, C. P., Kane, L., & Anderson, L. (2014). *The elements of counseling children and adolescents.* New York, NY: Springer Publishing.

Courage, M. L., Bakhtiar, A., Fitzpatrick, C., Kenny, S., & Brandeau, K. (2015). Growing up multitasking: The costs and benefits for cognitive development. *Developmental Review, 35,* 5–41.

Emmons, R. A., & Stern, R. (2013). Gratitude as a psychotherapeutic intervention. *Journal of Clinical Psychology, 69,* 846–855.

David, D. S. (2009). *Mindful teaching and teaching mindfulness: A guide for anyone who teaches anything.* Boston, MA: Wisdom Publications.

Fredrickson, B. L. (2001). The role of positive emotions in positive psychology: The broaden-and-build theory of positive emotions. *American Psychologist, 56,* 218–226.

Grabovac, A. D., Lau, M. A., & Willett, B. R. (2011). Mechanisms of mindfulness: A Buddhist psychological model. *Mindfulness, 2*(3), 154–166. doi:10.1007/s12671-011-0054-5

Greenland, S. K. (2010). *The mindful child: How to help your kid manage stress and become happier, kinder, and more compassionate.* New York, NY: Atria, A Division of Simon & Schuster, Inc.

Gunaratana, B. H. (2001). *Eight mindful steps to happiness: Walking the Buddha's path.* Somerville, MA: Wisdom Publications.

Hanh, T. N. (1975). *The miracle of mindfulness: An introduction to the practice of meditation.* Boston, MA: Beacon Press.

Hanh, T. N. (2002). Clouds in each paper. *Awakin.com: Waking up to wisdom in stillness and community.* Retrieved from http://www.awakin.org/read/view.php?tid=222

Hanson, R., & Mendius, R. (2009). *Buddha's brain: The practical neuroscience of happiness, love, and wisdom.* Oakland, CA: New Harbinger Publications.

Kabat-Zinn, J. (2013). *Full catastrophe living: Using the wisdom of your body and mind to face stress, pain, and illness.* New York, NY: Bantam Books.

Morita, S., Morita, M., Kondo, A., & LeVine, P. (1998). *Morita therapy and the true nature of anxiety-based disorders (Shinkeishitsu).* New York, NY: SUNY Press.

Olson, K. (2014). *The invisible classroom: Relationships, neuroscience, and mindfulness in school.* New York, NY: W. W. Norton.

Price, T. F., Peterson, C. K., & Harmon-Jones, E. (2012). The emotive neuroscience of embodiment. *Motivation and Emotion, 36,* 27–37.

Rechtschaffen, D. (2014). *The way of mindful education: Cultivating well-being in teachers and students.* New York, NY: W. W. Norton.

Shapiro, S. L., & Carlson, L. E. (2009). *The art and science of mindfulness: Integrating mindfulness into psychology and helping professions.* Washington, DC: American Psychological Association.

Stahl, B., & Goldstein, E. (2010). *A mindfulness-based stress reduction workbook.* Oakland, CA: New Harbinger Press.

Ullrich, P. M., & Lutgendorf, S. K. (2002). Journaling about stressful events: Effects of cognitive processing and emotional expression. *Annals of Behavioral Medicine, 24,* 244–250.

Willard, C. (2016). *Growing up mindful: Essential practices to help children, teens, and families find balance.* Boulder, CO: Sounds Trues

Wood, A. M., Froh, J. J., & Geraghty, A. W. A. (2010). Gratitude and well-being: A review and theoretical integration. *Clinical Psychology Review, 30,* 890–905.

CHAPTER 8

SCHOOL-BASED MINDFULNESS PROTOCOLS: MANUALIZED AND STRUCTURED MINDFULNESS PROGRAMS FOR SCHOOLS

He who does not research has nothing to teach.

Proverb, Author Unknown

Schools need practical, feasible, and acceptable interventions that work. Researchers are charged to assess each of these perspectives. Research in the field of mindfulness has been increasing for a few decades, with research conducted in schools evolving more recently. Currently, there are only a few research papers that have aggregated the findings but there are many papers that review specific interventions. Understanding the quality of the evidence as well as the findings is critical. Building on the conceptual, formal mindfulness, and informal mindfulness chapters, this chapter reviews several key issues in research and quality of evidence, risks, the outcomes on mindfulness in schools, and several structured programs for implementing mindfulness in schools.

KEY ASPECTS OF RESEARCH

No matter how many checks and balances we put into place, all research has some form of bias. Researchers want to find positive effects for their interventions. Journals tend to only publish studies with significant findings and participants tend to respond to surveys in socially acceptable ways. It is likely, too, that participating in a study creates bias, as those who do and those who do not participate may be inherently different in an important way related to mindfulness. These and many more variables can be sources of bias. With respect to quantitative research, it is important to be mindful of the differences in quality of evidence provided by a study. At higher quality levels, there is less chance of bias, or influence of other variables on the outcomes. At lower quality levels, there is an increased chance of bias. Distinctly, qualitative studies serve a different function (e.g., theory development) and provide an intentionally subjective view of the experiences of the participants within the frame of reference of the researchers.

As seen, there are many nuances that can deeply affect the way that researcher outcomes are determined and how they are framed for dissemination. Often when research is shared in popular culture, little attention is paid to the quality of the evidence being shared. As school personnel, it is important that you attend both to the outcomes and to the quality of the study providing the outcomes. There are many issues to which you should attend; I offer a few critical ones here.

Feasibility and Acceptability

Typically, research begins with looking at the feasibility and acceptability of an intervention (Zenner, Herrnleben-Kurz, & Walach, 2014). That is, researchers study if a program can practically, or feasibly, be carried out within a school (Zenner et al., 2014). Implementation is an important aspect of feasibility (Zenner et al., 2014). As educators know all too well, it will not matter if the intervention is highly effective in a lab or during a trial. If it cannot be carried out easily during the school day or as part of the school schedule (e.g., after school program, academic intervention services), teachers and school administrators won't use it (Lawlor, 2014). Another critical aspect is acceptability (Zenner et al., 2014). Researchers also need to make sure that school personnel and students will accept the program, find it suitable, satisfying, and interesting (Zenner et al., 2014). A program may be very feasible and effective, but if the students, teachers, or administrators do not like it or do not find it acceptable it won't work (Lawlor, 2014). Only after feasibility and acceptability, do educators look at effectiveness.

Understanding the Range in the Quality of Research

The quality of research studies ranges substantially from weak to strong. Studies that are empirically rigorous tend to be associated with less bias from influences outside of the intervention. Analyses that aggregate the work of many rigorous studies are believed to reduce bias even more and be at the highest level of evidence (e.g., systematic literature reviews, meta-analyses). Research of lower quality is more vulnerable to bias and we can be less sure that the outcomes are strictly associated with the intervention (e.g., anecdotal evidence, expert opinions, studies using surveys and questionnaires collected at one point in time; Figure 8.1).

Researchers exploring effectiveness have many challenges when working in schools. Ideally, researchers conduct a randomized controlled trial (RCT; Greenberg & Harris, 2012). This means that the students are assigned randomly to the intervention group, an active control group, or a passive control group. The intervention group takes part in the mindfulness program. The active intervention group receives a program that involves some action; yet they are not engaged in the activities that are essentially *active ingredients* for the intervention. Active ingredients are the aspects of the practice that are believed to help students improve. For example, an active control group might sit quietly or engage in silent reading. Last, a passive control group engages in life as usual and does not take part in the intervention or the active control group activities.

Each of these groups takes a pre-test or baseline measure of the variables the researchers are looking to study. Some researchers are very interested in academic engagement

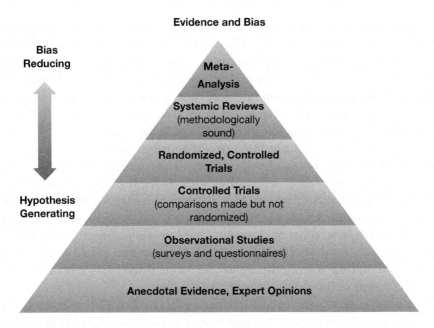

FIGURE 8.1 Evidence and bias.

and school achievement. Those researchers will look at grades, maybe a self-report of students' academic engagement, and other measures that help them know if these things change across time as students engage in mindfulness practices, the active control activity, or school as usual. As you will see, researchers are interested in a variety of student outcomes including attention, self-regulation, behaviors, academic achievement, and engagement. Some researchers take measurements along the way, while some researchers wait until after the intervention has ended to do a posttest. The best studies do all of those things and do a follow-up after several weeks, at a few months post intervention, at 6 months post intervention, and perhaps even a year or more later to see if the intervention effects remained intact over time.

As a doctoral student, I thought, "Why would anyone do anything other than an RCT?" As an assistant and now associate professor, I now understand. RCTs are very challenging to conduct, even in the most controlled environments. Schools provide a host of challenges including the need to deliver the academic curricula, state and federal tests, teacher performance assessment, children with a variety of behavior and learning problems that may or may not be included in the study, complex schedules, limited free or elective time, and more. School districts and schools are complex systems with one of the most important mandates in our culture—to educate our youth. School personnel must put that charge first. School-based research comes second. I have watched my own studies and those of my colleagues devolve from the most beautifully planned RCT, to a shadow of the original vision as the many challenges of delivering research in schools were negotiated. This is not due to anyone acting as an intentional obstacle. Rather, schools and school systems are extremely complex systems with a primary charge, other than research, that they must take as their highest priority.

I now read each study with substantial empathy and respect for the researchers as well as the administrators who took the risk to approve the study in their district and schools;

for the teachers who are already time constrained and challenged with heavy workloads who added research to their load; and to the students and their families who agreed to add research to their commitments. To participate in research and help researchers conduct a high-quality study is a generous act of civic philanthropy. It is a gift to future school districts, schools, teachers, students, families, and generations. I am so grateful for each and every school who has worked hard to support my team's research and for all the schools who help us better understand mindfulness and yoga in the schools.

There are other options that can yield results to help inform what we do in schools. There are some RCTs that do not randomly assign individual students to the various groups; rather they assign whole classes or schools randomly to the treatment group, active control group, or school as usual control group. This process carries with it some complications as it is difficult to sort out the effects of the classroom teacher, or the school environment, or the cohort of students in a school or classroom and how they already function together in a group. You probably remember being in a class or group that didn't work well together or a class that did and the teacher saying to you, "This is the best class I have ever had." Sometimes, these sorts of influences can affect study data.

Another option is a controlled trial. Controlled trials are like RCTs in that there is a comparison group. However, who is in the intervention group and who is in the other groups are not randomly decided. In order to make sure that the groups are equal, researchers sometimes match the control and treatment groups according to variables such as socioeconomic status, race and ethnicity, and age. This way, even though participants were not randomly assigned, researchers can analyze data based on inferences that the groups were comparable in many ways. This is called a matched controlled trial.

Sometimes, even with the best-laid plans, researchers are not able to secure control groups or enough participants for an active control group (e.g., a group doing calisthenics or something else physically active) or a school-as-usual control group (i.e., doing nothing special for the study). In such situations, researchers create a simpler design with only one control group, or do a study with the intervention-only group. These studies are less compelling as we cannot be sure that the intervention yielded the results because there is no group to compare the results against. It could be that the intervention group, and all of the kids in the school, began working harder because of some other variable: Maybe the school shifted the schedule around so all of the students were able to sleep in longer in the morning. Maybe the school rolled out iPads for everyone that year. Or maybe there was a dramatic event (e.g., a student killed in a car accident or the death of a beloved teacher) that affected all of the students and the researchers' intervention group got worse as did everyone else. In the latter case, it looks as if the intervention had a negative effect, rather than the school-wide or community-wide stressors.

When a field of research is new or evolving in an important way, researchers engage in correlational studies to better understand how variables might be associated and affect each other. This type of research is not considered causal. That is, we cannot infer that just because two things tend to correlate together (e.g., mindfulness and fewer behavior problems) that one causes the other. An example is a child who is maturing neurodevelopmentally who has been placed in a healthier, more nurturing foster home, and is now also better able to sit for meditation class. Note, however, that there are some ways to analyze the data to understand the relations among variables in a causal manner. For example, in a study my research team recently conducted, we collected data across 14 different middle schools all in one semester. We aggregated and cleaned the data and analyzed the variables to see how they tended to associate. We hypothesized that self-compassion and eating disorder thoughts and behaviors were inversely related. We then looked at the role anxiety played in predicting eating disorder behaviors and how self-compassion might influence that relationship. We conducted an analysis that helped us confirm our hypothesis; that is, that those with high anxiety were at more risk for eating disorder thoughts and behaviors. However, for those who engaged in self-compassion, such risk was reduced. That is, self-compassion appears to predict a weaker relationship between anxiety and eating disorder thoughts and behaviors (Cook-Cottone, Rovig, & Guyker, manuscript in preparation). This is compelling. The next step would be to create an intervention that taught self-compassion to middle school students and see if that group experiences an increase in self-compassion and decreased eating disorder risk while the control group remains unchanged or experiences increased risk. In this way, the latter design gives us more confidence in terms of the protective influence of self-compassion.

Case studies are another way to begin to test out hypothesized relationships among variables. There are also some very interesting case study designs. Depending on the design and the statistical measures done, case studies and case series can also vary substantially. Because there are fewer students involved in the case study it can be difficult to make generalizations about the success or lack of success and apply it to larger groups of students. Case studies are often good to show that an intervention may have some positive effects and should be explored on a larger level. Also, because there is more attention paid to the intervention's influence on students, the case study can provide insight into what the active ingredients are. So, the take-away is that while case studies have some drawbacks in terms of generalizability, they can provide valuable information in terms of answering the larger research questions of, "Can this work?" and "How does it work?"

Another design that has a similar generalizability challenge, yet offers a lot in terms of insight, is qualitative research. Qualitative research focuses on the lived-experience of the participants and explores in detail the perceptions of the participants. There are many different subtypes of qualitative research. They share the commitment of amplifying the voice and experiences of participants and the effort to reduce research bias in terms of the researcher's perceived expectations or views. For example, my team just completed a study of the Encinitas School District lawsuit in which a group of parents asserted that the yoga program being taught at the school was religious in nature and therefore should not be taught (Cook-Cottone, Lemish, & Guyker, 2016). Having read and watched all of the news reports on the lawsuit, my team went in with a few preconceptions regarding the experiences of the teachers, administrators, and researchers who were involved in the yoga intervention during the time of the lawsuit. As a team, we discussed how stressful and disruptive the lawsuit must have been to the day-to-day operations of the schools and classrooms, and were ready to handle resistance, anger, and anything that came up as we conducted the study. At the end of our week of collecting data, we were surprised to find that very few people reported extreme stress, negative feelings, or tensions. Nearly all of the people we interviewed supported the right of the families to engage in the lawsuit and believed that it spoke to the quality of our society that these families could have a voice and ask questions. Across the board, no matter their beliefs in terms of the religious nature of yoga, school personnel supported the legal process and the importance of creating a school environment in which students felt safe and supported. Teachers, administrators, and researchers were kind and respectful. Because we were doing a qualitative study, we were able capture the authentic respectful experience of those who worked for the school district.

Manualizing: Detailing the Practice

Researchers and practitioners serve the larger effort to share and study mindfulness when they detail the interventions that they are doing (Greenberg & Harris, 2012). There are many aspects to the intervention that should be detailed including the "dosage" (e.g., frequency and duration of each session, the length of the overall intervention, and home practice; Cook-Cottone, 2013), exactly what specific activities are part of the intervention (e.g., focused meditations, guided meditation, metta meditation, body scans), and teacher specifics (e.g., training of teachers, experience of teachers, supervision). The highest form of detailing the intervention is creating a manual that details specific statements, intervention activities, assessment points, and resources. Manuals should be updated and revised during the early years of an intervention. A formally published manual should be well vetted via feedback from those who have implemented the program. With a detailed account of what was done, other researchers and practitioners can replicate the program and assess how well it works in other areas with other populations (Greenberg & Harris, 2012). Here is a list that includes many of the specifics that should be detailed during an intervention (Zeller et al., 2014):

- The theoretical basis for the study (Greenberg & Harris, 2012; Zeller et al., 2014)
- The specific intervention details (e.g., activities, types of mindfulness taught and led, leader statements and scripts, steps of implementation; Greenberg & Harris, 2012; Zeller et al., 2014)
- Dosage (e.g., frequency, duration, and length of each aspect of the intervention—15 minutes guided meditation [with script], 20 minutes mindful stretching [with sequence], and 10 minutes body scan [with script] for 10 weeks, three times a week during homeroom; home practice; Greenberg & Harris, 2012; Cook-Cottone, 2013)
- Teacher details (e.g., training, experience, support, supervision; Zeller et al., 2014)
- Treatment or intervention integrity (e.g., a checklist or more detailed accounting system noting the aspects of the program and how effectively they were implemented at each session)
- Program context (e.g., the room, distractions, challenges, time of day, competing programs)

Types of Outcome Measures

As you will see in the research detailed in the following, there are many ways to explore the effects of mindfulness. Some researchers are looking at health and well-being and their measures assess those constructs. Other researchers believe that the important effects are on student engagement and academic success. Accordingly, they measure and assess those areas. There are many other perspectives that researcher have taken. If you look back to Chapters 1, 2, and 3, you will see a variety of outcomes that are believed to be associated with constructs such as mindfulness—stress reduction, improved health, reduced impulsivity, emotional regulation, self-regulation, and academic functioning. In good research, the outcomes are measured by assessment tools that can effectively detail the changes in the variable from pre- to posttest, and at follow-up.

Often when research is presented in popular culture and even in textbooks, the quality or type of the measures used is not discussed. The field of assessment is an evolving field and the measures used to detect changes associated with mindfulness practice are sometimes as young as the mindfulness field itself. Other research measures are tried, tested, and well-established, yet the details are too much for a press release or Facebook post. In these cases, the quality of measure is often ignored. Currently, researchers believe that objective measures are of the highest quality. That is, measures that objectively measure school performance such as an achievement test, grades, class rank, and attendance. There are also measures that objectively measure stress such as salivary cortisol or markers of inflammation or behavior such as discipline referrals and suspensions. Still others turn to neuropsychological measures and brain scans. As many of these direct measures can be costly and difficult to administer across large populations, many researchers turn to self-report measures. Self-report measures are either surveys or structured interviews in which the participant reports on his or her own progress, stress, well-being, emotional health, and so on. It is believed that although there are many quality self-report measures, they are all inherently biased via the perspective of the participant.

Generalizability: Who Participated and What Does That Tell Us?

Generalizability is a term used to describe the usefulness of research. It refers to the degree to which the outcomes of a particular study can be used to understand individuals who were not in the study. For example, if a study were conducted exploring the effects of meta meditation (i.e., loving kindness meditation; see Chapter 6), and was done for 4 weeks, 3 times a week among children with *attention difficulties*, to whom would the findings apply? We could answer that question by looking at how many participants were included in the study, how old they were, and how representative the sample seems to be of all kids with attention difficulties. We would want to ask if the children were formally diagnosed with an attention disorder and if so, which one? Who made the diagnosis? What criteria were used? We would want to know the participants' ethnicity, race, socioeconomic status, school success, and many other demographic variables so that we would know how this sample of students compares to the student with whom we are working. A study done on 20 upper socioeconomic class students from a private school in California with mild attention concerns (as indicated by a teacher checklist) does not help us know if the technique will work for poor children attending a public, inner-city school where the teacher indicated attention concerns. A study of high school students may not help us understand first graders. A study of high school students struggling with addiction in a suburban middle class area, may not help us understand students at risk in the inner city. And so it goes (Vonnegut, 1991).

As you continue to learn more about mindfulness and the research on mindfulness interventions, look carefully at the research. Consider the students with whom you are working, their demographics, context, and their school. Compare the students in the study to your students and ask how much of the information can be generalized to your students. Look carefully at the design of the study. Notice if the researchers detailed what they were doing, how long, how often, and in what sequence. Look over the limitations section of the study (all good studies have one) and consider that the editors of the journal found these limitations to be valid concerns worth reporting.

RESEARCH ON MINDFULNESS IN SCHOOLS

The next two sections of this chapter will detail the current state of mindfulness in school research as well as review several mindfulness programs and interventions for school-age children and adolescents used in the school settings. There is a growing body of evidence supporting mindfulness programs in schools.

Reviews and Meta-Analyses

In 2014, Zenner et al. systematically reviewed the evidence regarding the effects of school-based mindfulness interventions on psychological outcomes, using a comprehensive search strategy designed to locate both published and unpublished studies. The team performed systematic searches in 12 databases and further studies were identified via hand search and contact with experts. In order to reduce bias, two reviewers independently extracted the data, also selecting information about intervention programs, feasibility, and acceptance (Zenner et al., 2014). The team identified 24 studies of which 13 were published. Fourteen of the studies were conducted in North America, seven in Europe, one in Australia, and two in Asia. Overall, of the 24 studies, 19 studies used a controlled design. When taken together, 1,348 students were instructed in mindfulness and 876 students served as controls (Zenner et al., 2014). The students in the studies ranged from grades 1 to 12 reflecting ages 6 to 19. The sample sizes of the studies varied substantially from 12 to 216. Eight of the studies were implemented in elementary school (grades 1–5), two in middle school (grades 6–8), and four studies in high school (grades 9–12).

Zenner et al. (2014) found the descriptions of the schools, neighborhoods, or participants not very detailed. For those who did offer descriptions, the researchers reported that there was a wide variety of school types including public schools in both urban and suburban settings. The groups of studies also included a private residential school, a Catholic school for girls, a for-fee boy's school, a rural high school, and a public alternative high school (Zenner et al., 2014). Of the characteristics reported, described samples were from low performing and at-risk schools. The authors noted that it was possible that studies that did not report socioeconomic status could have included students from higher socioeconomic backgrounds. As you know, the lack of these data makes it difficult to generalize from the findings.

The reported theoretical frameworks for studies' programs were mindfulness ($N = 24$), positive psychology (including social emotional learning [SEL]; $N = 9$), and executive functioning ($N = 6$; Zenner et al., 2014). Many of the mindfulness-oriented programs cited previously existing programs such as Mindfulness-Based Stress Reduction (MBSR), Mindfulness-Based Cognitive Therapy (MBCT), Dialectic Behavior Therapy (DBT), and Acceptance and Commitment Therapy (ACT; Zenner et al., 2014). Only two of the programs reported using manuals that existed for more than 5 years. Thirteen of the programs used a manual that was less than 5 years old. Nine of the programs were run ad hoc with no manual (Zenner et al., 2014). Two thirds of the studies used manualized programs such as *Mindful Schools* and *Learning to BREATHE* (L2B); both programs are detailed in the next section of this chapter. According to Zenner et al., (2014), the programs defined similar objectives related to the assessment methods and reflected the targeted areas: cognitive performance (e.g., attention tests, creativity tests, mind wandering paradigm, grades), emotional problems (e.g., maladaptive emotion, cognition, behavior, clinical symptoms such as anxiety, depression, test anxiety, somatic reactions, ruminative thinking styles, emotion regulation difficulties), stress and coping (e.g., perceived stress, coping, cortisol samples with stress test), resilience (e.g., well-being, positive and constructive emotions or affect, resiliency, social skills and positive relationships, self-concept, self-esteem), and third-person rating (i.e., aggressive or oppositional behavior, social skills, emotional competence, well-being, attention, self-regulation).

Seven of the programs were taught by the teacher, 15 by an outside trainer, and two by a teacher and outside trainer (Zenner et al., 2014). The programs varied in length from

4 weeks to 24 weeks with a median length of 8 weeks (Zenner et al., 2014). Programs were typically offered once per week for 45 minutes. Some program split the time over several sessions per week (Zenner et al., 2014). Most programs offered more than one component with observation of breath noted as the essential exercise (Zenner et al., 2014). Groups also frequently included psycho-education and group discussion (Zenner et al., 2014). The intervention components were as follows (Zenner et al., 2014):

- Breath awareness ($N = 24$)
- Working with thoughts and emotions ($N = 21$)
- Psycho-education ($N = 20$)
- Awareness of senses and practices of daily life ($N = 20$)
- Group discussion ($N = 18$)
- Body scan ($N = 14$)
- Home practice ($N = 12$)
- Kindness practice ($N = 11$)
- Body practices (e.g., yoga; $N = 6$)
- Mindful movement ($N = 5$)
- Additional material ($N = 10$)

Zenner et al. (2014) conducted a study quality assessment. Overall, 19 of the 24 studies used a control design and five used a pre/post design. Randomized designs were used in 10 studies in which mindfulness training was offered as an alternative to extracurricular activities at school (Zenner et al., 2014). One study used a matched control group. Eight of the studies used a quasi-experimental design teaching mindfulness in a classroom setting with another parallel class serving as control, and in one study reading training took place at the same intensity level (Zenner et al., 2014). Allocation to mindfulness or control was mainly decided upon by department heads and classroom teachers (Zenner et al., 2014). Four of the studies randomly assigned mindfulness interventions to classes or schools. Five of the studies collected follow-up data (Zenner et al., 2014).

Zenner et al. (2014) reported that those studies that reported feasibility data described how the mindfulness program was integrated into the school routine. The researchers reported collecting these data through questionnaires, focus groups, or interviews. About one third of the studies reported acceptability data (Zenner et al., 2014). Results yielded from the interviews and focus groups (including both teachers and students) indicated positive experiences. Large percentages (greater than 80%) of students would recommend the training to others, found the program extremely useful, and rated the program as satisfying. Over three fourths of the students said they would like the program to continue and wished it had lasted longer. The programs that included a home practice found that about one third of students practiced at least three times a week and two thirds practiced once a week or less (Zenner et al., 2014).

Zenner et al. (2014) found that overall effect sizes were Hedge's $g = 0.40$ among groups and $g = 0.41$ within groups ($p < .0001$). The significant between-group effect sizes for domains were: cognitive performance $g = 0.80$, stress $g = 0.39$, and resilience $g = 0.36$ (all $p < .05$). Of note, both emotional problems ($g = 0.19$) and third-person ratings ($g = 0.25$) were found to be not significant. The authors concluded that mindfulness-based interventions in children and youth hold promise (Zenner et al., 2014). Further, Zenner et al. (2014) also concluded that mindfulness interventions for children and youth might hold the most promise in relation to improving resilience to stress and cognitive performance. The authors noted that there were several limitations to their study. First, Zenner et al. (2014) reported that the diversity of study samples, variety in implementation and exercises, and wide range of instruments should be explored with careful and discerned investigation of data. Second, Zenner et al. (2014) indicated that they found great heterogeneity across studies with many studies underpowered. Last, the authors also reflected on the challenging nature of researching mindfulness in a school setting.

Mindfulness Interventions With Youth

Zoogman, Goldberg, Hoyt, and Miller (2015) conducted a meta-analysis on mindfulness interventions on youth. This analysis included those studies done outside of the school setting. Overall, they included 20 quantitative studies in the analyses. The age range was 6 to 21 years old. Three studies used MBSR, three used MBCT for children, five used one component of MBSR, and nine used another type of mindfulness intervention (Zoogman et al., 2015). Programs ranged from 4 to 24 weeks, with a majority of the programs running 8 to 12 weeks in length.

Overall, mindfulness interventions with youth were found to be helpful and not to carry iatrogenic harm, with the primary omnibus effect size (*del*) in the small to moderate range (0.23, $p < .0001$), indicating the superiority of mindfulness treatments over active control comparison conditions (Zoogman et al., 2015). Of note, *del* is a measure of the difference in pre-/post-effect sizes among groups (Zoogman et al., 2015). A significantly larger effect size was found on psychological symptoms (e.g., anxiety and depression) compared to other dependent variable types (0.37 vs. 0.21, $p = .028$), and for studies drawn from clinical samples compared to non-clinical samples (0.50 vs. 0.20, $p = .024$). Mindfulness appears to be a promising intervention modality for youth. Authors report that as of 2011, the majority of studies on mindfulness with youth engage generally healthy participants recruited from schools (Zoogman et al., 2015).

Meditation Interventions in Schools

In a review of meditation interventions in schools, Waters, Barsky, Ridd, and Allen (2015) reviewed evidence from 15 peer-reviewed studies with respect to three student outcomes: well-being, social competence, and academic achievement. The researchers calculated 76 effect sizes, with 1,797 participants. Overall, 61% of findings were statistically significant, with 76% having small effects, 24% medium effects, and 9% large effects. The type of meditation program mattered. Transcendental meditation programs (i.e., silently repeating a word or mantra to achieve a meditative state, refocusing when distracted) had a higher percentage of significant effects than mindfulness-based and other types of meditation programs (e.g., loving-kindness, Zen, Yoga Nidra; Waters et al., 2015). Program elements such as duration, frequency of practice and type of instructor influenced student outcomes (Waters et al., 2015). Setting may also play a role. A conceptual model is put forward positing that meditation positively influences student success by increasing cognitive functioning and by increasing emotional regulation (Waters et al., 2015).

School Faculty and Staff

Weare (2013) describes the benefit of mindfulness implementation in schools for faculty and staff. Given the requirement for those who teach mindfulness to be experienced and regular practitioners, a desire to teach mindfulness to students often supports an ongoing practice or initiates a practice. Weare (2013) reports that teachers experience improvements in physical and mental health and reductions in burnout as they integrate mindfulness into their lives and classrooms. She cites research on teachers in training and outcomes of mindfulness education programs for teachers (Weare, 2013). Teaching mindfulness in your school and/or your classroom will likely help you feel better and experience less burnout.

Can Mindfulness Do Harm?

In general, mindfulness-based studies are believed to be salutogenic. That is, they promote health and come with little if any risk. However, there is currently no conclusive body of evidence to confirm this is the case. To answer this question, Dobkin, Irving, and Amar (2012) reviewed literature pertaining to attrition and adverse effects following participation in MBSR and MSCT. Overall, after their extensive review of programs, the authors reported that they could not provide an empirically based answer to the question. The authors hypothesize that those who may not benefit from programs like MBCT may be more likely to drop out. Dropping out was associated with history of suicide, chronic pain, higher obsessive-compulsive scores, brooding, cognitive and emotional reactivity, stress, and a number of medical symptoms (Dobkin et al., 2012). They also noted that there are some case studies of individuals who manifested various mental health issues after meditation experiences; however, details on this were lacking.

In a qualitative study of 30 male participants (aged 20 to 60-plus), with experience in meditation ranging from 1 to 20 or more years, Lomas, Cartwright, Edginton, and Ridge (2015) found that along with outcomes associated with well-being, meditation was also associated with substantial difficulties. Specifically, four main problems were uncovered, listed in order of increasing severity: Meditation was a challenging skill to learn and practice (e.g., feeling trapped, self-doubt, ongoing struggle, inattention, back pain, early attempts very challenging, a skill that needed to be constantly practiced); participants were met with troubling thoughts and feelings that were difficult to manage (e.g., engagement with troubling thoughts, stuck in negative quality of thoughts, surprise at uncovered emotions); meditation reportedly worsened mental health issues (e.g., depression, anxiety, increases awareness of sensitivity); and in a few cases, meditation was associated with psychotic episodes (e.g., alienation, fixation on extreme emotions; Lomas et al., 2015). It is important to note that the authors placed these negative experiences within the context of the meditators reporting a majority (75%) of positive experience and outcomes. Further, participants reported that experiencing negative emotions, thoughts, and discomfort seems to be part of the process of connecting with self and growth (Lomas et al., 2015).

These findings reported among adult populations shed light on the risks and negative experiences that may arise for some. More research is needed exploring risk among children and adolescents with attention to high-risk groups detailing the type of meditation, dosage, and context of practice. Dobkin et al. (2012) suggest the following:

• Screen potential participants for psychiatric problems, addiction, and posttraumatic stress disorder.
• Ensure that those with psychopathology (e.g., anxiety or mood disorder) are being treated appropriately by a qualified mental health professional.

- Prime participants with regard to the type of commitment needed, what the program will be like, and the homework that is required.
- Inform participants of the potential challenging nature of the practice and how to respond when disconcerting emotions or thoughts arise.
- Establish a referral system for participants who experience emotional or psychiatric problems.
- Emphasize that participants should prioritize well-being in both the present moment and long term, giving permission and time for students to take breaks and check in with instructors.

Aggregated Research

Generally, aggregated research on mindfulness in schools suggests that mindfulness helps students in schools. The results are mild to moderate and may matter most for those students, teachers, and schools that are struggling. Meditation and mindfulness techniques appear to help both cognitive functioning and stress management. There is also some evidence that mindfulness helps with self-regulation and, particularly, emotion regulation. Many studies rely on self-report and teacher report. Few use direct measures of behavior or physiological measures. Many studies self-describe as pilot and/or feasibility studies. Currently, researchers believe that the key mechanisms of mindfulness are focused attention, decentering (i.e., a self-reflective stance toward inner and outer experiences), and emotion regulation (Zoogman et al., 2015). Remember that many studies are at a lower quality level and school personnel should read carefully the studies they use to make decisions and those used to support packaged programs for schools.

EARLY MINDFULNESS PROGRAMS

Mindfulness programs were originally implemented among adult populations. The first empirically supported programs were utilized to support patients who were not responsive to typical Western medical and psychological approaches. Early mindfulness programs include MBSR, DBT, MBCT, and ACT. Across studies the main outcomes include increased subjective well-being, reduced psychological symptoms and emotional reactivity, and improved behavioral regulation (Cook-Cottone, 2015; Keng, Smoski, & Robins, 2011). Many of the current school-based and youth programs have been inspired by these early programs (Obrien, Larson, & Murrell, 2008; Zoogman et al., 2015).

Mindfulness-Based Stress Reduction (MBSR)

MBSR was the first mindfulness-based protocol (Black, 2014; Cook-Cottone, 2015; Obrien et al., 2008; Shapiro & Carlson, 2009; Zoogman et al., 2014). It was developed by John Kabat-Zinn in 1979 specific to a behavioral medicine setting to help patients with chronic pain and stress (Baer & Krietemeyer, 2006; Black, 2014; Cook-Cottone, 2015; Felver, Doerner, Jones, Kay, & Merrell, 2013; Shapiro & Carlson, 2009; Zoogman et al., 2014). Briefly, MBSR is a standardized protocol with a duration of 8 weeks with weekly sessions from 2.5 to 3.0 hours with an all-day intensive occurring on the sixth week (Baer & Krietemeyer, 2006; Black,

2014; Cook-Cottone, 2015; Felver et al., 2013; Shapiro & Carlson, 2009; Zoogman et al., 2014). Participants are asked to complete extensive home practice of at least 45 minutes a day at least 6 days a week (Baer & Krietemeyer, 2006). Program content is, in part, psycho-educational covering education on stress and its effects. There is also an experiential component with time devoted to mindfulness exercises and processing these experiences in a group format (Baer & Krietemeyer, 2006; Cook-Cottone, 2015). Experiential activities include formal and informal mindfulness practices such as the body scan, mindful eating, sitting meditation, hatha yoga, walking meditation, and incorporating mindfulness into daily life (Baer & Krietemeyer, 2006; Cook-Cottone, 2015; Felver et al., 2013; Shapiro & Carlson, 2009). For training, resources, and further information on MBSR, go to the Center for Mindfulness in Medicine, Health-care and Society at the University at Massachusetts Medical School (www.umassmed.edu/cfm/stress-reduction/). For an easy to read and useful resource on specific techniques see *The Relaxation and Stress Reduction Workbook,* Sixth Edition, by Davis, Eshelman, and McKay (2008).

Mindfulness-Based Cognitive Therapy

Now over 20 years in existence, MBCT is considered to be almost mainstream. It was originally developed to prevent the relapse of major depression (Obrien et al., 2008; Zoogman et al., 2014). It is based on MBSR and utilizes many of its components including mindful eating, body scan, sitting meditation, yoga, walking meditation, and informal daily mindful practices (Baer & Krietemeyer, 2006; Cook-Cottone, 2015; Felver et al., 2013; Obrien et al., 2008; Shapiro & Carlson, 2009). Like MBSR, MBCT includes the observing of pleasant and unpleasant events (Baer & Krietemeyer, 2006; Cook-Cottone, 2015). The didactic components of MBCT addresses depressive symptoms rather than stress (Baer & Krietemeyer, 2006; Felver et al., 2013; Obrien et al., 2008). Specifically, MBCT utilizes cognitive techniques to disrupt depressive thought patterns (Zoogman et al., 2014). As in MBSR, homework and group discussions are critical factors in implementation. The format is a group-based, 8-week intervention delivered in 2-hour weekly sessions (Cook-Cottone, 2015; Shapiro & Carlson, 2009; Zoogman et al., 2014).

There are added components to the MBCT protocol. For example, participants are taught to ask themselves, "What is my experience right now?" (Baer & Krietemeyer, 2006, p. 14). They are encouraged to scan their bodies and minds for thoughts, sense impressions, and feelings and to experience and accept them without judgment (Baer & Krietemeyer, 2006; Shapiro & Carlson, 2009; Zoogman et al., 2014). Next, patients are asked to move their awareness to their breath and then to the whole body. The breathing space is designed to increase awareness and give space for new behavioral choices rather than default to maladaptive, automatic responses (Baer & Krietemeyer, 2006; Zoogman et al., 2014). Addressing cognitive aspects of the treatment, the MBCT protocol includes thoughts and feelings exercise, discussion of automatic thoughts, de-centering work, and an exercise that focuses on mood, thoughts, and alternative viewpoints (Baer & Krietemeyer, 2006; Cook-Cottone, 2015; Zoogman et al., 2014). Weare (2013) describes several adaptions for children and adolescents yielding reduced anxiety, depression, somatic distress, problem behaviors, and improved happiness, sleep quality, self-esteem, academic performance, attention, self-regulation, and social skills. For more on MBCT, see Baer's (2006) *Mindfulness-Based Treatment Approaches: A Clinician's Guide to Evidence-Base and Applications.* For more on MBCT resources, and training go to mbct.com.

Dialectic Behavioral Therapy

DBT was developed by Marsha Linehan for patients with borderline personality disorder (BPD; Linehan, 1993; Obrien et al., 2008). The term "dialectic" refers to the central tenet of the therapy—an emphasis on balance and integration of opposing ideas such as acceptance and change (Baer & Krietemeyer, 2006; Cook-Cottone, 2015; Obrien et al., 2008). Specifically, DBT provides psychosocial skills training in four modules: core mindfulness skills, interpersonal effectiveness skills, emotional regulations skills, and distress tolerance skills (Linehan, 1993). The core mindfulness skills module includes didactic information that provides a rationale for practicing mindfulness and controlling attention (Baer & Krietemeyer, 2006; Cook-Cottone, 2015). Linehan (1993) refers to the integration of the cognitive (i.e., reasonable) mind and the emotional mind as *wise mind*. The specific skills include teaching patients what to do when being mindful (i.e., observe, describe, and participate [attend to activity in the present moment]; Linehan, 1993). Patients are all taught how to be mindful (i.e., nonjudgmentally, one-mindfully, and effectively; Linehan, 1993). The emotional regulation and distress tolerance modules of DBT also integrate mindfulness skills (Baer & Krietemeyer, 2006). Within the distress tolerance module, patients are taught to notice the rising and passing away of distressful or uncomfortable feelings or urges (Linehan, 1993). Patients are taught other skills such as distraction and breath work to assist in tolerating distress (Obrien et al., 2008). There are many adapted manuals for DBT. See Fleischhaker et al. (2011) for a description of a DBT adaption for adolescents (DBT-A). For a detailed description of DBT see *Skills Training Manual for Treating Borderline Personality Disorder* (Linehan, 1993) and for more on DBT training, and resources, go to the Linehan Institute at behavioraltech.org/index.cfm.

Acceptance and Commitment Therapy

ACT is viewed as a general approach to psychotherapy designed to increase psychological flexibility in terms of an individual's current context (Baer & Krietemeyer, 2006; Felver et al., 2013; Obrien et al., 2008; Wilson, Schnetzer, Flynn, & Kurz, 2012). Psychological flexibility has been defined as "the willingness to accept all aspects of one's experience without engaging in unnecessary avoidance behaviors, when doing so serves the development of patterns of values-congruent activity" (Wilson et al., 2012, p. 27). Specifically, ACT addresses mindfulness and acceptance skills and behavioral changes needed to help patients engage in a life that is vital and meaningful (Baer & Krietemeyer, 2006; Obrien et al., 2008).

Central to ACT is the negotiation of experiential avoidance of feelings, sensations, cognitions, or urges (Baer & Krietemeyer, 2006; Cook-Cottone, 2015; Felver et al., 2013). Present moment awareness is encouraged and experiential avoidance is seen as a root cause of many forms of psychopathology (Baer & Krietemeyer, 2006; Cook-Cottone, 2015; Obrien et al., 2008). Present moment awareness in ACT is consistent with present moment awareness activities described throughout this text. Specifically, ACT involves a series of mindfulness activities that encourage observation of present moment experience, accompanying internal and external sensations, labeling experiences without judgment or evaluation, and acceptance (Baer & Krietemeyer, 2006; Cook-Cottone, 2015). Values and committed action is a feature unique to ACT (Baer & Krietemeyer, 2006). The ACT protocol includes activities that help patients address goals and values related to areas of their lives (e.g., career, relationships, personal growth, and health; Baer & Krietemeyer, 2006). Goals and values are used to organize intentions and behaviors around meaning (Baer & Krietemeyer, 2006). Obrien et al. (2008) suggest that ACT may be especially suited for children since it relies so heavily on experiential exercise and metaphors much like the teaching methods used in educational settings. For a text on ACT for children and adolescents, see Greco and Hayes (2008) *Acceptance and Mindfulness Treatments for Children and Adolescents: A Practitioner's Guide.*

MINDFULNESS PROGRAMS FOR SCHOOLS

During the preparation of this book, three school psychology students engaged in an extensive search for all the mindfulness-based programs for schools (thank you to Heather Cahill, Jillian Cherry, and Rebeccah Sivecz for your hard work). They used academic search tools and web-based search tools in an effort to provide the extant information on the mindfulness programs available. I have contributed to their work by integrating their research and my own search to present what we know to date. What we found was a wide variety of programs, some with a large body of research specifically on the program and others reported to be based on research with no specific program research reported or found. Often self-described, research-based programs provide references and citations that refer to research done on other mindfulness programs or on components of the program (e.g., mindfulness meditation, loving-kindness meditation, or mindful eating). In this section I provide descriptions of a few high-quality programs to give a sense of what is available for your school. I included web and/or contact information, and a brief description of the research base associated with the program. Please note, this is not an exhaustive list of all of the research on each program; rather, key articles are highlighted. The programs are presented in alphabetical order by name of the program. At the end of the chapter, I have provided a list of additional programs we found with their web information as a resource.

CARE for Teachers

Cultivating Awareness and Resilience in Education (CARE) is a professional development program designed to reduce stress and improve teachers' performance (Jennings, Snowberg, Coccia, & Greenberg, 2011; Weare, 2013). The program was developed by the Garrison Institute (www.garrisoninstitute.org) to meet the specific needs of K–12 teachers by Richard C. Brown, Patricia Jennings, Christa Turksma, and Kari Snowberg. That is, the program strives to improve teachers' overall well-being and their effectiveness in providing support for students (Weare, 2013). The CARE intervention utilizes three primary instructional components: (a) emotional skills, (b) mindfulness and stress reduction practices, and (c) listening and compassion exercises (Jennings, 2011). According to the program developers, the CARE for Teachers program is based upon current research on the neuroscience of emotion. That is, CARE introduces emotion skills instruction to promote understanding, recognition, and regulation of emotion (Jennings, 2011). The program introduces basic mindfulness activities (e.g., short periods of silent reflection, mindful listening) to reduce stress and to promote awareness and presence applied to teaching. The program also includes activities that demonstrate how to bring mindfulness to challenging situations teachers often encounter (Jennings, 2011). The CARE program is presented in four day-long sessions spread out over 4 to 5 weeks. It includes intersession coaching via phone and Internet to support teachers' practice and application of new skills. The program involves a blend of didactic instruction and experiential activities, including time for reflection and discussion. CARE for Teachers is also offered annually as a 5-day summer retreat at the Garrison Institute (www.care4teachers.com). Program developers report that teachers who have completed the program say they found it relaxing, enjoyable, and inspiring). According to the program developers, the CARE curriculum has been piloted in several sites across the United States—Colorado, California, Pennsylvania, and New York.

Published articles and chapters include Jennings et al. (2011), Jennings (2011), Schussler, Jennings, Sharp, and Frank (2015), and Jennings, Frank, Snowberg, Coccia, and Greenberg (2013). The Jennings et al. (2011) paper reviews two pilot studies examining program feasibility and attractiveness and preliminary evidence of efficacy. In study 1 researchers assessed educators from a high-poverty urban setting ($n = 31$) and in study 2 researchers worked with student teachers and 10 of their mentors working in a suburban/semi-rural setting ($n = 43$) with both treatment and control groups. The sample sizes were small. Researchers found that while urban educators showed significant pre/post improvements in mindfulness and time urgency, the other sample (i.e., suburban/semi-rural) did not. Researchers concluded that these findings suggest that CARE may be more effective in supporting teachers working in high-risk settings (Jennings et al., 2011).

Jennings et al. (2013) report on a RCT that examined CARE program efficacy and acceptability among a sample of 50 teachers randomly assigned to CARE or a waitlist control condition. Participants completed a battery of self-report measures at pre- and postintervention to assess the impact of the CARE program on general well-being, efficacy, burnout/time pressure, and mindfulness (Jennings et al., 2013). In addition, participants in the CARE group completed an evaluation of the program after completing the intervention (Jennings et al., 2013). To analyze the data, ANCOVAs were computed between the CARE group and control group for each outcome, and the pretest scores served as a covariate (Jennings et al., 2013). Overall, researchers found that participation in the CARE program resulted in significant improvements in teacher well-being, efficacy, burnout/time-related stress, and mindfulness when compared with controls (Jennings et al., 2013). Evaluation data showed that teachers viewed CARE as a feasible, acceptable, and effective method for reducing stress and improving performance. Overall, the researchers concluded that the CARE program has promise to support teachers working in challenging settings and can consequently improve classroom environments (Jennings et al., 2013).

Qualitative findings were similar in terms of the program's ability to support teachers (Schussler et al., 2015). Results suggest that participants (i.e., teachers) developed greater self-awareness, including somatic awareness and the need to practice self-care (Schussler et al., 2015). Participants also reportedly improved their ability to become less emotionally reactive. However, the authors noted that the participants were less likely to explicitly articulate an improvement in their teaching efficacy (Schussler et al., 2015).

Inner Kids Program

The Inner Kids program was developed by Susan Kaiser Greenland for students in Pre-K to 12th grade (Greenberg & Harris, 2012; Weare, 2013; Zoogman et al., 2014). Kaiser calls mindfulness the New ABCs: Attention, Balance, and Compassion. Aligned with the Mindful and Yogic Self as Effective Learner (MY-SEL) model (see Chapters 1, 2, and 3 of this text), the new ABCs are taught via games, activities, instruction, and sharing to develop: (a) awareness of inner experience (awareness of thoughts, emotions, and physical sensations); (b) awareness of outer experience (awareness of other people, places, and things); and (c) awareness of both together without blending the two (www.susankaisergreenland.com/inner-kids.html). The program can be found at www.susankaisergreenland.com/inner-kids.html. Greenland is author of *The Mindful Child: How to Help Your Kid Manage Stress and Become Happier, Kinder, and More Compassionate*, a text for parents and professionals that teaches techniques of mindful awareness to children and teens (Greenland, 2010). It includes simple activities for families that help children and parents become more mindful and develop confidence, concentration, and an ability to regulate their emotions. Many of these techniques were described in the formal and informal chapters of this book (Chapters 6 and 7, respectively).

The Inner Kids program emphasizes paying attention to inner and outer experiences with compassion (Greenberg & Harris, 2012; Weare, 2013; Zoogman et al., 2014). Attention, balance, and compassion are taught through games, activities, instruction, and sharing. The program length and frequency varies based on the age of the students. For Pre-K through third grade, students meet twice a week for 8 weeks, in one-half hour sessions. Older students meet once a week for 10 to 12 weeks, in 45-minute sessions. The program can be offered during the school day, after the school day, or in a sleep-away camp. It has been taught in one or more classrooms in Los Angeles schools every year between 2000 and 2009 (www.susankaisergreenland.com/inner-kids.html). Each session has three sections: beginning (i.e., introspective period, sitting practice), middle (i.e., games and activities that address the themes for the week [e.g., breath awareness]), and end (i.e., inspective period, lying down and friend wishes practice for kindness and compassion). Over the 8- to 12-week course, the length of the beginning and end sections increases (www.susankaisergreenland.com/inner-kids.html).

Training for this program consists of two weekend residential retreats in Santa Barbara, California, with instruction from a core faculty, periodic webcasts and office hours, self-paced online study, small group interaction online, and meditation instruction with online practice opportunities (www.susankaisergreenland.com/inner-kids.html). Upon completion of the training program, teachers receive a diploma certifying that they completed Inner Kids Level 1 training, which comes with peer support and training material benefits. A copy of *The Mindful Child* text is included with the training program.

A school-based version of the Inner Kids program was evaluated in a randomized control study of 64 second- and third-grade children ages 7 to 9 years (Flook et al., 2010). The program was delivered for 30 minutes, twice per week, for 8 weeks (Flook et al., 2010). Before and following the intervention, teachers and parents completed questionnaires assessing the children's executive function (EF; Flook et al., 2010). Multivariate analysis of covariance on teacher and parent reports of students' EF indicated an interaction effect baseline EF score and group status on posttest EF (Flook et al., 2010). That is, researchers found that students in the group that received mindful awareness training (Inner Kids) who were less well regulated showed greater improvement in EF compared with controls (Flook et al., 2010). As well, researchers found that students who started the Inner Kids program with poor EF showed gains in behavioral regulation, metacognition, and overall global executive control (Flook et al., 2010). As seen in other research studies, students who are struggling frequently show the greatest improvements. In this case, results indicate a stronger effect of mindful awareness training on children with EF difficulties (Flook et al., 2010). Finally, the authors hypothesize that both the teachers' and parents' reported changes suggest that improvements in children's behavioral regulation was generalized across settings (Flook et al., 2010).

Learning to BREATHE (L2B)

L2B is a mindfulness-based curriculum created for classroom or group settings based on MBSR (Greenberg & Harris, 2012; Weare, 2013). The L2B group defines mindfulness as the practice of becoming aware of one's present-moment experience with compassion and openness as a basis for wise action (learning2breathe.org; Greenberg & Harris, 2012). This curriculum is intended to strengthen attention and emotion regulation, cultivate wholesome emotions such as gratitude and compassion, expand the repertoire of stress management skills, and help students integrate mindfulness into daily life (learning2breathe .org). According to the program developers, each lesson includes age-appropriate discussion, activities, and opportunities to practice mindfulness in a group setting (learning-2breathe.org). The L2B curriculum has been recognized in the 2015 CASEL (Collaborative for Academic, Social, and Emotional Learning).

The curriculum is comprised of six themes built around the acronym BREATHE (Broderick, 2013). The *B* represents listening to the body, which is an introduction to mindful awareness of physical sensations. The *R* represents reflections, the idea that thoughts are just thoughts. Students discuss and practice so that they can explore automatic self-talk and mindfulness as an antidote. The *E* represents surfing the wave of emotions (Broderick, 2013). The content in this area is done in two parts. First, it involves discussion and practice to explore emotions and their interconnection with thoughts and bodily sensations. Second, students discuss and practice in order to uncover and learn how to handle emotion-triggered responses and coping behaviors (Broderick, 2013). The *A* represents attention to body sensations, thoughts, and emotions as the foundation of effective stress management. The content includes discussion and practice to understand stress and its effects. The *T* represents taking things as they are or a nonjudgmental approach to daily life stressors (Broderick, 2013). The content includes discussion and practice of loving-kindness to increase a sense of social responsibility and connectedness to others. The *H* reflects healthy mind habits leading to reduced stress and stronger inner power. Here the content involves an overview of previous sessions and discussion about the use of mindfulness in daily life. Last, the *E* reflects the overall program theme—empowerment (Broderick, 2013). The curriculum can be purchased: *Learning to BREATHE: A Mindfulness Curriculum for Adolescents to Cultivate Emotion Regulation, Attention, and Performance* (Broderick, 2013).

Teachers can choose to deliver the curriculum in 6, 12, 18, or more sessions. Included in the curriculum are the main messages and sample teacher narratives for both 6- and 18-session versions. There are in-depth descriptions of group activities, in-class mindfulness practice scripts, suggested home practices, links to state and national assessment standards, sample outcome assessments, program process evaluation, teacher resources about mindfulness, background information on stress processes and adolescent development, a message to mindfulness teachers, four practice audio files, posters, wallet cards, and workbook pages (can be downloaded and personalized). There are three training opportunities offered including an introduction workshop, a 2-day workshop, and a 3-day intensive.

There have been several studies conducted on the curriculum. The latest published study was conducted by Bluth et al. (2016). Bluth et al. (2016) conducted a randomized, school-based pilot study of L2B, with ethnically diverse at-risk adolescents. Twenty-seven students were randomly assigned to a mindfulness or substance abuse control class that met for 50 minutes, once a week, over one school semester (Bluth et al., 2016). The authors reported that adjustments were made to increase acceptability of the mindfulness class, including enhanced instructor engagement in school activities (Bluth et al., 2016). At post-test, reductions in depression were seen for students in the mindfulness class compared to controls. Interestingly, the authors reported that, initially, the students' perceived credibility of the mindfulness class was lower than that of the substance abuse class (Bluth et al., 2016). Remarkably, over the course of the semester, perceived credibility of the mindfulness class increased while that of the substance abuse class decreased (Bluth et al., 2016). Acceptability was measured qualitatively. This assessment revealed that the mindfulness class reportedly helped students relieve stress and that students favored continuing the class (Bluth et al., 2016).

In 2013, Metz et al. published quasi-experimental pretest/posttest comparison group design to study L2B. Researchers utilized a convenience sample of students attending two public high schools matched on school-level demographics in the same Eastern suburban school district (Metz et al., 2013). The study included 216 regular education public high school students participating in the program or instruction-as-usual comparison condition students (Metz et al., 2013). According to the authors, program participants reported statistically lower levels of perceived stress and psychosomatic complaints and higher levels of efficacy in affective regulation (Metz et al., 2013). Program participants also demonstrated statistically larger gains in emotion regulation skills (e.g., emotional awareness, access to regulation strategies, and emotional clarity; Metz et al., 2013). More research on L2B can be found at learning2breathe.org/curriculum/research.

Mindfulness in Schools Program

The Mindfulness in Schools Program (MiSP) curriculum is a set of nine scripted lessons tailored to secondary schools, supported by tailored teacher training (Kuyken et al., 2013; Lawlor, 2014; Weare, 2013). The lessons are designed to teach mindfulness or "learning to direct attention to immediate experience, moment by moment, with open-minded curiosity and acceptance" (Kuyken et al., 2013, p. 2). The program teaches new skills in a practical way through the practice of mindfulness and applications in everyday life (Kuyken et al., 2013). The MiSP program purports to be drawn from MBSR and MBCT. The main teaching principles include explicit teaching of skills and attitudes; shortening and adapting mindfulness lessons for students; using age-appropriate, interactive, and experienced teaching methods; providing age-appropriate resources that bring mindfulness to life (such as a book, downloadable audio files); intensive and focused teacher education that enhances teachers' effectiveness and well-being; and program implementation that attends to implementation fidelity (i.e., a manual and script; Kuyken et al., 2013).

The program's webpage is mindfulnessinschools.org. The co-founders are Richard Burnett and Chris Cullen. There are two levels of curricula: .b (dot be) and Paws b. Specifically, .b is a 10-week course for ages 11 to 18 delivered in the classroom or small groups in other youth-related settings. The name refers to the process—stop, breathe, and be (Lawlor, 2014). The lessons include a brief presentation by the teacher with visuals, film, sound (audio), practical exercises, and demonstrations. The 10 lessons include:

- An Introduction to Mindfulness
- Playing Attention: Training the Muscle of Your Mind
- Taming the Animal Mind: Cultivating Curiosity and Kindness
- Recognizing Worry: Noticing How Your Mind Plays Tricks on You
- Being Here Now: From Reacting to Responding
- Moving Mindfully
- Stepping Back: Watching the Thought-Traffic of Your Mind
- Befriending the Difficult
- Taking in the Good: Being Present With Your Heart
- Pulling It All Together

Paws b is a program for children ages 7 to 11. It consists of either six 1-hour lessons or 12 30-minute lessons taught by school teachers or by an external Paws b teacher. The curriculum contains PowerPoint lessons with film clips, short meditation practices, discussion and exploration of experiences, and home practice encouragement and support. It is related to some other aspects of the school curriculum such as music, sports, art, drama, how to be mindful lining up to come into a classroom. Tabitha Sawyer's, co-creator of Paws b, TED Talk can be found here youtu.be/bT5UFU9ZGnI. She gives a background and overview of what the program does.

There are several steps to bring the MiSP program to your schools. First, the school staff learns mindfulness via an 8-week course, taught by a MiSP instructor—school staff learns about mindfulness before learning how to teach the students. Next, the teachers learn how to teach the students. The training is 3 days for Paws b and 4 days for the .b curriculum. In order to train to be a MiSP teacher, you must complete the 8-week mindfulness course (or an equivalent training such as MBSR or MBCT) and then practice mindfulness on a regular basis for at least 6 months (mindfulnessinschools.org). The training includes all materials necessary to teach the curriculum: student booklets; the how to teach .b/Paws b; teacher's notes on each lesson; PowerPoint slideshow of each lesson; audio and video files; and a period of membership in the MiSP Teachers' Network. Note, materials are not sold—you must be trained in order to receive the curriculum.

In a study of 522 students aged 12 to 16 across 12 secondary schools, Kuyken et al. (2013) found that overall rates of acceptability were high compared to controls (usual school curriculum). At post intervention, students who participated in the intervention reported significantly fewer depressive symptoms. Interestingly, at follow-up, intervention students showed continued fewer depressive symptoms, lower stress, and greater well-being. Aligned with what we know from other research, the students who practiced mindfulness skills experienced better well-being and less stress at the 3-month follow-up (Kuyken et al., 2013).

Mindful Schools

Mindful Schools is an organization that offers a series of courses and year-long certification designed for those who are interested in integrating mindfulness with youth education (www.mindfulschools.org). Content includes the basics of mindfulness meditation; how to work with thinking that arises while practicing mindfulness; techniques for meeting and navigating intense emotions; and practices that cultivate positive states of mind such as gratitude, kindness, joy, and compassion (www.mindfulschools.org). Coursework is online with continuing education units available for mental health professionals. The program offers a K–5 curriculum (30 modules for ages 5–12), a middle and high school curriculum (25 modules for ages 12–17), student workbooks, a manual on facilitation and classroom management, summaries of neuroscience concepts, and program evaluation tools. This certification program is designed for educators interested in deepening their personal practice and playing an active role as a mindful leader in their school community.

The research on this program includes one small published pilot study and a larger unpublished program report. In the smaller 2010 pilot study, Liehr and Diaz (2010) found that the Mindful Schools elementary grades curriculum (studies on ages 8–11) reduced depressive symptoms among minority children. Researchers randomized 18 minority children at a summer camp to either mindfulness or health education (Liehr & Diaz, 2010). An instructor led ten 15-minute lessons from the Mindful Schools curriculum. The mindfulness group showed significantly more reduction in depressive symptoms than the control group. Anxiety results were in the same direction but not significant ($p = .07$).

Mindful Schools partnered with the University of California, Davis, to conduct a randomized-controlled study involving 937 children and 47 teachers in three Oakland public elementary schools (Smith, Guzman-Alvarez, Westover, Keller, & Fuller, 2012). The Mindful Schools curriculum was taught to educators (Smith et al., 2012). The in-class program included 15 lessons, lasting 15 minutes, taught two to three times per week over 6 weeks. Content included mindful breathing, listening, test-taking, and empathy. The program report indicated that the intervention produced statistically significant improvements in paying attention and participation in class activities versus the control group. The full program report is available at www.mindfulschools.org/pdf/Mindful-Schools-Study-Highlights.pdf.

Other Mindfulness Program for Schools

The following table provides an additional reference list of mindfulness programs for schools (see Table 8.1). As you research programs that might work for your district, look carefully at the research considerations listed at the beginning of this chapter. Think about acceptability and feasibility. Look at costs and what resources you might have to adapt or create your own program using a combination of formal and informal techniques.

TABLE 8.1 Additional Mindfulness Programs for Schools and Youth

PROGRAM	WEBPAGE	BRIEF DESCRIPTION
Attention Academy Program Intervention	www.stressbeaters.com/mbsr-education/the-attention-academy-program/	*The Attention Academy*® Program offers classes, workshops, and seminars on developing attention skills for students, teachers, and parents. The program mixes mindfulness and relaxation. The mission of *The Attention Academy*® Program is to help students improve their quality of life through practicing mindfulness. The goal of the program is to help students learn to (a) increase their attention to the present experience, (b) approach each experience without judgment, and (c) view *each* experience as novel and new with a "beginner's eye." There is some research support (Weare, 2013).
Growing Minds	www.growingmindstoday.com/-our-curriculum.html	The Growing Minds curricula is rooted in the areas of self-awareness, self-management, social awareness, relationship skills, and responsible decision-making. Lessons are broken into themes: sustained attention, self-awareness and impulse control, and social awareness and relationship skills.
Inward Bound Mindfulness Education	ibme.info/	A nonprofit that offers in-depth mindfulness programming for young adults, adolescents, and the parents and professionals who support them. The program develops self-awareness, compassion, and ethical decision-making, and empowers participants to apply these skills in improving their lives and communities. They offer staff training prior to and experiential training during retreat. Teen retreats are held in the summer and during school breaks; student retreats are held during the school year.
Lineage Project	www.lineageproject.org	The Lineage Project offers mindfulness practices for youth at risk. The program utilizes yoga and meditation techniques with disenfranchised youth in New York City to help break the cycle of poverty, violence, and incarceration. Workshops and training are offered.
Mind Body Awareness Project	www.mbaproject.org/about-mindfulness-3/our-curricula/	This is a rehabilitation program designed to meet the social and emotional needs of highly at-risk youth. The curriculum utilizes a universal class structure that includes periods of check-ins, meditation practice, and group discussion.

(continued)

TABLE 8.1 Additional Mindfulness Programs for Schools and Youth (*continued*)

PROGRAM	WEBPAGE	BRIEF DESCRIPTION
Mindful Life	mindfullifetoday.com/	Mindful Life is a weekly wellness program for individual teachers offering a six-module online training program; 1-day intensive retreat; and 60-minute workshop. The curriculum includes: scripts for lessons, a workbook, and classroom and extended curriculum for Pre-K to eighth grade.
Mindfulness Without Borders	mindfulnesswithoutborders .org/our-programs/ youth-education/	Mindfulness Without Borders offers educational programs in mindfulness-based social and emotional learning that help individuals flourish socially, emotionally, academically, and professionally. Creates space for personal reflection and the development of human potential by nurturing self-awareness, healthy social and emotional behavior, and important life skills. It includes workshops and continuing education.
MindUP	thehawnfoundation.org/ mindup/	MindUP combines mindfulness, SEL, and positive psychology, and draws from neuroscience (Lawlor, 2014; Weare, 2013). The program teaches social and emotional learning skills that link cognitive neuroscience, positive psychology, and mindful awareness training utilizing a brain-based approach. There are three curricula available (grades K to 2, 3 to 5, and 6 to 8). Two training programs exist: (a) District Wide/Government/Public and Private Institution Implementation, where MindUP staff works with your district's educational leaders to implement the MindUP curriculum in your school district. Training includes onsite workshops, virtual support, and ongoing coaching and mentoring. (b) MindUP School Based On-Site Training: MindUP staff works with on-site principals and staff and includes a 12-month support plan with a program coordinator. Ongoing interactive forums are created both in person and online. A parent workshop is also offered. There is some research support (see Lawlor, 2014; Schonert-Reichl & Lawlor, 2010; Weare, 2013).

(*continued*)

TABLE 8.1 Additional Mindfulness Programs for Schools and Youth (*continued*)

Program	Webpage	Brief Description
Modern Mindfulness	www.modmind.org/	This is an interactive online mindful program that strengthens executive functioning skills, resulting in a focused and relaxed student with only 5 minutes of practice per day. It was created by mindfulness experts in collaboration with teachers in a public school (Center for Mindful Learning). The program trains teachers and gives them access to an interactive online curriculum that supports them while teaching mindfulness to youth (applications). Training is for educators of children 5 to 18 years old.
Move-into-Learning Program	www.youtube.com/ watch?v=aukqfWGYeoA	Provides eight weekly 45-minute sessions of yoga, meditation, and breathing exercises set to music along with opportunities for self-expression through writing and visual arts. Focus is on children's hyperactive behavior and symptoms of attention-deficit/hyperactivity disorder (ADHD), and results in a decrease in inattentiveness, according to teacher observations.
Movement and Mindfulness	move-with-me.com/shop/ movement-mindfulness -curriculum/	The program integrates stories, exercise, and self-regulation to build fitness, focus, and learning readiness. The curriculum includes lesson plans for 30 weeks with over 200 movement and mindfulness-building activities (stories, cooperative games, mindfulness activities, music). It also includes nine yoga/ movement video classes, 16 skill flash cards, a poster, and three CDs for K and first grades.
Niroga	www.niroga.org/education/ school/	Niroga offer 15-minute transformative life skills in in-class sessions—a simple and proven intervention that integrates mindful yoga, breathing techniques, and meditation.
Quiet Time Program	www.davidlynchfoundation .org/schools.html	This program provides training for students and faculty in the Transcendental Meditation technique at school and with follow-up support. Training to become a teacher of Transcendental Meditation is open to everyone and involves 5 months of in-residence training. Designed to become a permanent, ongoing part of a school's curriculum.

(continued)

TABLE 8.1 Additional Mindfulness Programs for Schools and Youth (*continued*)

Program	Webpage	Brief Description
Still Quiet Place	www.stillquietplace.com/	A book that outlines a mindfulness curriculum, it outlines an 8-week mindfulness-based stress reduction (MSBR) program that therapists, teachers, and other professionals can use to help students manage stress and anxiety in their lives and to develop their natural capacities for emotional fluency, respectful communication, and compassionate action. The mindfulness practices in the program's guide are said to be designed to help increase attention, learning, resiliency, and compassion by showing students how to experience the natural quietness that can be found within oneself. For K–12 educators, focusing on grades 4 to 7. There is some research support (see Weare, 2013).
SMART: Stress Management and Relaxation Techniques in Education	passageworks.org/courses/smart-in-education/	SMART in Education is an evidence-based personal renewal program designed especially for faculty and staff working in early childhood education through grade 12 settings. It is modeled after the MBSR program (Weare, 2013). It is designed to increase teacher attention, awareness of emotion, empathy, and compassion. The program involves experiential activities in mindfulness including meditation, emotional awareness, and movement. Weekly meetings also include presentations and group discussions. There is some research support for the program (see Weare, 2013).
Stop, Breathe, Think	www.toolsforpeace.org/programs-events/programs-for-schools/stop-breathe-think/	This is a step-by-step mindfulness curriculum that guides participants through a variety of mindfulness activities, personal reflections, and group discussions. It is designed to be integrated into advisory classes, character- and leadership-building classes, and enrichment electives.
With Pause	www.withpause.com/work-with-renee/for-schools/	With Pause offers a variety of programs from a short workshop to an in-depth 8-week training series. The programs offer mindfulness tools and exercises that can be used immediately to manage classroom stressors, and offer exercises and techniques to enhance your focus, become more in-tune with your emotions, better live in line with your personal values, and help students and teachers deal with stress, handle emotional situations, and expand self-awareness. Focused on Pre-K to high school.

Source: Black, Milam, and Sussman (2009), Burke (2010), Meiklejohn et al. (2012), Sprengel and Fritts (2012); Weare (2013), Zenner et al. (2014)
ADHD, attention-deficit hyperactivity disorder; MBSR, mindfulness-based stress reduction; SEL, social emotional learning.

CONCLUSION

As the body of research on mindfulness in schools and for youth grows, it becomes increasingly more difficult to capture the nuances of all that is happening. There is a wide range of quality across programs with research to assess these programs. There are gorgeous web pages citing extensive studies and plastered with pictures of the brain with catchy graphics seeming as if they are entirely research-based and supported by program-specific research. Yet, like the old saying goes, when you lift the hood and kick the tires, you realize that the program is nothing more than a car with a fancy paint job. We can think back to the proverb at the beginning of the chapter, "He who does not research has nothing to teach." Research is difficult, and even more difficult when done in schools. As educators, we must commit to moving the field forward by keeping up with the research, by supporting research efforts in your own school, and by partnering with universities and researchers to make the research happen.

Research must be carefully vetted for its quality. Some of the studies described in this chapter offered small sample sizes, were self-described pilot studies, and lacked objective measures. And each study carries with it a bias from the researchers, the researchers' possible alliance with mindfulness practices, as well as all of the other biases listed in this chapter. Although the findings suggest that mindfulness practice may be helpful in classrooms and schools, we are far from a solid understanding of exactly how well mindfulness practices work across practices, student populations, dosages (i.e., durations, frequencies) and in what contexts. There is much we still need to understand.

REFERENCES

Baer, R. A. (2006). *Mindfulness-based treatment approaches: A clinicians guide to evidence base and applications.* New York, NY: Academic Press.

Baer, R. A., & Krietemeyer, J. (2006). Overview of mindfulness- and acceptance-based treatment approaches. In R. A. Baer's (Ed.). *Mindfulness-based treatment approaches: A clinician's guide to evidence base and applications.* New York, NY: Academic Press.

Black, D. S. (2014). Mindfulness-based interventions: An antidote to suffering in the context of substance use, misuse, and addiction. *Substance Use & Misuse, 49,* 487–491.

Black, D. S. Milam, J., & Sussman, S. (2009). Sitting meditation interventions among youth: A review of treatment efficacy. *Pediatrics, 124,* e532–e541.

Bluth, K., Campo, R. A., Pruteanu-Malinici, S., Reams, A., Mullarkey, M., & Broderick, P. C. (2016). A school-based mindfulness pilot study for ethnically diverse at-risk adolescents. *Mindfulness, 7,* 90–104.

Broderick, P. (2013). *Learning to breathe: A mindfulness curriculum for adolescents to cultivate emotion regulation, attention, and performance.* Oakland, CA: New Harbinger Press.

Burke, C. A. (2010). Mindfulness based approaches with children and adolescents: A preliminary review of current research in an emergent field. *Journal of Child and Family Studies, 19,* 133–144.

Cook-Cottone, C. P. (2013). Dosage as a critical variable in yoga research. *International Journal of Yoga Therapy, 2,* 11–12.

Cook-Cottone, C. P. (2015). *Mindfulness and yoga for self-regulation: A primer for mental health professionals.* New York, NY: Springer Publishing.

Cook-Cottone, C. P., Guyker, W., & Lemish, E. (2016). *Secular yoga in schools: A qualitative study of the Encinitas Union School Distract lawsuit.* Presented at the Yoga in Schools Symposium, April, Kripalu, Lenox, MA.

Cook-Cottone, C. P., Rovig, S., & Guyker, W. (manuscript in preparation). Anxiety, self-compassion, and eating disorder risk among middle school students.

Davis, M., Eschelman, E. R., & McKay, M. (2008). *The relaxation and stress reduction workbook* (6ᵗʰ ed.). Oakland, CA: New Harbinger Publications, Inc.

Dobkin, P. L., Irving, J. A., & Amar, S. (2012). For whom may participation in a mindfulness-based stress reduction program be contraindicated?. *Mindfulness, 3*, 44–50.

Felver, J. C., Doerner, E., Jones, J., Kaye, N. C., & Merrell, K. W. (2013). Mindfulness in school psychology: Applications for intervention and professional practice. *Psychology in the Schools, 50*, 531–547.

Fleischhaker, C., Böhme, R., Sixt, B., Brück, C., Schneider, C., & Schulz, E. (2011). Dialectical behavioral therapy for adolescents (DBT-A): A clinical trial for patients with suicidal and self-injurious behavior and borderline symptoms with a one-year follow-up. *Child and Adolescent Psychiatry and Mental Health, 5*, 1.

Flook, L., Smalley, S. L., Kitil, M. J., Galla, B. M., Kaiser-Greenland, S., Locke, J., ... Kasari, C. (2010). Effects of mindful awareness practices on executive functions in elementary school children. *Journal of Applied School Psychology, 26*, 70–95.

Greenberg, M. T., & Harris, A. R. (2012). Nurturing mindfulness in children and youth: Current State of the Research. *Child Development Perspective, 2*, 161–166.

Greenland, S. K. (2010). *The mindful child: How to help your kid manage stress and become happier, kinder, and more compassionate.* New York, NY: Atria Paperback.

Jennings, P. A. (2011). Promoting teachers' social and emotional competencies to support performance and reduce burnout. In A. Cohan & A. Honigsfeld (Eds.), *Breaking the mold of preservice and inservice teacher education: Innovative and successful practices for the twenty-first century* (chap. 13, pp. 133–143). New York, NY: Rowman & Littlefield.

Jennings, P. A., Frank, J. L., Snowberg, K. E., Coccia, M. A., & Greenberg, M. T. (2013). Improving classroom learning environments by Cultivating Awareness and Resilience in Education (CARE): Results of a randomized controlled trial. *School Psychology Quarterly, 28*, 374–390. doi:10.1037/spq0000035

Jennings, P. A., Snowberg, K. E., Coccia. M. A., & Greenberg, M. T. (2011). Improving classroom learning environments by Cultivating Awareness and Resilience in Education (CARE): Results of two pilot studies. *Journal of Classroom Interaction, 46*, 37–48.

Keng, S. L., Smoski, M. J., & Robins, C. J. (2011). Effects of mindfulness on psychological health: A review of empirical studies. *Clinical Psychology Review, 31*, 1041–1056.

Kuyken, W., Weare, K., Ukoumunne, O. C., Vicary, R., Motton, N., Burnett, R., ... Huppert, F. (2013). Effectiveness of the mindfulness in schools programme: Non-randomized controlled feasibility study. *British Journal of Psychiatry*, 1–6. doi:10.1192/bjp.bp.113.126649

Lawlor, M. S. (2014). Mindfulness in proactive: Consideration for implementation of mindfulness-based programming for adolescents in school context. *New Directions for Youth Development, 142*, 83–95.

Liehr, P., & Diaz, N. (2010). A pilot study examining the effect of mindfulness on depression and anxiety for minority children. *Archives of Psychiatric Nursing, 24*, 69–71.

Linehan, M. (1993). *Skills training manual for treating borderline personality disorder.* New York, NY: The Guilford Press.

Lomas, T., Cartwright, T., Edginton, T., & Ridge, D. (2015). A qualitative analysis of experiential challenges associated with meditation practice. *Mindfulness, 6*, 848–860.

Meiklejohn, J., Phillips, C., Freedman, M. L., Biegel, G., Roach, A., Frank, J., ... Saltzman, A. (2012). Integrating mindfulness training into K-12 education: Fostering the resilience of teachers and students. *Mindfulness, 3*, 291–307.

Metz, S. M., Franz, J. L., Reibel, D., Cantrell, T., Sanders, K., & Broderick, P. C. (2013). The effectiveness of the Learning to BREATHE Program on adolescent emotion regulation. *Research on Human Development, 10*, 252–272.

O'Brien, K. M., Larson, C. M., & Murrell, A. R. (2008). Third-wave behavior therapies for children and adolescents: Progress, challenges, and future directions. In L. A. Greco & S. C. Hayes (Eds.),

Acceptance and mindfulness treatments for children and adolescents: A practitioner's guide (pp. 15–35). Oakland, CA: New Harbinger Press.

Schonert-Reichl, K. A., & Lawlor, M. S. (2010). The effects of a mindfulness-based education program and pre and early adolescents' well-being and social emotional competence. *Mindfulness, 1*, 137–151. doi:10.1007/s12671-010-0011-8

Schussler, D. L., Jennings, P. A., Sharp, J. E. & Frank, J. L. (2015). Improving teacher awareness and well-being through CARE: A qualitative analysis of the underlying mechanisms. *Mindfulness, 7*(1), 130–142. Published online. doi:10.1007/s12671-015-0422-7

Shapiro, S. L., & Carlson, L. E. (2009). *The art and science of mindfulness: Integrating mindfulness into psychology and the helping professions.* Washington, DC: American Psychological Association.

Smith, A., Guzman-Alvarez, A., Westover, T., Keller, S., & Fuller, S. (2012). *Mindful schools program evaluation.* Retrieved from http://www.mindfulschools.org/pdf/Mindful-Schools-Study -Highlights.pdf

Sprengel, M., & Fritts, M. (2012). Utilizing mind-body practices in public schools: Teaching self-regulation skills and fostering resilience in our next generation. *BMC Complementary and Alternative Medicine, 12*, 050.

Vonnegut, K. (1991). *Slaughterhouse-five or the Children's Crusade: A duty dance with death.* New York, NY: Dell Publishing.

Waters, L., Barsky, A., Ridd, A., & Allen, K. (2015). Contemplative education: A systematic, evidence-based review of the effect of meditation interventions in schools. *Educational Psychology Review, 27*, 103–134.

Weare, K. (2013). Developing mindfulness with children and young people: A review of the evidence and policy context. *Journal of Children's Services, 8*, 141–143.

Wilson, K. G., Schnetzer, L. W., Flynn, M. K., & Kurz, A. S. (2012). Acceptance and commitment therapy for addiction. In Steven C. Hayes & Michael E. Leven's (Eds.). *Mindfulness and acceptance for addictive behaviors: Applying contextual CBT to substance abuse and behavioral addictions.* Oakland, CA: New Harbinger Publications, Inc.

Zeller, C., Herrnleben-Kurz, S., & Walach, H. (2014). Mindfulness-based interventions in schools: A systematic review and meta-analysis. *Frontiers in Psycholgy, 5*, Article 603.

Zoogman, S., Goldberg, S. B., Hoyt, W. T., & Miller, L. (2015). Mindfulness interventions with youth: A meta-analysis. *Mindfulness, 6*, 290–302.

PART III

YOGA FOR EDUCATING FOR
SELF-REGULATION AND ENGAGEMENT

CHAPTER 9

YOGA AS EMBODIED SELF-REGULATION AND ENGAGEMENT: FROM TRADITIONAL PRACTICES TO SCHOOL

I can
control my destiny,
but not my fate.
Destiny means there are opportunities to turn right or left,
but fate is a one-way street.
I believe we all have the choice
as to whether we fulfill our destiny,
but our fate is sealed.

Paulo Coelho (2014; emphasis added)

Yoga is a set of tools for well-being that integrate the mind and body through physical postures, breathing exercises, relaxation, and meditation (Cook-Cottone, 2015; Flynn, 2013; Harper, 2013). Lisa Flynn, author of *Yoga for Children* (2013), defined it this way, "[Yoga], the 5,000-year-old discipline[,] was designed to empower health, happiness, and a greater sense of self" (p. 14). Yoga is rooted in the belief that human suffering is a result of our minds continually thinking about the past, worrying about the future, and not being simply present, tuned in to this current moment and the world around us (Harper, 2013). Research indicates that yoga can help manage stress, improve focus, regulate emotions, increase positive behaviors, enhance learning outcomes, and support physical fitness (Butzer, Bury, Telles, & Khalsa, 2016; Cook-Cottone, 2015; Douglass, 2010; Felver, Butzer, Olson, Smith, & Khalsa, 2015; Flynn, 2013; Harper, 2010; Khalsa, Hickey-Schultz, Cohen, Steiner, & Cope, 2012; Serwacki & Cook-Cottone, 2012). Because of these findings, yoga is taught at growing rates in schools across the United States. From school to school and district to district, the type of yoga being delivered varies substantially (e.g., Flynn, 2013; Harper, 2013). With all of the possible options, it can be difficult for yoga teachers and school personnel to sort out what is best for their students, schools, and families. The next few chapters give you the context and background, and provide a review of the practices and programs to support your integration of yoga into your district, school, and classroom.

I CAN: AN EMBODIED, EMPOWERED HOME

The embodied self-regulation that occurs in yoga can be described in two words: I can. These words are filled with possibility and empowerment. I'll start with an example. Today, I co-taught a yoga class for Yogis in Service, Inc. (an all-ages, community-based yoga program; www.yogisinservice.org). We warmed up with sun salutations and a lunge sequence and moved into some partner work to lead up to a handstand practice. I noticed how many times participants were saying, "I can't" before we tried an exercise or a pose. Noticing this, I stopped the class and asked the group to participate in an activity. Upon request, the participants paired up. One of the individuals in the pair placed the hands out with palms facing up (i.e., Yogi A). The other person (i.e., Yogi B) placed the hands, palms facing down, on top Yogi A's hands. Yogi A, with palms facing up, was asked to look into the eyes of Yogi B and repeatedly say "I can't" while resisting Yogi B's efforts to push his or her hands down. Because of the way our arm muscles work, Yogi B's pressing down had an advantage; Yogi A did not have a chance. With effort and resistance being paired with "I can't," Yogis B's work was fast and easy. Next, I asked the all of the Yogi As, with palms up, to do that same thing, except this time, I asked them to look into their partner's eyes and say, "I can" and resist. The difference was remarkable. All of the class members were laughing, shocked by the difference between embodying, "I can't" and "I can."

Philosophers suggest it goes even deeper than that. In 2014, when I was writing the book, *Mindfulness and Yoga for Self-Regulation: A Primer for Mental Health Professionals* (Cook-Cottone, 2015), I experienced one of those moments that we all hope to have a few times in our lives. I found a piece of writing, a journal article written by a philosopher, which changed how I consider things. It is titled, "Anorexia Nervosa and the Body Uncanny: A Phenomenological Approach" (Svenaeus, 2013). I found the term *uncanny* in the title compelling and curious. To explain the term, we must first understand its relationship to the body. In his article, Svenaeus (2013) described our typical relationship with our bodies. He described how most of us live every day with our bodies, in our bodies, without a conscious sense of our bodies (Svenaeus, 2013). Although we can always turn toward our bodies with awareness (e.g., thinking about your breath rather than just breathing) as we go through the day, most of us do not do this (Svenaeus, 2013). Svenaeus (2013) suggests that the body lives in a preconscious field of attention in which it engages in many autonomic (e.g., heartbeat, breathing, digestion) and voluntary (e.g., reaching for someone's hand, opening a door) functions of which we have no awareness. We simply do these things. This is what it is like to be embodied.

> *The body is my place in the world—the place where I am that moves with me—which is also the zero-point that makes space and the place of thing that I encounter possible. The body, as a rule, does not show itself to us in our experiences; it withdraws and so opens up a focus in which it is possible for things in the world to show up to us in different meaningful ways.*
>
> Svenaeus (2013, p. 83)

The term *uncanny* comes from the root word *can*, a word that is first understood via its meaning as a verb. To say that you *can* is to both know how to do something and to be able to do it. It portends both knowledge and ability. The second definition of the word *can* is its function as a noun. A *can* is a container or vessel. If you take the dual meaning, or these meanings together, to say "*I can*" references an embodied sense of empowerment.

So what does *the body uncanny* mean? Svenaeus (2013) explains the term *uncanny* citing the German etymology of the word and Sigmund Freud. From this perspective, the term *uncanny* refers to something being fearful and not feeling like home (Svenaeus, 2013). Throughout out the many years I have worked on prevention of eating disorders and the enhancement of embodied self-regulation via my research, private practice, and yoga teaching, I have a sense that many of us, kids to adults, feel this way about our bodies. In today's culture, bodies are objectified, judged, measured, weighed, and undervalued in terms of their function and overvalued in terms of their appearance. Further, chronic stress creates a sensation of constant tension and agitation, triggering efforts to leave the embodied self through distraction and addiction (Cook-Cottone, 2015). Our bodies are objectified or seen as machines (Horton, 2012). In the past, work and life tasks demonstrated that we must be in our bodies (Horton, 2012). In contemporary society, we must carve out time to spend there (Horton, 2012).

When I teach yoga, I watch as yoga students, from the early elementary years to all ages of adults, shift back into a settled sense of themselves. I watch how their bodies shift from places of uncanny objectification to their safe, settled, and empowered home. In this way, yoga is a pathway to embodied self-regulation, to "I can." Self-regulation is the skill of engaging in thoughts and behaviors that allow you to be effective in your life. Embodied self-regulation is doing that while staying attuned to your physiological and emotional experience of self. Essentially, you work toward effectiveness in your life while honoring your body and your feelings. You can. You not only think you can, your lived, physical experience shows you that you can. It is embodied self-regulation. Gard, Noggle, Park, Vago, and Wilson (2014) describe it this way:

> . . . *yoga may function through top-down and bottom-up mechanisms for the regulation of cognition, emotions, behaviors, and peripheral physiology, as well as for improving efficiency and integration of the processes that subserve self-regulation.* (p. 77)

This chapter covers the definition of yoga, traditional forms and structures of yoga, and addresses general considerations related to the provision of yoga in schools. To provide context, the traditional view of yoga and connection with yoga's historical roots are reviewed. This also includes a discussion on the provision of secular yoga in schools and a brief discussion of the Encinitas lawsuit in which a group of parents sued the Encinitas Union School District (EUSD) purporting that yoga is a religion and therefore not appropriate for schools. Last, a trauma-sensitive approach to schools and the utility of yoga practice as trauma-informed tools for the classroom are introduced. The chapter provides school personnel with the context needed to discuss the historical roots of yoga, the secular approach, and the larger context of yoga practices in schools. The specific formal and informal practices of yoga as well as the body of research on yoga in schools are reviewed in Chapters 10, 11, and 12, respectively.

WHAT IS YOGA?

In a traditional sense, yoga is a philosophy, a way of understanding the fundamental nature of human existence. Yoga philosophy views the experience of self as inhabiting two domains: an inner experience of thoughts, emotions, and sensations, and an outer experience with which we interact (Anderson & Sovik, 2000; Cook-Cottone, 2015; Strauss, 2005). The yogic view of self is one of the root underpinnings of the mindful and yogic self as an effective learner (MY-SEL) model (see Figure 1.3). Successful self-regulation and academic engagement is contingent on the ability to live capably in both domains (Anderson & Sovik, 2000; Cook-Cottone, 2015; Gard et al., 2014). Accordingly, the term *yoga* is derived from the Sanskrit verb *yuj*, which means to join or unite (Anderson & Sovik, 2000; Cook-Cottone, 2015; Flynn, 2013; Iyengar, 1996; Strauss, 2005). The essential goals of traditional yoga involve these three aspects: (a) integration of the inner experience, (b) attunement with the outer experience, and (c) embodiment and expression of the best version of ourselves (see Figure 9.1). As you read about the different types and schools of yoga, you will see that although they vary in content and process, they all hold to these three major foci.

The definition of yoga also answers the question, "How does yoga work?" Flynn (2013) explains that yoga is a system of connecting mind, body, and spirit (derived from the Greek word *spirare*, meaning "to breathe"; p. 14). Flynn (2013) says that you can think of yoga as the union and integration of mind, body, and breath. The practice of postures strengthens, stretches, and relaxes the body (Flynn, 2013). The focus on the breath during practice brings the body and mind into balance (Flynn, 2013). Yoga practice helps students develop self-awareness and create attunement within the context of their external experiences (Anderson & Sovik, 2000; Cook-Cottone, 2015). Over time, the practice helps students develop an internal mind and body connection (Flynn, 2103). With this connection, students can counteract the effects of stress and come to a more centered place (Flynn, 2013). The evidence related to the benefits is growing—findings in the field of neuroscience support the use of yoga to foster a healthy, natural balance and integration of the mind–brain system (Cook-Cottone, 2015; Harper, 2013; Simpkins & Simpkins, 2011).

The way we practice yoga today is informed by knowledge passed down through oral transmission through the ages, ancient texts, modern books, and lineages of yoga masters (i.e., gurus) to yoga students (Stephens, 2010). The tradition of yoga is that true knowledge must be gained through one's own experience (Anderson & Sovik, 2000; Cook-Cottone, 2015). Traditionally, it is believed that yoga practices work like a mirror (Cook-Cottone, 2015). Yoga is a tool for examining yourself directly (Anderson & Sovik, 2000;

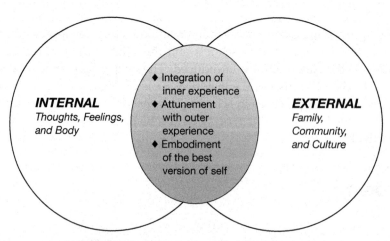

FIGURE 9.1 The essential goals of yoga.

Cook-Cottone, 2015). Further, yoga provides a structure of strengthening the body, relaxing the nervous and emotional systems, and bringing one-pointed, bare awareness to the present moment (Anderson & Sovik, 2000; Cook-Cottone, 2015).

THE EIGHT LIMBS OF YOGA

Most people think of yoga poses or the yoga asanas when they think of yoga (Harper, 2013). For many of us, we are surprised to learn that yoga poses are only one of the eight limbs or practices of yoga. Those who practice yoga in studios today often view yoga as the poses, breath work, and some relaxation and meditation (Gard et al., 2014) but these practices reflect only a portion of what yoga is. The eight limbs of yoga are described in the Yoga Sutras (Cook-Cottone, 2015; Gard et al., 2014; Harper, 2013; Strauss, 2005). The eight-limbed path is a sequential pathway to contentment, happiness, and embodied sense of self; that is, Raja yoga as outlined by Patanjali (Bryant, 2009; Cook-Cottone et al., 2015; Gard et al., 2014; Harper, 2013; Iyengar, 1996; Prabhavananda & Isherwood, 2007; Roach & McNally, 2005). The first five limbs are considered the external limbs of yoga (Cook-Cottone, 2015). They are practices associated with the outer world, the external aspects of the self (Anderson & Sovik, 2000). They are intended to serve as the preliminary steps to strengthen the mind and body in preparation for the three later steps of meditation (Anderson & Sovik, 2000; Cook-Cottone, 2015; Weintraub, 2004). The external pathway provides guidance of negotiating people in our lives, navigating decisions and challenges, and care and conditioning of the physical body. The final three limbs are considered the internal limbs and the pathway to self-awareness (Anderson & Sovik, 2000; Cook-Cottone, 2015; Stephens, 2010). Each of them is described in the following (Table 9.1).

TABLE 9.1 The Eight Limbs of Yoga

Foundational, External Limbs (Daily practices for coping, centering, and self-awareness)			
Limb 1	Traditional Practice	**Yama** (Conduct of self in society)	**The Five Restraints**
		Ahimsa	Non-harming
		Satya	Truthfulness
		Asteya	Non-stealing
		Brahmacharya	Moderation of the senses
		Aparigraha	Non-possessiveness
Limb 2	Traditional Practice	**Niyama** (Conduct of self)	**The Five Observances**
		Saucha	Cleanliness
		Santosha	Contentment
		Tapas	Self-discipline
		Svadhyaya	Self-study
		Ishvara Pranidhana	Self-surrender

(continued)

TABLE 9.1 The Eight Limbs of Yoga (*continued*)

Limb 3	Traditional/ Contemporary, School-Based Practice	**Asana**	**Posture**
Limb 4	Traditional/ Contemporary School-Based Practice	**Pranayama**	**Breath Regulation** (Diaphragmatic breathing, other breath work)
Limb 5	Traditional/ Contemporary School-Based Practice	**Pratyahara**	**Sense Withdrawal** (Relaxation techniques, inward focus, reduction of sensory Input)
Meditative, Internal Limbs (Daily practices cultivating awareness of the authentic self)			
Limb 6	Traditional/ Contemporary School-Based Practice	*Dharana*	*Concentration* (Focused attention, object-based focus)
Limb 7	Traditional/ Contemporary School-Based Practice	*Dhyana*	*Meditation* (Bare-awareness of attention, open monitoring)
Limb 8	Advanced Traditional Practice	*Samadhi*	*Self-awareness* (Complete self-awareness)

Source: Anderson and Sovik (2000), Bryant (2009), Cook-Cottone (2015), Gard et al. (2014), Harper (2013), Iyengar (1996), McCall (2007), Prabhavananda and Isherwood (2007), Roach and McNally (2005), Simpkins and Simpkins (2011), Stephens (2010), and Weintraub (2004)

The Foundational External Limbs

The foundational external limbs include the yamas (limb 1), niyamas (limb 2), asana (limb 3), pranayama (limb 4), and pratyahara (limb 5) (Cook-Cottone, 2015; Gard et al., 2014). The five yamas are ahimsa, satya, asteya, brahmacharya, and aparigraha (Cook-Cottone, 2015; Gard et al., 2014; Iyengar, 1996; Simpkins & Simpkins, 2011; Weintraub, 2004). These are considered traditional practices and are not typically included in many contemporary yoga studios or school-based yoga. Yamas (limb 1) help us get along in society and within our relationships with others (Gard et al., 2014; Harper, 2013; Stephens, 2010). First, ahimsa is nonviolence or non-harming toward self or others and reverence for all (Cook-Cottone, 2015; Harper, 2013; Iyengar, 1996; Weintraub, 2004). The next yama is satya, which means truth, integrity, and honesty (Cook-Cottone, 2015; Harper, 2013; Simpkins & Simpkins, 2011; Stephens, 2010; Weintraub, 2004). Next, asteya requires generosity and honesty (Harper, 2013). It refers to abstinence from stealing anything including property, time, or attention (Cook-Cottone, 2015; Simpkins & Simpkins, 2011; Stephens, 2010; Weintraub, 2004). Brahmacharya is the yama of overall restraint or self-regulation (Cook-Cottone, 2015; Harper, 2013; Roach &

McNally, 2005; Simpkins & Simpkins, 2011). Last, aparigraha requires the awareness of abundance and fulfillment (Harper, 2013). It is the yama of greedlessness, or the abstinence from greed and cultivation of non-attachment (Cook-Cottone, 2015; Bryant, 2009; Iyengar, 1996; Simpkins & Simpkins, 2011; Weintraub, 2004).

The niyamas (limb 2) are five personal observances (Bryant, 2009; Cook-Cotttone, 2015; Gard et al., 2014; McCall, 2007; Harper, 2013; Iyengar, 1996; Simpkins & Simpkins, 2011). These are also considered traditional practices and are not typically included in many contemporary yoga studios or school-based yoga (Gard et al., 2014). They include: saucha, santosha, tapas, svadhyaya, and ishvara pranidhana (Cook-Cottone, 2015). The first is saucha, which means cleanliness of body and mind (Iyengar, 1996; Stephens, 2010). The observance of purity ranges from self-care practices of physiological cleanliness to being careful about speech and actions (Iyengar, 1996; Simpkins & Simpkins, 2011; Weintraub, 2004). Santosha is the niyama referring to contentment (Bryant, 2009; Simpkins & Simpkins, 2011; Weintraub, 2004). Next, the observance of tapas refers to a commitment to personal growth or the "fires of change" (Weintraub, 2004, p. 76). Ancient yogis saw the body like an unbaked clay pot (McCall, 2007). Yoga practice was like the kiln that strengthened the pot making it durable enough to withstand challenge and distress (McCall, 2007). The niyama svadhyaya refers to self-education, or the pursuit of self-improvement via learning (Cook-Cottone, 2015; Iyengar, 1996; Simpkins & Simpkins, 2011; Weintraub, 2012). Last, ish-vara pranidhana is dedication and surrender to something bigger than oneself, to finding meaning in one's life (Cook-Cottone, 2015; Simpkins & Simpkins, 2011; Weintraub, 2004). A critical aspect of self-care (see Chapter 13), meaning, or a reason for being, can make all the difference (Cook-Cottone, 2015).

Asanas (limb 3) are the yoga postures that have evolved over centuries (Iyengar, 1996). The Sanskrit root *as* connotes being or living in one's body, with the full term *asana* referring to taking one's seat (Cook-Cottone, 2015; Stephens, 2010). Considered secular practices, the yoga postures are part of school-based yoga programs and are the focus of many studio classes. The practice of asana is intended to integrate body, mind, and breath within the context of holding postures and moving from one posture to the next (Cook-Cottone, 2015). The asanas are named after natural phenomena (e.g., tree pose), animals (e.g., fish and frog poses), and heroes (e.g., Hanumasana; Cook-Cottone, 2015). Iyengar (1996) posits that by taking the shapes of all creatures and things, the practitioner develops empathy and compassion for all things. Kraftsow (1999) worries that current interpretations of yoga have overemphasized the achievement of precise, fixed poses and preconceived, external standards of perfection. This is not the true intention of yoga (Cook-Cottone, 2015).

Pranayama is limb four. *Prana* means respiration, breath, vitality, life, wind, energy, and strength (Iyengar, 1996). *Ayama* refers to expansion, stretching out, length, and restraint (Iyengar, 1996). Pranayama is the practice of breath work to calm down and energize the body (Cook-Cottone, 2015; Simpkins & Simpkins, 2011). With practice, students begin to notice that as their experiences shift (e.g., they are startled, anxious, excited), their breathing shifts. Importantly, they learn the reverse is true, too. As students work with their breathing, their body and feelings can change (Harper, 2013). Breath work is included in many school-based programs due to its benefits in stress reduction and self-regulation (e.g., Harper, 2013). According to Weintraub (2012), control of breath allows for control of emotions and mood. Iyengar (1996) identifies three ways to control the breath: (a) inhalation, inspiration, or filling up; (b) exhalation, expiration, or emptying; and (c) retention. Breath work typically begins with simple observation of the breath and the qualities of breath (Sovik, 2005; see Table 9.2).

TABLE 9.2 The Qualities of Good Breathing

Quality	Description
Depth	Breath is deep and driven by firm, steady contractions of the diaphragm
Flow	Flow is smooth, without pause, agitation, or hesitation
Constancy	Exhalations and inhalations are equal in length
Sound	Breath is silent, without sound
Continuity	Breath is continuous with smooth transitions between exhalations and inhalations

Source: Sovik (2005) and Cook-Cottone (2015).

The last of the external practices, pratyahara (limb 5) is the practice of turning inward (Bryant, 2009; Cook-Cottone, 2015; Gard et al., 2014; Harper, 2013; Simpkins & Simpkins, 2011; Stephens, 2010). Pratyahara exercises prepare you for meditation by quieting the senses, withdrawing them from outward objects, so that the senses and the mind can rest (Sovik, 2005). Stephens (2010) put it this way, "As we sense, so we think, and as we think, so we tend to act" (p. 11). Systematic relaxation is an example of this type of practice. Relaxation techniques are frequently used as part of school-based yoga programs.

The internal limbs are dharana, dhyana, and samadhi (Bryant, 2009; Cook-Cottone, 2015; Harper, 2013; Simpkins & Simpkins, 2011). The five external limbs prepare the yogi for these practices. The internal limbs can be thought of as the stages of meditation. First, dharana is the practice of one-pointed focus of attention (Bryant, 2009; Cook-Cottone, 2015; Gard et al., 2014; Iyengar, 1996; Simpkins & Simpkins, 2011; Stephens, 2010). Next, dhyana is the practice of focusing on inner thoughts and feelings as you focus on the object of attention (Cook-Cottone, 2015; Gard et al., 2014; Simpkins & Simpkins, 2011). These forms of meditation are frequently used as part of school-based yoga programs. Samadhi is the deepest form of meditation and is seen as complete self-awareness (Cook-Cottone, 2015). This is considered an advanced traditional practice (Gard et al., 2014) and is not part of school-based yoga programs.

A BRIEF HISTORY OF YOGA

Understanding the nature of the origins of yoga is important (Cook-Cottone, 2015; Strauss, 2005). When I first learned about yoga and began practicing, I had no sense of the history. I simply loved the way I felt when I was practicing on a regular basis. Perhaps blinded by both my love of yoga and by naiveté, I did not understand the resistance that I occasionally experienced when I was working to bring yoga as a prevention intervention to schools. As my intellectual interest grew, I delved into the history to gain a better understanding of what others were thinking and feeling about yoga that might create resistance. Understanding their concerns and where they were coming from, I became empowered by my historical knowledge to ease worries and concerns, as well as to respect and have authentic empathy for their decision to choose not to participate.

I offer this brief history to you so that you will be able to effectively field inquiries, as well as have a sense of the history, religious tensions, and concerns over authenticity of various yogic practices (Cook-Cottone, 2015). Since ancient times, yoga has been evolving, adapting to meet the needs of individuals with different cultures, traditions, and applications (Cook-Cottone, 2015; Horton, 2012; Kraftsow, 1999; McCall, 2007; Simpkins & Simpkins, 2011; Strauss, 2005). The challenge lies in writing about yoga as an intervention for schools, ensuring that it is being implemented in a way that honors the extensive history of yoga practice, yoga culture, and mentorship and the philosophical foundations and ancient texts (Cook-Cottone, 2015; McCall, 2007). Current manifestations and applications of yoga are considerably different than early forms. It is believed that yoga has been practiced in India for more than 40 centuries, before recorded history (Anderson & Sovik, 2000; Cook-Cottone, 2015; Horton, 2012; Simpkins & Simpkins, 2011; Stephens, 2010; Weintraub, 2004). In its historical essence, yoga is a philosophy. It has been passed down and integrated by many, across a wide range of applications. If you look, elements of yogic philosophy can be found in Hinduism, Jainism, Buddhism, Christianity, therapy, self-improvement, coaching, and even fitness (Cook-Cottone, 2015; Simpkins & Simpkins, 2011; Stephens, 2010; Strauss, 2005). This is because yoga's unique integration of focused concentration, deliberate body positioning (i.e., asana), and control of the breath provides an enduring practical system that is not limited to any particular philosophical or religious system (Cook-Cottone, 2015; Simpkins & Simpkins, 2011).

Yoga scholars have identified several ancient texts that are the early foundations of today's yoga: the Vedas (i.e., Rig, Yajur, Sama, and Atharva), Upanishads, Bhagavad Gita, Vedanta, and Yoga Sutras (Cook-Cottone, 2015; Simpkins & Simpkins, 2011; Stephens, 2010). Horton (2012) describes the "Pashupati Seal," a stone originating from the Indus Valley civilization thought to date back 5,000 years. Horton's (2012) report reviews several theories as to its meaning and relevance to yoga (Horton, 2012): Is it Shiva sitting in an asana mediating? Is it a god of fertility? Is it an archaic god engaged in a shamanic rite? Historians are not sure. Accordingly, a 5,000-year-old link to yoga practice is conjecture at this point.

The Vedas were written approximately 1,200 BCE. They reflect the context of their times expressing some of yoga's root philosophical themes and what we would see today as eccentric, esoteric practices (Cook-Cottone, 2015; Stephens, 2010). The Upanishads were written between 800 and 600 BCE. Themes expressed include: We are all part of something greater, answers lie within, and the knowledge of the true nature of self can be found through consciousness (Cook-Cottone, 2015; Simpkins & Simpkins, 2011; Stephens, 2010). The Bhagavad Gita is the sixth book in a larger Indian text (i.e., the Mahabharata) written sometime between the fifth and second centuries BCE. It was written as the dialogue between a warrior named Arjuna and the god Krishna, Arjuna's charioteer (Cook-Cottone, 2015; Simpkins & Simpkins, 2011; Stephens, 2010). This text addresses the yoga of managing the inner experience of self within the context of the challenges and pressures presented by our external world (Cook-Cottone, 2015). In the text, Krishna teaches Arjuna yoga philosophy as he faces the dilemmas of battle (Cook-Cottone, 2015; Gandhi, 2011). If you are interested in reading this text, I have found that this version is especially easy to understand; see *The Bhagavad Gita According to Gandhi*, (Gandhi, 2011).

The Yoga Sutras were written between the second century BCE and the fourth century CE. This text is considered to be fundamental to modern yoga philosophy (Cook-Cottone, 2015; Iyengar, 1996; Simpkins & Simpkins, 2011; Stephens, 2010). The Yoga Sutras are a series of concise sentences, or aphorisms, conveying the essential concepts of yoga theory and practice (Anderson & Sovik, 2000; Cook-Cottone, 2015; Iyengar, 1996; Simpkins & Simpkins, 2011; Weintraub, 2004). The Yoga Sutras originated as an oral tradition presenting the practice of yoga in eight limbs (Anderson & Sovik, 2000; Cook-Cottone, 2015; Stephens, 2010; Weintraub, 2004). It is believed that the Yoga Sutras were originally written by someone named Patanjali, although it is unclear who or what Pantanjali may have been. He has been described in many ways including a mythological figure and a professor of grammar and linguistics (Simpkins & Simpkins, 2011). Interestingly, there are few references in the Yoga Sutras to the physical postures of yoga. As you can see, today's yoga, focused primarily on postures, is far from its original philosophical roots (Cook-Cottone, 2015).

Yoga was introduced to Europe via a translation of the *Bhagavad Gita* from Sanskrit to English in 1785, eventually making its way to America by 1845 (Cook-Cottone, 2015; Douglass, 2007). Fitting for schools, the initial interest in yoga was intellectual and academic. According to Douglass (2007), Ralph Waldo Emerson enthusiastically embraced the translation, inspiring serious inquiry into Hinduism and yoga. In the 1850s, the first signs of a critical shift emerged (Cook-Cottone, 2015). That is, what were considered oriental religions were being viewed as potential forms of practice rather than mere objects of study (Cook-Cottone, 2015; De Michelis, 2008). According to Douglass (2007), Henry David Thoreau, Emerson's student, a progressive educator, abolitionist, and poet, was the first to transition from the intellectual study of yoga to active practice. In fact, in a letter to a friend, Thoreau described himself as a *yogin* (Douglass, 2007; Horton, 2012).

It is believed that tensions developed as academic scholars struggled with their interest in yoga philosophy and practice, Asian religions, and the Christian belief that there is a single path to God (Douglass, 2007). Thoreau's continued practice of yoga begged the question that is still asked by some today: "Does the study and practice of yoga lead the practitioner away from Christianity?" (Douglass, 2007). Max Muller nearly personified these tensions with his scholarship on ancient texts such as the *Rig Veda* (Singleton, 2010). The negative tenor of his writings, which approached disgust, inspired a Hindu boycott of his lecture series in India (Douglass, 2007). Reports suggest that, perhaps, Muller saw the early roots of yoga as acceptable as they were more philosophical in nature (Singleton, 2010). However, he described later forms of yoga (e.g., hatha) as part of the degeneration of yoga toward crude practical applications. Ironically, it is the practical applications that are seen as more secular and acceptable today (Cook-Cottone, Lemish, & Guyker, 2016).

This split of yoga's philosophical and physical aspects continued. The 19th century witnessed a rise in the phenomena of the performing yogi (Cook-Cottone, 2015; Singleton, 2010). From some perspectives, yoga took a negative, even vulgar turn as yogis panhandled and performed advanced asanas (i.e., yoga postures) in sideshows reminiscent of European contortionism (Singleton, 2010). The argument continues today, as many view the present-day social media posting of asanas as a reverberation of this voyeuristic and perhaps excluding trend (Cook-Cottone, 2015). It is reported that some see these posts and think, "Only thin, athletic, and beautiful people do yoga," "Yoga is an art form to be observed and not practiced," or "I could never do that. Yoga is not for me" (Cook-Cottone, 2015, p. 172). There is little consensus as others argue that these photos and videos, including the historical photos, are inspiring (Cook-Cottone, 2015).

Another shift occurred at the end of the 19th century. In 1893, Swami Vivekananda, well versed in both Western philosophy and Indian traditions including yoga, spoke at the World Parliament of the World's Religions at the Chicago's World's Fair (Cook-Cottone, 2015; De Michelis, 2008; Douglass, 2007; Strauss, 2005). Although not embraced by academics, Vivekananda's framing of yoga as an approach to physical health accessible to everyone helped defuse tension around religion, opened the door to yoga as a subject for all, and stimulated a genuine interest in the health benefits of yoga (Douglass, 2007; Horton, 2012). Strauss (2005) notes that the cultural focus on health aspects of yoga was also a marker of the movement into modernity. According to Douglass (2007), scholars were critical of Vivekananda's reinterpretations of yoga and seemingly reckless blending of Eastern and Western religions and popular Western culture. Despite the intellectual debates, by the end of the 1880s, most American students of yoga circumvented religious conflict (Douglass, 2007). American students adapted a view of yoga as a method for enhancing physical and mental health (Douglass, 2007). Interestingly, Swami Vivekananda's success in the United States sparked a yoga renaissance in India. The time was ripe for revitalization. It had been over 100 years since the emergence from British colonialism, which exposed India to relentless cultural and religious humiliation (Horton, 2012).

From 1900 to 1940, the exploration of yoga took divergent paths in academia and popular culture (Cook-Cottone, 2015). De Michelis (2008) notes that this period was marked by the substantially disruptive and intellectually unsettling influences of World Wars I and II, as well as surges and intellectual debates in the field of psychology. At this point, academic literature highlighted exotic and magical aspects of classic yogic texts, discounting yoga's potential to enhance personal growth (Douglass, 2007). Still, popular culture continued to embrace the health aspects (Douglass, 2007). English translations of yogic texts were becoming increasingly available. Perhaps one of the biggest moves toward accessibility of yoga for all occurred in 1966 when B. K. S. Iyengar's 544-page book, *Light on Yoga*, was published with complete descriptions and illustrations of yoga postures and breathing techniques (Cook-Cottone, 2015). Also, Americans were studying yoga in India in growing numbers, setting the stage for the personal exploration of yoga (Douglas, 2007).

Throughout the 1960s and 1970s, yoga was popular and being practiced by rock stars such as the Beatles. In fact, Swami Satchidananda opened the legendary Woodstock music festival (Douglass, 2007). It was around this time that the history of yoga took another interesting turn. I think this is the point when my parents, like many others, began to see yoga as a practice of the hippy and drug culture. At this point, the practice and study of yoga became intertwined with the infamous LSD studies conducted by Harvard psychologists Richard Alpert and Timothy Leary (Douglass, 2007). These studies and the behavior of the professors appropriately inspired ethical concerns across the country. Ultimately, the two left Harvard. According to Douglass (2007), Alpert departed to study Buddhist meditation in India, returning as Ram Dass to propagate new ideas on consciousness. As a doctoral student at University of Buffalo, I saw Ram Dass speak. With the charisma of a practiced storyteller and free from conflict regarding the blending of substance use and yoga and mindfulness practice, he spoke of his journey from the LSD experiments to a life-long practice of meditation (Cook-Cottone, 2015). Leary's path led him to urging the youth of America to: "Turn on, tune in, and drop out" (Douglass, 2007, p. 40). For many, yoga's association with drugs and rock music solidified their concerns, further setting the association of yoga with a long list of deviant behaviors (Douglass, 2007). Notably, a majority of yoga teachers and practitioners strongly believe that substance use has no place in the practice and teaching of yoga (Cook-Cottone, 2015). I am among them.

In the 1970s, an increasingly sound research began to emerge. Simultaneously, there was a gradual, nation-wide adoption of yoga as a pathway to health and well-being. Today, we see yoga studios in nearly every city. Yoga is practiced in gyms, prisons, treatment centers, and schools (Cook-Cottone, 2015). As yoga has evolved in Western culture, there was yet another twist in its history. Both scholars and practitioners began to raise concerns over yoga's *authenticity*. Some hold that an *authentic Indian yoga practice* should be held as the standard by which all yoga should be compared and contrasted (Cook-Cottone, 2015; Singleton & Byrne, 2008). Conversely, others suggest that contemporary practices of yoga should "not be dismissed or condemned simply on account of their dislocation from perceived tradition" (Singleton & Byrne, 2008, p. 6). Still others say that this tension may be a misunderstanding of the history of yoga. For example, Liberman (2008) argues that there never was an *authentic Indian yoga practice*, or pure yoga, as some imagine, and that the concept of pure yoga is a social construction. Liberman (2008) argues further that asana practice, as we know it now, did not manifest until the 10th to 12th centuries with the earliest forms of yoga consisting primarily of contemplation and mantra (Liberman, 2008). Strauss (2005) refers to the *pizza effect*. This is an anthropological term that refers to the phenomenon of certain elements of a nation or culture being transformed or more completely embraced elsewhere, ultimately to be re-imported back to the culture of origin. That is, the yoga that we debate is not the yoga that came from India. Today's yoga, in all its diversity and complexity, is something new. "It is extraordinarily different from its counterparts in antiquity" (Horton, 2012, p. 23).

Over the past 30 years we have seen the emergence of the medicalization of yoga. In this paradigm, researchers and practitioners advocate for the practice of yoga to address health concerns through prevention and intervention (Cook-Cottone, 2015). This shift toward medicalization has somewhat relieved religious and cultural tensions by providing validity of the practice from another source—the field of medicine (Cook-Cottone, 2015; De Michelis, 2008; Strauss, 2005). Horton (2012) called the contemporary yoga paradoxical: "a modern invention with ancient roots, a fitness fad with spiritual sustenance, a $6 billion 'industry' with non-material values" (p. xi). As incarnations of its forms come and go, it is increasingly clear that yoga is a creative process, always evolving as its central, core feature—the integration of physical engagement, breath, and intention—weaves its way through the centuries. And so the debate continues questioning secularism, religious content, authenticity, and cultural appropriation. There is so much more to know about the rich history of yoga, along with its many nuances, that are not within the scope of this text. I encourage you to access the papers I have cited. Read them in their entirety. See also Sarah Strauss's (2005), *Positioning Yoga: Balancing Acts Across Cultures* and Carol Horton's (2012) *Yoga Ph.D.: Integrating the Life of the Mind and the Wisdom of the Body.*

TRADITIONAL AND CONTEMPORARY TYPES OF YOGA

There are many forms of yoga. In Chapter 10, I review many of the current styles of yoga that have originated from these early forms (e.g., Vinyasa, Power, Ashtanga, and Yin). Traditionally, yoga is described in older texts in terms of seven main paths (i.e., Hatha, Raja, Jnana, Mantra, Karma, Bhakti, and Tantra [with Kundalini]; Anderson & Sovik, 2000; Cook-Cottone, 2015; Simpkins & Simpkins, 2011; Stephens, 2010). No path is considered entirely separate and the final goal remains the same across all paths: integration of the inner world, harmony with the outer world, and connection with the true nature of self (Anderson & Sovik, 2000). I think of the true nature of self as the version of self that comes from a deep connection with your inner experience (i.e., thoughts, feelings, and the needs and strengths of your body) and intentional, authentic engagement with your outer experience (i.e., family, friends, community, and culture). The true nature of self honors inner experiences and carefully cultivates and nurtures external experiences. This version of self is different from the version of self that might ignore or be reactive to feelings, get caught in obsessive or negative thinking, fail to care for or attempt to harm the body, engage in invalidating or hurtful relationships, or internalize cultural values that are in conflict with health and positive relationships. Yoga allows you to practice checking in and cultivating positive attunements inside and out. The traditional schools of yoga were the first yogic pathways to this attunement. Typical secular, school-based yoga practices are quite distinct from these traditional forms. It is good for school personnel to know what these traditional forms are called and to what they refer. The traditional forms of yoga are very briefly described here (see Table 9.3).

Over the past 150 years, many styles of contemporary yoga have emerged from various traditions and for a variety of functions including stress relief, fitness, community, and spirituality. The list and brief descriptions in Table 9.4 are offered to provide a brief overview of some of the main styles of yoga. It is important to note that there are so many different types of yoga that it is not feasible for all of them to be listed here. Several of the more popular styles of yoga are listed and described in alphabetical order. Note that there is no generally accepted source that delineates all types of yoga (Cook-Cottone, 2015). Sources and discrepancies and similarities between and among sources are cited in Table 9.4 (Cook-Cottone, 2015).

TABLE 9.3 Traditional Forms of Yoga

Raja Yoga	The first form of yoga; Raja yoga is focused on the mind, consciousness, and character. Rather than reliance on rational thought, it is the pursuit of wisdom through the techniques of focused attention, concentration, and contemplation with the intention of discipline of the mind.
Hatha Yoga	Hatha yoga, or post-classical yoga, is the yoga of health, integrating postures (i.e., asanas), breath work, and meditation as a path to physical health and well-being as a preparation for meditation.
Jnana Yoga	Jnana is referred to as the yoga of knowledge, wisdom, awareness, and discrimination. This yogic path involves meditation and contemplation using conceptual, rational thought to bring the mind toward higher consciousness.
Mantra Yoga	In Mantra yoga, the practitioner uses a focus on mantra (i.e., sounds and words) as a tool for self-regulation of the mind.
Karma Yoga	Karma yoga is considered the yoga of service for everyday life. Karma yoga emphasizes an intentional focus on cultivating good deeds in action without expectation or attachment to reward, outcome, or acknowledgment.
Bhakti Yoga	Bhakti yoga is the yoga of devotion. The practice involves devotion, compassion, and selfless love for something bigger than yourself. It is believed that a life of work devoted to others facilitates the journey through the personal self toward the experience of the authentic self.
Tantra Yoga	Tantra yoga is the yoga of symbolic experiences designed to weave mind and body into one. Closely associated with spirituality, Tantra has a long history with roots in Hinduism and Tibetan Buddhism.
Kundalini Yoga	Also spiritual in nature, Kundalini yoga involves awakening and assimilation of the energy of consciousness. Kundalini yoga targets mind-body-spirit integration through cultivation and regulation of energy.

Source: Anderson and Sovik (2000), Cook-Cottone (2015), Gard et al. (2014), Simpkins and Simpkins (2011), and Stephens (2010).

TABLE 9.4 Contemporary Styles of Yoga

Anusara	Anusara yoga was developed by John Friend, a student of B. K. S. Inyengar (McCall, 2007). This style of yoga emphasizes limb alignment in asana, uses props to facilitate alignment, and integrates a positive philosophy. The main philosophical tenet is that an intrinsic energy of oneness underlies everyone and everything. Each class is taught with a centering theme and includes asana and meditation. Learn more about anusara yoga at www.anusarayoga.com. It is known for free-flowing, Vinyasa movements (Field, 2011).
Ashtanga	Ashtanga yoga is based on the teachings of K. Pattabhi Jois (kpjayi.org; McCall, 2007). Taught by Krishnamacharya, Jois is the founder of the Ashtanga Yoga Research Institute in Mysore, India (kpjayi.org/the-institute; Swenson, 1999). It is considered one of the more challenging and vigorous styles of yoga and is one of the foundational roots of power yoga (see the following; McCall, 2007). Ashtanga involves specialized sequencing of postures, practiced in a continuous flow, and a set of breathing exercises (McCall, 2007; Swenson, 1999). Ujjayi breath is used during practice. Ashtanga teachers sometimes offer a Mysore class in which students practice at their own pace and can secure individual guidance from the teacher on the poses on which they are working (McCall, 2007). See Swenson (1999) for a detailed practice manual.
Bikram/Hot Yoga	Brikram yoga was created and founded by Choudhury Bikram (www.bikramyoga.com; McCall, 2007). Bikram yoga is practiced in higher temperature (i.e., over 100 degrees; Field, 2011; McCall, 2007). It is a challenging practice that involves 26 postures done in a standard sequence (McCall, 2007). Postures are held for 30 seconds and nearly all of the asanas are repeated twice (McCall, 2007). People who like the Bikram style enjoy the heat, sweating, the predicable sequence, and the standardization across studios. It is not recommended for those with high blood pressure, chronic illness such as multiple sclerosis or fibromyalgia, cardiovascular disease, or other medical illnesses that can be exacerbated by intense exercise in heat (Field, 2011; McCall, 2007).
Himalayan Institute Yoga	The Himalayan Institute was founded in 1971 by Swami Rama of the Himalayas. The asana practice emphasizes the therapeutic benefits of the poses, alignment, and physical and mental health. The Himalayan Institute offers teacher training that includes advanced studies in sequencing, verbal and hands-on assists, subtle body anatomy, pranayama, mantra meditation, therapeutic applications of yoga, and the study of sacred yoga texts. See the Institute's web page for more information: www.himalayaninstitute.org.
Integral Yoga	Integral yoga is considered to be a gentle style of yoga founded by Swami Satchidananda who studied under Swami Sivananda (McCall, 2007). The practice includes asana, pranayama, chanting, meditation, and discussions of ancient yogic texts (McCall, 2007). The school reflects a commitment to selfless service encouraged in karma yoga, which is attributed to the lineage (McCall, 2007). Dean Ornish's early studies on yoga and cardiovascular health stylized this type of yoga (McCall, 2007). For more on integral yoga, see the Integral Yoga Institute's web page (iyiny.org).

(continued)

TABLE 9.4 Contemporary Styles of Yoga (*continued*)

Iyengar Yoga	Iyengar yoga is known for longer holding of poses and inclusion of more strenuous poses (www.bksiyengar.com; Field, 2011). B. K. S. Iyengar is the founder of Iyengar yoga and author of several books on yoga and the seminal work, *Light on Yoga* (Iyengar, 1966). Iyengar yoga focuses on alignment as the primary meditative focus of practice (McCall, 2007). Pranayama (i.e., breath work) is taught after a certain level of proficiency is attained in asana—a process that takes, on average, about 2 years of steady practice (i.e., postures; McCall, 2007). B. K. S. Iyengar is thought to be a pioneer in yoga in both use of props and in the development of restorative yoga. Props such as blocks, bolsters, straps, benches, and ropes mounted on the wall are used to enhance practice (McCall, 2007). Restorative yoga is useful for students, who are in need of respite, recovery, and have other physiological challenges (e.g., illness). Teacher training in Inyengar yoga is believed to be among the most rigorous (McCall, 2007).
Kripalu Yoga	Kripalu yoga was created by a group of yogis who followed Yogi Amrit Desai in the 1970s (McCall, 2007). Kripalu yoga emphasizes emotional release, spiritual growth, and self-acceptance (McCall, 2007; www.kripalu.org). There is a focus on creating a space for yoga students that is emotionally safe (McCall, 2007). The practice is presented in different levels of intensity ranging from gentle to more vigorous practices (McCall, 2007). Sequences stress coordination of movement and breath, awareness of energy in the body, and working to find your edge in postures (McCall, 2007). Sometimes teachers integrate breathing techniques and postures to elicit specific energy experiences (McCall, 2007). It includes asana, chanting, pranayama, and meditation (McCall, 2007). Kripalu yoga is associated with the Kripalu Center for Yoga and Health in Lenox, Massachusetts (www.kripalu.org; McCall, 2007)
Mindful Yoga	Mindful yoga focuses on raising a practitioner's awareness of the patterns in his or her mind (Douglass, 2011). The methodologies include postures, breathing, deep relaxation, and concentration techniques (Douglass, 2011). Mindful yoga emphasizes embodied experience and mental responses and checking with students as they move through poses and engage in breathing and relaxation techniques. Students are encouraged to bring awareness to thoughts, feelings, and physical postures and how they feel in the body, to discern thoughts and bodily sensations, and to notice that they can have multiple reactions to single sensations. Mindful yoga emphasizes awareness of sensations and the choice that follows (Douglass, 2011). Notably, it is not prescriptive but a form of inquiry in which negation and embracing of multiple meanings over experience, perceptions, sensations, and thoughts are encouraged (Douglass, 2011).
Power Yoga	Power yoga evolved during the 1980s as a physical practice with a focus on personal empowerment. Its roots are in Vinyasa flow, Ashtanga, and Bikram yoga. In Baptiste methodology, there is a standard sequence emphasizing 12 different energetic foci including: integration, awakening, vitality, equanimity, grounding, igniting, stability, opening, release, rejuvenation, and deep rest (Baptiste, 2003). Physical and mental integration is reinforced via a central teaching tenet referred to as *true north alignment*, a continuous guidance to bring awareness and focus to the core of the physiological body and a grounded, mindful mental state. The power yoga emphasis is on inquiry and personal achievement. Some power yoga classes use heat (around 90 degrees) and a standard sequence of poses (e.g., Baptiste, 2003). Others have more flexibility in the sequences and vary the use of heat. See the Baptiste Power Vinyasa Yoga webpage for more information: www.baronbaptiste.com.

(*continued*)

TABLE 9.4 Contemporary Styles of Yoga (continued)

Viniyoga	Viniyoga was disseminated by T. K. F. Desikachar, the son of the guru Krishnamacharya (McCall, 2007). In the yogic culture, many find the lineage of teachers important; that is, who studied under whom. This helps people understand the emphasis, style, and general sense of the yogic culture a particular style might manifest. For example, B. K. S. Iyengar and Pattabhi Jois, two well-known yogis and founders of their own yoga methodologies, studied under the guru Krishnamacharya (McCall, 2007). Viniyoga focuses on breath, includes pranayama and chanting, and integrates pranayama techniques and chanting into asana practice (McCall, 2007). Consistent with the belief that yoga practice should be tailored to individual needs and challenges, yoga postures are typically practiced one-on-one, in a gentle, therapeutic manner (Kraftsow, 1999; McCall, 2007).
Vinyasa Yoga	The Vinyasa style of yoga has its roots is Ashtanga yoga. This style of yoga emphasizes flow, breath, and energy work. There are many different forms of Vinyasa yoga. Seane Corn, a modern Vinyasa teacher who emphasizes self-acceptance, self-love, energy work, spirituality, and activism, is one example this type of practice (see www.seanecorn.com/about.php). As another example, Shiva Rae created Prana Flow, an energetic, creative, full-spectrum approach to embodying the flow of yoga. In Prana Flow yoga, practitioners learn classical and innovative approaches to Vinyasa yoga and the state of flow drawn from Krishnamacharya's teachings, tantra, ayurveda, bhakti, and somatics. For more information, see shivarea.com/about-prana-flow.
Yoga Nidra	Yoga nidra means sleep in Sanskrit (McCall, 2007). Yoga nidra is a guided meditation technique that involves a series of relaxation exercises beginning with the body, moving to the breath, then to the mind, and to total relaxation and meditation (Rybak & Deuskar, 2010). Yoga nidra is typically done while the practitioner lies in savasana (i.e., lying down on the floor or mat, face up, with the feet slightly more than hip distance apart and the palms a few inches from the sides of the body, palms facing up. Eyes are closed). The instructor guides you through attentional focus to different areas of your body (McCall, 2007). For a step-by-step Yoga nidra practice, see Weintraub (2012).

Source: Cook-Cottone (2015), informed by Baptiste (2003), Douglass (2011), Field (2011), Kraftsow (1999), McCall (2007), Rybak and Deuskar (2010), and Weintraub (2012).

SCHOOL-BASED YOGA

Yoga in schools is a set of mind-body practices for well-being and student engagement: postures, breathing, relaxation, and meditation (Butzer et al., 2016; Childress & Harper, 2015; Cook-Cottone, Childress, & Harper, 2016; Serwacki & Cook-Cottone, 2012). The word *yoga* means *to yoke* or integrate. Yoga in schools helps students develop and practice a set of mind-body tools that support well-being (i.e., stress management, self-regulation, and enhanced health) so that they are ready to engage in learning in the classroom (Cook-Cottone et al., 2016a; Felver et al., 2015; Khalsa et al., 2012; Serwacki & Cook-Cottone, 2012). In fact, Horton (2012) refers to yoga as a *technology of consciousness*.

The notion of mind-body tools can be traced to theoretical work in the field of educational psychology (Cook-Cottone et al., 2016a; Cook-Cottone et al., 2016b). The concept of a mental tool was most effectively introduced by Lev Vygotsky (1962) in his book *Thought and*

Language. While there is still so much more for researchers and educators to understand, current research and experience suggest that the basic practices of school-based yoga (i.e., poses, breathing exercises, relaxation, and meditation) offer students the opportunity to develop their inner mental tools via the integration of mind and body (Cook-Cottone et al., 2016a; Cook-Cottone et al., 2016b).

Mental tools extend mental faculties in the same way that a physical tool can extend human physical faculties (see Chapter 1 for the MY-SEL model; Baron, Evangelou, Malmburg, & Melendez-Torrez, 2015; Cook-Cottone et al., 2016a; Karpov, 2014). For example, many years ago Vygotsky described how students can be taught to use private inner speech to concentrate even when there are distractions around them (Baron et al., 2015; Cook-Cottone et al., 2016a; Cook-Cottone et al., 2016a; Karpov, 2014). For example, as described in our paper, "What is Secular Yoga in Schools: Conceptual Review and Inquiry," a student named Mathilde might say to herself, "Mathilde, yes, your friends are talking; really listen to the teacher. Breathe and focus. Physically engage. Press your feet into the floor, connect through your seat, and take notes so you are sure you are listening to each thing she is saying" (Cook-Cottone et al., 2016a). Here, the student uses her *mental tool* of inner, private speech and her yoga skills to enhance her baseline ability to focus and engage (Cook-Cottone et al., 2016a). In this way, school-based yoga focuses on the teaching and practice of mind-body tools that help students manage stress, self-regulate, and engage in learning. More on the formal and informal practices of school-based yoga in Chapters 11 and 12 of this text.

A SECULAR APPROACH TO YOGA FOR SCHOOLS

At the 2015 National Kids Yoga Conference, a panel presentation of the text, *"Best Practices for Yoga in Schools,"* included a discussion on the best practice, *"Offer Secular Programs"* (Childress & Harper, 2015, p. 21). More specifically, the editors and contributors of the book agreed that best practice holds that yoga service providers working in schools have both a legal and ethical obligation to recognize and uphold the principles of secularism (Childress & Harper, 2015; Cook-Cottone et al., 2016a). What followed was a deep and thoughtful discussion on keeping yoga in schools secular with strong beliefs, feelings, and arguments for integrating spirituality and working toward absolute secularism. These types of discussions are exactly why it is so important to be at the conferences. Following the conference, a few of us spent several months working on a paper addressing the key issues related to offering secular yoga programs. There were a variety of ideas and concerns presented. Next, Traci Childress, Jennifer Cohen Harper, and I began developing a working paper to offer as a guide or placeholder to generate further discussion and perhaps to begin to develop a set of guidelines (i.e., Cook-Cottone et al., 2016a, manuscript in preparation).

To be secular, yoga instruction should follow several key grounding principles: (a) teach practices that are research based, (b) prioritize access and inclusion, (c) eliminate religious content, and (d) align with legal imperatives and secular ethics (Cook-Cottone et al., 2016a; Cook-Cottone et al., 2016b). A secular approach to yoga shares the core features of yoga with traditional and spiritual approaches to yoga (i.e., physical postures, breathing exercises, relaxation, and meditation; see Figure 9.2; Cook-Cottone et al., 2016b).

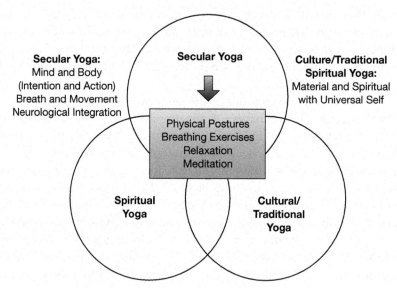

FIGURE 9.2 A secular approach to yoga.
Source: Cook-Cottone et al. (2016b).

Yet, it does not share many other features found in traditional and spiritual yoga including religious dogma, spiritual language or belief, use of Sanskrit, and traditional yoga artifacts, such as mala beads. In more traditional, philosophical approaches to yoga, the yoking, or integration, is viewed as occurring between the material and the universal, spiritual self. Distinctly, in a secular approach, the yoking or integration is mind and body, intention and action, breath and movement, and neurological integration (Cook-Cottone et al., 2016b; see Figure 9.2). An explication of the four main features of a secular approach to yoga follow.

First, secular yoga for schools is informed by and responsive to yoga research (Cook-Cottone et al., 2016a; Cook-Cottone et al., 2016b). For many decades now, schools have been moving toward best practices and empirically supported practice mandates. Teachers and administrators view instructional time as a precious resource that should be used only for intervention and methodologies known to work for their populations (Cook-Cottone et al., 2016b). As will be reviewed in Chapter 13, yoga researchers are investigating how yoga can best support positive school behaviors, self-regulation, stress management, and learning outcomes (Cook-Cottone et al., 2016a; Cook-Cottone et al., 2016b). Further, researchers are exploring how to administer yoga in schools looking at issues related to optimal frequency and duration of yoga sessions, gender differences, safe practices and risks, effective teaching methodologies, and optimal teacher training (Cook-Cottone et al., 2016a). Each year we learn more about what it means to teach yoga effectively. School-based yoga teachers attend conferences, read publications, and stay up to date in order to deliver the most effective yoga possible for their schools.

Second, secular yoga instruction in schools prioritizes access and inclusion for all students (Cook-Cottone et al., 2016a; Cook-Cottone et al., 2016b). Specifically, a secular approach to yoga creates access by respecting diverse religious and nonreligious beliefs, maintaining separation of church and state in principle and practice, and recognizing religious equality before the law (Childress & Harper, 2015; Cook-Cottone et al., 2016a;

Cook-Cottone et al., 2016b). Notably, this is consistent with the legal requirements of the First Amendment, which, as Childress and Harper (2015) remind us, maintain that there be religious neutrality in public schools and their associated activities.

Third, a secular approach to yoga is not religious, spiritual, or comprised of practices, symbols, or narratives from historical, religious traditions (Cook-Cottone et al., 2016a; Cook-Cottone et al., 2016b). Specifically, the term *secular* means "not pertaining to or connected with religion" (Jennings, 2015, p. 167). Published literature on the topic in both the fields of mindfulness and yoga agree that it is important to draw a clear line between secular and religious practices (e.g., Childress & Harper, 2015; Greenburg & Mitra, 2015). Secular yoga has evolved from the traditional forms of yoga with roots in Indian philosophy and religion (Cook-Cottone et al., 2016a; Cook-Cottone et al., 2016b). It is perfectly acceptable to acknowledge and study the roots of yoga—it is a fascinating history. Yet, like the modern clock, a technology initially used to time and regulate prayer, the methodology has been brought forward for modern, secular use. As articulated in our paper, secular yoga utilizes the effective yoga methodologies (i.e., physical postures, breathing techniques, relaxation, and meditation) and does not integrate the religious or spiritual dogma of traditional yoga practice and philosophy (i.e., Hinduism, Jainism, and Buddhism; Cook-Cottone et al., 2016a; Cook-Cottone et al., 2016b; Masters, 2014).

There is a nuance here: spirituality. At the 2016 Yoga in the School Symposium at Kripalu, my team led a deep and passionate discussion among all of the yogis, researchers, and school personnel in attendance (Cook-Cottone et al., 2016b). On nearly every other point, we were able to find consensus. However, the closest we could get to consensus here is that we all agree that it is at exactly this point at which we were most conflicted. Spirituality is defined in many ways. If you do an Internet search you will find all of these things associated with spirituality: expression of the sacred, a search for transcendent meaning, simply a search for meaning, an effort to be part of something bigger than ourselves, and inspiration. Flynn (2013) in her book on yoga for children, emphasizes spirituality (pp. 23–24). She explains that spirituality is not defined by religious practices (Flynn, 2013). Rather, it is a student's ability to find meaning and value in his or her own life and deeply engage in purposeful relationships with others (Flynn, 2013). Cobb, McClintock, and Miller (2016) write of the importance of mindfulness and spirituality in positive youth development across a variety of critical domains. Spirituality may be protective and connected with reduced risk for concerns such as substance use, mood disorder, and anxiety. Nevertheless, given the broad and multifaceted understanding of the term, the room for misperception and misunderstanding is seen as too great for the risk tolerance of many school personnel. Many feel that the focus should remain on the core practices of yoga, which are currently viewed as the key mechanisms of change (i.e., physical poses, breath work, relaxation, and meditation).

Next, a secular approach to yoga does not integrate the cultural artifacts often associated with traditional yoga (e.g., mandalas, chanting "om," and Sanskrit terms; Cook-Cottone et al., 2016a; Cook-Cottone et al., 2016b; Masters, 2014). Integration of yoga culture into any form of yoga practice can give the impression that the practice is religious and/or spiritual (Cook-Cottone et al., 2016a; Cook-Cottone et al., 2016b; Jennings, 2015). Note, however, that there are several perspectives on this and some differences of opinion within the field of school-based yoga. It is acknowledged that within the appropriate developmental and educational contexts, it is important to share histories as histories (Cook-Cottone et al., 2016a). For example, Herrington (2012) makes a case for integrating Sanskrit, yoga history, and artifacts into her classes as a way of honoring the heritage of the practices.

Fourth, a secular approach to yoga is aligned with legal imperatives and secular ethics (Cook-Cottone et al., 2016a; Cook-Cottone et al., 2016b). There is a legal imperative for school-based yoga teachers to comply with federal law. Accordingly, publicly funded schools in the United States must practice separation of church and state (Cook-Cottone et al., 2016b). Specifically, the Establishment Clause of the First Amendment prohibits public schools from advancing any particular religious belief over another, or over non-belief (Cook-Cottone et al., 2016b). Further, the Free Exercise clause requires public schools to accommodate the religious beliefs and practices of teachers and students where such practices do not interfere with the daily operation of the school. Because secularism maximizes inclusivity, this approach is recommended for private as well as public schools (Childress & Harper, 2015; Cook-Cottone et al., 2016a).

A secular approach to yoga aligns with secular ethics. By definition, secular ethics is a branch of moral philosophy in which moral ethics are separated from religion and spirituality (Cook-Cottone et al., 2016a). A yoga teacher using a secular approach to yoga can address important social-emotional values that enhance emotional and relational well-being within the context of a purely secular program (Cook-Cottone et al., 2016a; Greenburg & Matri, 2015; Jennings, 2015). Note that secular ethics do not come from a spiritual or religious source and include concepts such as gratitude, integrity, self-inquiry, loving-kindness, honesty, hope, caring for others, compassion for others, self-compassion, equanimity, non-harming, and joy (Cook-Cottone et al., 2016a; Greenburg & Matri, 2015; Jennings, 2015). In fact, several of the Principles of Embodied Growth and Learning reflect this approach (see Chapter 3; e.g., compassion, principle 10 and kindness, principle 11). Aligned with a research-based approach, many of these constructs are currently being studied in the field of positive psychology (Bolier et al., 2013).

As well articulated by Childress and Harper (2015), yoga service providers working in schools have an obligation to recognize and uphold the principles of secularism, and respect the diverse religious and nonreligious beliefs of the school community, both in principle and practice. As research shows, secular yoga practices—postures, breath exercises, relaxation, and meditation—have effects that enhance the mind–body connection, giving students tools for facing stress, enhancing their capacity for control over the physical body, emotions, and thoughts, as well as supporting overall physical well-being (Butzer, et al., 2016; Felver et al., 2015; Khalsa et al., 2012; Serwacki & Cook-Cottone, 2012). Such *transformative experiences* have obvious merit (Cook-Cottone et al., 2016a; Cook-Cottone et al., 2016b). Failure to adhere to the key components of secular yoga in publicly funded schools threatens to undermine the success of the field, as well as access to practices that have positive effects on young people (Cook-Cottone et al., 2016a; Cook-Cottone et al., 2016b). Given the sensitivity and complexity of this issue, it will serve you to be intentional, transparent, and collaborative in how you plan to handle this in your teaching of yoga. Be sure that your administrators, parents, and peers know exactly how you will handle these issues.

THE COURT RULES: YOGA IN SCHOOLS IS OKAY

Many had thought the tensions surrounding religion were to continue to slowly dissipate only to be seen as part of the long history of yoga (Cook-Cottone, 2015). In Encinitas, a coastal beach city in San Diego County, California, the religion debate resurfaced and went to the court systems. The lawsuit emerged from a set of concerned parents within the

Encinitas Union School District (Baird, 2014). The district had received a grant from the Jois Foundation to offer Ashtanga yoga (i.e., a style of contemporary yoga) practice to the students. In an effort to accommodate concerned parents, the yoga was presented free of Sanskrit terms and Hindu references. For example, postures were given different names (e.g., sukhasana was called crisscross applesauce; Cook-Cottone, 2015; Cook-Cottone et al., 2016b). Still concerned, a group of parents moved forward with the lawsuit demanding that the school district suspend its unconstitutional religion-based physical education program (Cook-Cottone, 2015; Cook-Cottone et al., 2016b). The school district argued that they were offering a contemporary physical education program that included stretching, breathing techniques, and relaxation strategies for children and they were *not offering* a religious program (Baird, 2014). On July 1, 2013 the court system agreed with the school district ruling that the practice of yoga in schools neither endorses nor inhibits any religion (Baird, 2014; Cook-Cottone, 2015; Cook-Cottone et al., 2016b). In 2015, the California Court of Appeals upheld the lower court's ruling that the Encinitas program was constitutional, stating that while the practice of yoga may be religious in some contexts, the classes in question were "devoid of any religious, mystical, or spiritual trappings" (*Sedlock v. Baird*, 2015). Note that, in order to be considered constitutional, a government practice must pass the Lemon test: (a) the governmental program must have a secular purpose, (b) the program's primary effect must be one that neither advances nor inhibits religion, and (c) the program must not foster an excessive government entanglement with religion (*Lemon v. Kurtzman*, 1971).

TRAINING FOR TEACHERS: HAVING THE TOOLS FOR SUCCESS

"Any education program is only as effective as its teachers" (Childress & Harper, 2015, p. 33). That said, the success and effectiveness of the yoga program in your school or classroom is highly dependent of the quality, enthusiasm, and training of the teachers who deliver it. The following issues are important to consider: specific training for teaching yoga in schools, supervision, classroom management, training specific to students with disabilities, and training specific to trauma (Childress & Harper, 2015).

Teachers should be specially trained and mentored to deliver yoga in schools (Childress & Harper, 2015). Teaching yoga to children in school is wholly different from teaching yoga to children in a studio or community center and, more obviously, from teaching adolescents and adults in a studio setting. With experience only from studios or centers in which families sign-up for yoga classes with intention and interest, yoga teachers are frequently ill prepared to teach school-based yoga where students sometimes lack interest and motivation to engage. School-based yoga teachers, at best, should have school-specific yoga teacher training credentials (see Kripalu Yoga in the Schools Teacher Training at kripalu.org/kyis-teacher-training or Little Flower: The School Project at littlefloweryoga.com/programs/the-school-yoga-project). It is also acceptable, although school-specific content will be missed, to secure training programs specific to children (see The Baptiste Institute: Kids Yoga Teacher Training at www.baptisteyoga.com/pages/kids-yoga-teacher-training; for an overview of programs see Chapter 13 of this text). The Yoga Alliance has a set of Children's Yoga Standards. A school that meets these standards is called a Registered Children's Yoga School (RCYS; see www .yogaalliance.org/Credentialing/Standards/ChildrensStandards). Once a teacher is credentialed, they are considered a Registered Children's Yoga Teacher (RCYT; see www.yogaalliance .org/Credentialing). Note that, with children's and not school-specific training, there will be a strong need for supervision as yoga teachers work to navigate the nuances of working within a school system and within the context of diversity of students and student needs.

Childress and Harper (2015) caution that school-based programs should be developmentally and school appropriate. In order to do this, yoga instruction should include specific training that addresses the nuances of the school system and how the classroom teachers, administration, and other school personnel work together to deliver the curriculum. The training should include developmental principles in all domains of child development: cognitive, emotional, physical, and social (Childress & Harper, 2015). To ensure that the program continues to be delivered with effectiveness, integrity, and fidelity, school-based yoga teachers should be offered routine supervision.

School-based yoga teachers need skills in classroom management (Childress & Harper, 2015). Over the 15 years that we studied our yoga prevention program for middle school girls, the most challenging aspect of the program delivery had nothing to do with yoga poses, the psycho-educational content, the relaxation techniques, or the journal reflections. The most difficult aspect was behavior management. No matter how wonderful your program is and how compelling it is to you, delivering it to students and getting them excited about it, while following directions and managing all the feelings and challenges that present during a yoga practice, takes some doing. As you can imagine, my research team meetings were filled with coaching for behavior management. For a great book on overall classroom management in schools read Wong, Wong, Jondahl, and Ferguson (2014), *The Classroom Management Book*. See also Childress and Harper (2015) and their thoughts on classroom management (pp. 36–37), Jennings (2015; pp. 40–50), and Herrington's (2012) yoga star chart (pp. 53–54).

Use the Principles of Embodied Growth and Learning (see Chapter 3) to help students make good behavioral choices (e.g., principle 7, I choose my focus and my actions). These principles provide a framework for embodiment, self-regulation, compassion, and kindness. On the yoga mat and in the classroom, if you reinforce the 12 principles, the students will be well on their way to self-regulation. Post the principles on your wall and refer to them as children struggle. For example, you can remind them to work toward awareness and presence in their bodies (principles 2 and 3). Remind them that in yoga and in life we allow feelings and use them carefully to make choices (principles 5 and 7). One of my favorites is self-determination (i.e., principle 8, I do the work). As all of the principles are written in the first person, the ownership is placed within the student to choose his or her actions. It is from that perspective (self-management from within) that behavioral management should stem. Over the years of the Girls Growing in Wellness and Balance Program, we came up with many tools (Cook-Cottone, Kane, Keddie, & Haugli, 2013):

- Prioritize personal responsibility and learning.
- Work with the group to develop ground rules (for discussion, yoga, and the sequence of the session).
- Present guiding principles (see Chapter 3); for example, respect for others, kindness, honoring confidentiality, keeping each other safe, and support.
- Use the borders of the mat to create personal boundaries.
- Prioritize safety first.
- Give students control and chances to lead.
- Place an assistant or teacher between challenging students (use proximity).

- Place the mats in a circle so students feel safe (no one behind anyone).
- Cycle between effort and rest.
- Follow a routine to create a predicable structure.
- Remember that school rules are always part of yoga rules.
- Model appropriate behavior always and in all ways.

Perhaps the last tip is the most important. Remember, you are always teaching. Remind the students they are worth the effort (principle 1, see Chapter 3). That is, they are worth their own effort to be present for themselves. Critically, you will show them through your intentional self-regulation that you think *they are worth your effort*, too. Harper (2013) also suggests that we remember this, "[Each] child is more important than yoga," (p. 30). Sometimes we get so wrapped up in our desire to share yoga and teach the tools of yoga that we forget to stay aware of and connected to the students' experiences (Harper, 2013). As school-based yoga teachers, one of the most important qualities we will model is connection to self and others (Cook-Cottone, 2016).

School-based yoga teachers need training specific to students with disabilities, to diversity and cultural responsiveness, and to students who experienced trauma (Childress & Harper, 2015). Childress and Harper (2015) cite statistics reminding us that across the United States, about 13% of students are receiving services due to a classification in special educational services. This percentage is higher in some cities and states and lower in others. These students and other students at risk for academic struggle have intellectual disability, developmental delay, autism, health impairments, emotional disturbance, hearing impairments, physical challenges (e.g., cerebral palsy, multiple sclerosis), traumatic brain injury, or blindness; some students have a combination of issues that make learning a challenge. More on trauma-sensitive approaches in Chapter 10.

CONCLUSION

As you can see, the history is long, complex, paradoxical, and ever-evolving. Consistent with its history, today's yoga continues to be multifaceted, heterogeneous, diverse, and, for those of us trying to define it, a moving target (Cook-Cottone, 2015; Cook-Cottone et al., 2016a). To know one type of yoga is *not* to know all types (Cook-Cottone, 2015). Generally, there is a movement toward academic and popular acceptance of yoga as a method for improving well-being, reducing stress, and enhancing mental and physical health as evidenced by insurance companies reimbursing members for classes in many states and the addition of federal funding streams supporting research on yoga and other complementary approaches to health (Cook-Cottone, 2015). As years pass, needs change, and cultures evolve, the goal of yoga stays the same—to integrate mind and body and bring growth (Cook-Cottone, 2015). In this way, what is known as yoga today, may look different and be different from yoga in the past; yet, it is in the exact form that we need right now (Cook-Cottone, 2015; Horton, 2012). History, as well as the legal, ethical, and social narrative all tell us this—it is quite likely that as we continue to study and practice yoga, it will continue to evolve in both form and content (Cook-Cottone, 2015). Moreover, we will continue debating and exploring issues such as authenticity, religious content, secular content, and efficacy. For an overview of the best practice of yoga in schools see Childress and Harper (2015).

REFERENCES

Anderson, S., & Sovik, R. (2000). *Yoga mastering the basics*. Honsedale, PA: The Himalayan Institute.

Baird, T. (2014). *Encinitas Union School District; yoga in the schools conference keynote*. A keynote presentation given at the Yoga in the Schools Conference (April 23–25) at Kripalu, Lenox, MA.

Baptiste, B. (2003). *Journey into power: How to sculpt your ideal body, free your true self, and transform your life with yoga*. New York, NY: Fireside.

Baron, A., Evangelou, M., Malmberg, L. E., & Melendez-Torres, G. J. (2015). *The tools of the mind curriculum for improving self-regulation in early childhood: A systematic review*. Oslow, Norway: The Campbell Collaboration.

Bolier, L., Haverman, M., Westerhof, G. J., Riper, H., Smit, F., & Bohlmeijer, E. (2013). Positive psychology interventions: A meta-analysis of randomized controlled studies. *BMC Public Health, 13*(1), 119.

Bryant, E. F. (2009). *The yoga stutras of Patanjali*. New York, NY: North Point Press.

Butzer, B., Bury, D., Telles, S., & Khalsa, S. B. S. (2016). Implementing yoga within the school curriculum: A scientific rationale for improving social-emotional learning and positive student outcomes. *Journal of Children's Services, 11*(1), 3–24.

Childress, T., & Harper, J. C. (2015). *Best practices for yoga in the schools*. Rhinebeck, NY: Omega Institute, Yoga Service Council.

Cobb, E. F., McClintock, C. H., & Miller, L. J. (2016). Mindfulness and spirituality in positive youth development. In Itia Ivtzan & Tim Lomas (Eds.), *Mindfulness in positive psychology: The science of meditation and wellbeing* (pp. 245–264). New York, NY: Routledge.

Coelho, P. (2014). This much I know. *The Guardian*. Retrieved January 25, 2014, from https://www.theguardian.com/books/2014/jan/25/paulo-coelho-this-much-i-know.

Cook-Cottone, C. P. (2015). *Mindfulness and yoga for self-regulation: A primer for mental health professionals*. New York, NY: Springer Publishing.

Cook-Cottone, C. P., Childress, T., & Harper, J. C. (2016). What is secular yoga in schools: Conceptual review and inquiry. Manuscript in preparation.

Cook-Cottone, C. P., Kane, L., Keddie, E., & Haugli, S. (2013). *Girls growing in wellness and balance: Yoga and life skills to empower*. Stoddard, WI: Schoolhouse Educational Services.

Cook-Cottone, C. P., Lemish, E., & Guyker, W. M. (2016). *Yoga is religion lawsuit: Phenomenological analysis of the Encinitas Union School District experience*. Yoga in the Schools Symposium, March, 2016, Kripalu Center, Stockbridge, MA.

De Michelis, E. (2008). Modern yoga: History and forms. In M. Singleton, & J. Byrne (Eds.), *Yoga in the modern world: Contemporary perspectives* (pp. 17–35). New York, NY: Routledge.

Douglass, L. (2007). The yoga tradition: How did we get here? A history of yoga in America, 1800–1970. *International Journal of Yoga Therapy, 17*, 35–42.

Douglass, L. (2010). Yoga in the public schools: Diversity, democracy and the use of critical thinking in educational debates. *Religion & Education, 37*, 162–174.

Douglass, L. (2011). Thinking through the body: The conceptualization of yoga as therapy for individuals with eating disorders. *Eating Disorders, 19*, 83–96.

Felver, J. C., Butzer, B., Olson, K. J., Smith, I. M., & Khalsa, S. B. S. (2015). Yoga in public school improves adolescent mood and affect. *Contemporary School Psychology, 19*, 184–192.

Field, T. (2011). Yoga clinical research review. *Complementary Therapies in Clinical Practice, 17*, 1–8.

Flynn, L. (2013). *Yoga for children: 200+ yoga poses, breathing exercise, and meditations for healthier, happier, more resilient children*. Avon, MA: Adams Media.

Gandhi, M. (2011). *The Bhagavad Gita according to Gandhi*. Blacksburg, VA: Wilder Publications.

Gard, T., Noggle, J. J., Park, C. L., Vago, D. R., & Wilson, A. (2014). Potential self-regulatory mechanisms of yoga for psychological health. *Frontiers in Human Neuroscience, 8*, 76–95.

Greenburg, M. T., & Mitra, J. L. (2015). From mindfulness to right mindfulness: The intersection of awareness and ethics. *Mindfulness, 6*, 74–78.

Harper, J. C. (2010). Teaching yoga in urban elementary schools. *International Journal of Yoga Therapy,* *20,* 99–109.

Harper, J. C. (2013). *Little flower yoga for kids: A yoga and mindfulness program to help your child improve attention and emotional balance.* Oakland, CH: New Harbinger Press.

Herrington, S. (2012). *Om Schooled: A guide to teaching kids yoga in real-world schools.* San Marcos, CA: Addriya.

Horton, C. A. (2012). *Yoga Ph.D.: Integrating the life of the mind and the wisdom of the body.* Chicago, IL: Kleio Books.

Iyengar, B. K. S. (1996). *Light on yoga.* New York, NY: Schocken Books.

Jennings, P. A. (2015). Mindfulness-based programs and the American public school system: Recommendations for best practices to ensure secuality. *Mindfulness, 7,* 176–178.

Karpov, Y. V. (2014). *Vygotsky for educators.* New York, NY: Cambridge University Press.

Khalsa, S. B. S., Hickey-Schultz, L., Cohen, D., Steiner, N., & Cope, S. (2012). Evaluation of the mental health benefits of yoga in a secondary school: A preliminary randomized controlled trial. *The Journal of Behavioral Health Services & Research, 39*(1), 80–90.

Kraftsow, G. (1999). *Yoga for wellness: Healing with the timeless teachings of Viniyoga.* New York, NY: Penguin Putnam.

Lemon v. Kurtzman. (1971) 403 U.S. 602 [29 L.Ed.2d 745, 91 S.Ct. 2105].

Liberman, K. (2008). The reflexivity of the authenticity of hatha yoga. In M. Singleton, & J. Byrne (Eds.), *Yoga in the modern world: Contemporary perspectives* (pp. 100–116). New York, NY: Routledge.

Masters, B. (2014). the (f) law of karma: In light of *Sedlock v. Baird*, would meditation in classes in public schools survive the First Amendment establishment clause challenge? *California Legal History, 9,* 225.

McCall, T. (2007). *Yoga as medicine: The yogic prescription for health and healing.* New York, NY: Bantam Dell, Random House.

Prabhavananda, S., & Isherwood, C. (2007). *How to know God: The yoga aphorisms of Patanjali.* Hollywood, CA: Vedanta Press.

Roach, G. S., & McNally, C. (2005). *The essential yoga sutras: Ancient wisdom for your yoga.* New York, NY: Three Leaves Press, Doubleday.

Rybak, C., & Deuskar, M. (2010). Enriching group counseling through integrating yoga concepts and practices. *Journal of Creativity in Mental Health, 5,* 3–14.

Sedlock v. Baird. (2015). 235 Cal. App. 4th 874 (Ct. App. 2015).

Serwacki, M., & Cook-Cottone, C. (2012). Yoga in the schools: A systematic review of the literature. *International Journal of Yoga Therapy, 22,* 101–110.

Simpkins, A. M., & Simpkins, C. A. (2011). *Mediation and yoga in psychotherapy: Techniques for clinical practice.* New York, NY: Wiley.

Singleton, M. (2010). *Yoga body: The origins of modern posture practice.* New York, NY: Oxford University Press.

Singleton, M., & Byrne, J. (2008). *Yoga in the modern world: Contemporary perspectives.* New York, NY: Routledge.

Sovik, R. (2005). *Moving inward: The journey to meditation.* Honesdale, PA: Himalayan Institute Press.

Stephens, M. (2010). *Teaching yoga: Essential foundations and techniques.* Berkeley, California: North Atlantic Books.

Strauss, S. (2005). *Positioning yoga: Balancing acts across cultures.* New York, NY: Berg/Oxford.

Svenaeus, F. (2013). Anorexia nervosa and the body uncanny: A phenomenological approach. *Philosophy, Psychiatry, & Psychology, 20,* 81–91.

Swenson, D. (2007). *Ashtanga yoga: The practice manual.* Austin, TX: Ashtanga Yoga Productions.

Vygotsky, L. S. (1962). *Thought and language.* Cambridge, MA: MIT Press.

Weintraub, A. (2004). *Yoga for depression: A compassionate guide to relive suffering through yoga.* New York, NY: Broadway Books.

Weintraub, A. (2012). *Yoga skills for therapists: Effective practice for mood management.* New York, NY: W. W. Norton.

Wong, H. K., Wong, R., Jondahl, S., & Ferguson, O. (2014). *The classroom management book.* California, CA: Harry K. Wong Publications.

CHAPTER 10

THE YOGA CLASSROOM: CREATING SUPPORTS AND STRUCTURE FOR YOGA-BASED SELF-REGULATION AND LEARNING

As goes your breath, so goes your heart.
As goes your heart, so go your thoughts.

(Cook-Cottone, 2015, p. 200)

Watch your thoughts;
they become words.
Watch your words; they become actions.
Watch your actions;
they become habit.
Watch your habits; they become character.
Watch your character;
it becomes your destiny.

(Barwick, 1983, p. 23)

The Barwick (1983) quote is one of my all-time favorites. The original version comes from an interpretation of an ancient yoga text by Eknath and Nagler (2007). I cite this quote along with a reminder I often give in yoga class, "As goes your breath, so goes your heart. As goes your heart, so go your thoughts" (Cook-Cottone, 2015). In each breath and each moment our destiny is created. Steadiness of breath yields steadiness of mind. From there, we intentionally self-regulate, choosing our actions as we engage in our lives and relationships. To me, this is yoga. It is well accepted that yoga enhances overall physiological health, strength, and flexibility (Cook-Cottone, 2015; McCall, 2007), but research tells us that yoga offers even more. Consistent with the quote "As a person acts, so he becomes in life..." (Eknath & Nagler, 2007, p. 114), yoga is the embodiment of intention and growth. That is, yoga gives you an on-the-mat and in-your-life opportunity for development.

As explicated by the principles for growth and learning in Chapter 3, teaching these skills begins with teaching competence in breath, awareness, presence, and feeling. Tantillo (2012) says that we honor the social and emotional needs of our students by including daily

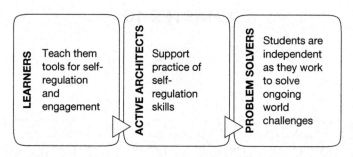

FIGURE 10.1 From learner to architect of the future.

relaxation, breathing, and yoga activity to help them relax, focus, and concentrate. Often discounted, a student who can intentionally breathe, cultivate awareness, stay physically present, and manage feelings has a substantial advantage in being the architect of his or her destiny (see Figure 10.1).

There is a critical shift in focus away from student self-control or an inhibition of impulses, toward a mindful and embodied self-regulation (Shanker, 2016). In mindfulness and embodied self-regulation, students are aware of their impulses and stresses (Shanker 2016). They explore what triggers their impulses and what might be keeping them chronically stressed or wound-up. They work with school personnel independently to create an environment and way of being that is conducive to mindfulness, engagement, and calm yet alert states. They know what calm feels like and have tools to get themselves there (Shanker, 2016). This chapter conceptualizes yoga as *embodied learning* of these tools and offers you the context and guidance to create supports and structure for yoga-based learning in your classroom and/or school. To do this, the concepts of neurological integration, intentional engagement, stress, and trauma are covered. Next, specific guidance for your classroom and school on how to bring yoga to various age groups, create a space for your tools and the accessories needed, as well as how to structure a lesson are given. Figures, case examples, and instructional stories are used to illustrate points.

YOGA AS EMBODIED LEARNING

We ask a lot of our students—we ask them to learn math, language arts, sciences, social and world studies, and the arts. We show them exactly how to do the math; construct a sentence, paragraph, and essay; ways to memorize the countries, cities, landscapes, and biospheres; and how to hold a paintbrush or make a musical instrument sing. We ask them to pay attention, to manage their emotions and behavior, and to be good friends to their classmates, but we often fall well short of teaching them how to do this (Harper, 2013).

Harper (2013) suggests that we don't always have a clear idea of what we are actually asking of students. She gives the example of asking students to pay attention. To pay attention our students must stop thinking about all the things that seem very important and interesting to them, no matter how they are feeling about them. Those other things might be scary, worrisome, exciting, and very compelling (e.g., a provocative text from a peer, mom's panic attack this morning, pizza for lunch, the kid that keeps flicking your head with a pencil and taunting you, or the guy flirting with the student you like). Still, we ask them to focus exclusively on what we are teaching, saying, or doing, no matter how complicated, difficult, lackluster, or frustrating. We ask them to focus and do so in a "way that is productive

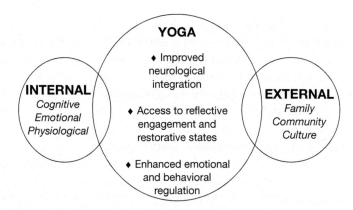

FIGURE 10.2 Neurological and physiological benefits of yoga.
Source: Cook-Cottone, 2015; used with permission.

and socially appropriate" (Harper, 2013). What we are asking when we ask our students to pay attention is something that is very hard to do, even for adults (Harper, 2013). What we want for them and for us is to become skilled at: (a) choosing what we are attending to, (b) filtering out distractions, (c) noticing when we leave ourselves and/or the moment, (d) reengaging, and (e) to keep doing so for a set period of time. That five-step process is the definition of paying attention and can be taught and practiced (Harper, 2013). So, too, can physical presence, emotion regulation, behavioral regulation, and compassion and kindness in friendships (see Chapter 3).

We exist as our bodies—nourishing, nurturing, challenging, attuning, and learning (Cook-Cottone, 2015). Douglass (2011) posits that thinking is only and always embodied. She holds that yoga is an educational tool and an embodied learning in which practitioners systematically engage "in the process and action of thinking through the body" (p. 85). Embodiment, as seen in yoga, promotes well-being at the neurological and physiological levels in these three ways: (a) enhances neurological integration (i.e., neurological differentiation and linkage); (b) reduces reactivity, increases reflective engagement, and improves access to restful and restorative states; and (c) improves emotional and behavioral regulation (Cook-Cottone, 2015; see Figure 10.2).

Supporting Improved Neurological Integration

First, formal yoga practices can help with self-regulation by facilitating mind–body integration (Cook-Cottone, 2015). Neurological integration allows for independent and effective self-regulation (Cook-Cottone, 2015). Students may lack neurological integration for a variety of reasons including their childhood environments and quality of familial relationships, a genetic or physiological background (i.e., physical or emotional trauma) that has resulted in a brain that needs more practice and support for integration than most brains, or there has been engagement in behaviors or practices that disrupted integration (Cook-Cottone, 2015; Siegel, 2012). A lack of integration along with a history of trauma can lead students to negative health, psychological, and relational outcomes (Ahlers, Stanick, & Machek, 2016; Telles, Singh, & Balkrishna, 2012; see *Childhood Disrupted: How Your Biography Becomes Your Biology and How You Can Heal* by Nakazawa [2015]). Our students are stressed

(Harper, 2013); students today have a tremendous amount of worry and anxiety. They feel the tensions and stressors of their parents, hear about the ongoing violence in our communities, hear talk of ongoing war, and feel tremendous pressure to succeed academically and to perform within the arts as well as physical realms (Harper, 2013). As students get older, they also feel pressure to look the right way (Cook-Cottone, Kane, Keddie, & Haugli, 2013). It seems that today's students do little for the sheer joy or play of it, living to negotiate stress and to perform, trying to live up to some set of standards academically, physically, and emotionally. Living in this way, students become disembodied.

Interpersonal neurobiologists posit a similar understanding of integration and healing of the mind-body system. They describe mental life as an *embodied* relational flow of energy and information (Siegel, 2012). That is, the mind is not separate from the body—it both arises from and regulates it (Levine, 2010; Siegel, 2012). Therefore, speaking both from a yogic and neurological point of view, self-regulation is, most certainly, an integrated, embodied experience (Cook-Cottone, 2015). Yoga practice integrates. When practiced as intended, it is believed that yoga brings all of the split-apart aspects of the self together allowing for integration and healing (Cook-Cottone, 2015).

Supporting Access to Reflective Engagement and Restorative States

Many students do not have knowledge of or a sense of regulating themselves emotionally, psychologically, or physically. They often feel as if they are subject to their external world and any stressors that come from it, their unsettled internal world, or both (Cook-Cottone, 2015). Access to reflective engagement and restorative states of being is critical for engaged learning and positive relationships (Cook-Cottone, 2015). Stephen Porges (2011), the author of *The Polyvagal Theory: Neurophysiological Foundations of Emotions, Attachment, Communication, and Self-Regulation,* suggests that yoga training may improve the ability to self-regulate, dampen physiological reactivity, and help students feel more comfortable in their bodies. The general physiological and neurological bases of self-regulation lie in the ability to respond to the outer world and to inner events (e.g., thoughts, memories) in a neurologically integrated and non-reactive manner (Cook-Cottone, 2015; Levine, 2010; Siegel, 2010). In part, this means that we have the capacity to access the reflective and relational aspects of the nervous system even when we are triggered, threatened, or challenged (Porges, 2011).

We need tools for bringing the body away from stressed, defensive reaction and toward healthier and more productive states such as calm, alert, and engagement and states of rest and restoration (Flynn, 2013; Levine, 2010; Porges, 2011). Many of us, and our students as well, get stuck in a stress-response cycle, with chronically activated stress hormones surging through us, causing tension, increased blood pressure, and diverting resources away from digestion, restoration, and healing (Flynn, 2013). Over time, this way of being leads to illness and may have cognitive and learning implications. To develop the skills that we and our students need to manage stress and calm our bodies and minds, we need to engage in practices that require active engagement of the central nervous system while in action, intention, and challenge. We must practice using tools that empower us to intentionally move from one state (e.g., activation, defensive reaction) to another (i.e., restoration and repair; Cook-Cottone, 2015).

Yoga can help students and school personnel to understand what is going on in their bodies and within their nervous systems. There are specific neurological systems that regulate aspects of the body critical to self-regulation (Cook-Cottone, 2015; Levine, 2010; Porges, 2011). Recent research suggests that these systems are a bit more complex than originally understood and are involved in the regulation of physiological, emotional, and relational aspects of self (Porges, 2011). Specifically, the nervous system comprises the central nervous system (the brain and spinal cord) and the peripheral nervous system (Levine, 2010), which comprises the autonomic nervous systems (maintains homeostasis and regulates organs and metabolism) and the somatic nervous systems (involves voluntary muscle control, touch, and proprioception; Levine, 2010). Feeling triggered and in reaction involves the autonomic nervous system, which comprises two systems, the sympathetic nervous system (fight or flight response) and the parasympathetic system.

The vagus nerve, the 10th cranial nerve, plays a substantial role in the dynamics of these systems and in self-regulation (Porges, 2011). The Latin word *vagus* means wandering. It is called the wandering nerve because it has multiple branches that begin in the cerebellum and brainstem and reach through the core of your body and connect to the heart and other major organs. The vagus nerve was named by the German physiologist, Otto Loewi, who discovered that stimulation of the vagus nerve released acetylcholine reducing the heart rate. Today, the vagus nerve is believed to play a role in the calming response from deep breathing, and the parasympathetic nervous system in the rest-and-digest and tend-and-befriend responses. When the vagus nerve is functioning well it is said to have higher vagal tone, which is associated with a decrease in inflammation, blood pressure, depression, and negative moods, and increase in positive emotion, physical health, and social connection.

More specifically, the parasympathetic nervous system functions through what is believed to be two subsystems: (a) the unmyelinated primitive vagus system associated with immobilization and shutdown, and (b) the myelinated vagus system associated with social engagement and muscles in the face, middle ears, and throat (Levine, 2010). When a person is in a safe environment, the parasympathetic nervous system also promotes functions that are associated with rest, growth, and restoration; the sympathetic nervous system promotes increases in metabolic output to negotiate challenges that come from outside of the body (Porges, 2011). It is believed that when threatened or challenged, the nervous system works in a problem-solving hierarchy (see Table 10.1).

It is believed that these systems activate in the face of both real danger and perceived dangers (Levine, 2010). Individuals who have been chronically traumatized, abused, or neglected can experience a domination of the immobilization or shut-down system (Cook-Cottone, 2015; Levine, 2010). Those who have experienced acute trauma or challenge may be more dominated by the fight-or-flight system (Levine, 2010). Choice is lost and self-regulation problems can follow. It is important for teachers to keep in mind that: (a) there are physiological foundations for emotional regulation and self-regulation, and (b) dysregulation of these systems can play a role in self-regulation challenges (Cook-Cottone, 2015). Yoga is an integrated system of tools that can support neurological integration, down regulation of sympathetic (i.e., defensive or reactive) and immobilizing parasympathetic responses, increases in reflective engagement, and promotion of health, strength, and flexibility (Cook-Cottone, 2015; Field, 2011; Levine, 2010). That is, yoga can help. Levine (2010) states, "Somatic approaches can be enormously useful, or even critical, in [the] healing effort" (p. 115). Embodied practices help move students from immobilization and reaction and toward equilibrium and social engagement (Cook-Cottone, 2015; Levine, 2010). For a review of interpersonal neurobiology, see Siegel (2012); for an extensive review of the research on the vagus nerve, see Porges (2011); and for an exploration of trauma and the body, see Levine (2010).

TABLE 10. 1 Hierarchy of Neurologically Based Response Strategies

Problem Stage	Response and Example
Problem or challenge presents	Social engagement, communication, and self-soothing systems are activated. The muscles of the face and throat are stimulated and social engagement is attempted (i.e., activation of the myelinated parasympathetic nervous system).
	Sonya's mom storms into the room, obviously drunk and enraged. Sonya asks, "Mom, are you okay? What happened?" Sonya says to herself, "You've got this. Everything is going to be okay."
Problem or challenge is unresolved or escalates	The body prepares for fight or flight. The nervous system activates the sympathetic nervous system sending information and energy to the limbs and away from rest and restorative processes such as healing and digestion.
	"No, Sonya, I am not okay. I just ran over your f%##@# bicycle in the driveway." She reaches for a belt, "Get over here. Let me show you how many hours I worked to pay for the %%#% bike."
	Sonya runs upstairs, slams her door, and pushes a chair against it. She tries to open the window. It's stuck. She hears her mom coming. Her mother beats her horribly when she's drunk. Sonya can't escape.
Problem or challenge is unresolved or escalates	The body is immobilized or freezes. The nervous systems activate the vagus nerve and dorsal vagal systems.
	Her mom gets through the door. She has the belt and she is enraged. Sonya has dropped to the floor. Unable to escape, she is immobilized, frozen.

Source: Adapted from Cook-Cottone, 2015; informed by Levine, 2010.

CALM BODY, CALM MIND: STRESS AND TRAUMA

As described in Chapter 2, today's students experience substantial stress and a significant subgroup of students have known personal, interpersonal, and/or community trauma (see Cook-Cottone [2004] for an overview of children and trauma). Part of being sensitive and responsive to the diversity among our students is being prepared to work with all levels of stress and trauma. Notably, some argue that the recent history of mass shootings, social tensions and civic unrest, along with ongoing war and international instability is creating a vulnerability among students that is unmatched in history. Most quality yoga teacher trainings have a component that informs teachers-in-training about trauma, trauma effects, and how to teach in a trauma-sensitive manner.

Trauma, Schools, and Yoga

School-based yoga can help students learn skills to self-regulate and calm. Harper (2013) calls this using the *thoughtful brain,* or integrated brain and letting the *protective brain* relax its control. Childress and Harper (2015) argue that all yoga teachers who work in schools should have a basic understating of the effects of trauma on children. With training, school-based yoga teachers will be prepared to respond to the needs and potential reactions of students who have been trauma exposed (Childress & Harper, 2015). They note that it is not within the scope of practice of yoga or for school teachers to treat trauma in school (Childress & Harper, 2015). Knowledge of symptoms and how to be sensitive and responsive creates a framework for better delivery of yoga and the school curriculum (Childress & Harper, 2015). Children who have experienced, or are currently experiencing, trauma (e.g., abuse, neglect, neighborhood violence, ongoing community stress) can experience outcomes that substantially affect their learning, emotional regulation, attentional systems, and relationship behaviors (Childress & Harper, 2015).

According to Telles et al. (2012), it is well recognized that severe psychological trauma is associated with substantial effects. It can cause impairment within the body's neuroendocrine systems, resulting in sympathetic activation and suppression of the parasympathetic nervous system (Telles et al., 2012). Researchers note that there is also an increase in the level of circulating cortisol that has adverse effects on different systems (Telles et al., 2012). Severe trauma occurring in early childhood may have especially serious consequences affecting all aspects of development (i.e., cognitive, social, emotional, physical, psychological; Telles et al., 2012).

In 2015, a lawsuit was filed in Compton, California (*Peter P. et al. v. Compton Unified School District*) in which the plaintiffs cite the empirical literature regarding trauma, its neurobiology and psychological effects (Ahlers et al., 2016). According to Ahlers et al. (2016), the lawsuit highlights complex trauma, or the experience of multiple or chronic trauma experiences, often involving caregiver systems. Specific to schools and learning, the suit alleges that the district does not accommodate students who were exposed to trauma, asking for: (a) immediate implementation of school-wide trauma training for school personnel, and (b) school-wide restorative practices to establish a safe and supportive campus (*Peter P. et al. v. Compton Unified School District*; Ahlers et al., 2016). The lawsuit is proceeding to trial. Ahlers et al. (2016) report that this lawsuit brings the possibility of making trauma training salient for all schools.

Calm Body, Calm Mind: Finding the Growth Zone

Calm body, calm mind is my research team's approach to trauma using yoga. We are in process of finalizing a school-personnel training program. Lindsay Travers, an elementary school teacher, and Melissa LaVigne, a trauma-trained social worker, are core curriculum developers. Through Yogis in Service, Inc. (www.yogisinservice.org; a community-based yoga access program), we have been piloting the curriculum with great success. The program is based on an extensive literature review of the extant research on yoga and trauma. We developed teacher guidelines as well as principles for growth.

When a student has been through severe stress and/or trauma, his or her systems can become highly sensitive. It can be helpful to think about three zones: (a) safe zone, (b) risk zone, and (c) growth zone. First, the place in which students feel safe and competent is their safety zone. Second is the risk zone, which is well outside of the safety zone and is where students may not experience emotional or physical safety. In the risk zone, the stress of the situation may be re-traumatizing. Between the two zones is the growth zone (see Figure 10.3). In the growth zone, students feel uncomfortable because they are learning and doing new things but they are safe. It is important to keep in mind that students who have been traumatized often feel like *any* experience outside of their comfort zones is unsafe. Olson (2014) emphasizes the distinction between *being safe* and *feeling safe*. Although schools can never

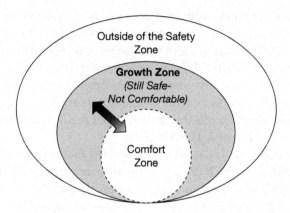

FIGURE 10.3 The growth zone.
Source: Adapted from www.yogisinservice.org.

assure students that they are 100% physically safe, Olson (2014) reinforces that we can, and should, create a school culture within which students and staff feel safe enough for learning to occur.

Teaching from a trauma-informed, yoga-based perspective, school personnel can help students learn how to expand competencies and feel safe within their growth zones. Yoga provides tools that allow students to connect through mindful embodiment (see Chapter 3, principles 1–4, mindful embodiment). Next, with awareness and presence, students practice tools such as inquiry, choice, self-determination, and sustainability (see Chapter 3, principles 6–9, embodied self-regulation). Last, in their growth zones, students work toward developing new competences and tolerances for distress as they practice compassion, kindness, and possibility (see Chapter 3, principles 10–12, mindful development). The tools for mindfulness and yoga-based teaching are effective for working with students who have experienced trauma because they help students develop mindful grit and the tools for mindful growing (see Chapter 3). Further, I encourage you to have a school-wide trauma training program and to attend trainings through conferences teaching mindfulness and yoga to youth in a trauma-sensitive manner.

In yoga practice, students notice that all things (e.g., thoughts, memories, triggers, sense impressions, situations, impulses, and cravings) arise in intensity, eventually decrease in intensity, and then pass away (Cook-Cottone, 2015). You also learn that you have a choice to either notice, attach, or avoid these things. B. K. S. Iyengar (1966) is often quoted as saying, "The pose begins the moment that you want to leave it." What is so powerful about yoga practice is that individuals can live the moments of triggers, intense emotional states, and urges and be in a practice of experiencing and breathing into them. Nakazawaw (2015) puts it this way, "Mending the body [by] moving the body" (p. 177). Emphasizing choice, self-determination, and sustainability (i.e., balancing effort and rest), students can practice moving in and out of their growth zones (see Chapter 3). Growth is found in learning how to try new things (e.g., yoga poses, math problems, or speaking in front of the class) and practicing the mindfulness and yoga skills that you have to navigate feelings and anxieties. There are some additional tips that you may also find helpful when working to be trauma sensitive:

• Provide a safe, stable, and predicable environment (Childress & Harper, 2015; Emerson & Hopper, 2011).

- Handle transitions carefully, letting students know what is happening next and if you will be presenting something new (Childress & Harper, 2015).
- Cultivate safety so that the students can challenge themselves when they are ready in ways that feel safe (Childress & Harper, 2015; Emerson & Hopper, 2011).
- Make sure *how* you are saying something matches the content of what you are saying (Emerson & Hopper, 2011).
- Use a steady, calm, authentic voice that fosters a calm environment (Emerson & Hopper, 2011).
- Use language that invites and provides options versus commands (i.e., "You may wish to …," You may choose to …"; Emerson, 2015).
- Remind students that they can come out of any form or activity at any time (Childress & Harper, 2015; Emerson, 2015).
- Create alternative safe and grounding options during any part of the yoga session that involves closing the eyes and vulnerable postures (e.g., lying on their backs may feel vulnerable, in which case students can assume a resting pose seated with back supported by the wall, eyes open; Childress & Harper, 2015).
- Make sure students are aware of opt out options by using reminders throughout each class (Childress & Harper, 2015).
- Avoid telling students what poses or experiences should feel like; rather, guide them toward what they may notice in a pose (i.e., "You may notice …"; Emerson, 2015).
- Note that praise can communicate a need to please the teacher above inner connection (Emerson & Hopper, 2011).
- Emphasize experience, feelings, and presence over getting the pose right (Emerson, 2015).
- Avoid overpraising students who are compliant or appear to have good form as the message of compliance and perfection for approval may be inadvertently communicated to the whole group (Childress & Harper, 2015).
- Choose verbal assists over physical assists (Childress & Harper, 2015; Emerson & Hopper, 2011).
- Place mats in a circle facing inward, so no one has anyone behind anyone else (Cook-Cottone et al., 2013).
- Remember that children who have experienced trauma may be in a state of flight or fight that may increase the likelihood that they perceive others' behaviors as a threat (Childress & Harper, 2015).
- Be aware of the scope of practice issues and refer students in need to the appropriate mental health professional in your school and/or community (Childress & Harper, 2015).
- Resource supplemental texts such as *Mindfulness and Yoga Skills for Children and Adolescents: 115 Activities for Trauma, Self-Regulation, Special Needs, and Anxiety*, by Barbara Neiman (2015).

GETTING READY FOR YOUR YOGA SESSIONS

To get ready for your yoga sessions you will need to be clear on your goals and objectives for yoga. You also need to be sure you are ready. See also Carla Tantillo's books and body of work (www.mindfulpracticesyoga.com). A trained and seasoned teacher and yoga teacher trainer, she consults with schools and teachers to help them provide curricula aligned with mindful and yoga practices.

Clarify Goals and Objectives

Students will take learning during yoga time seriously if you do. Research is currently being conducted to look at the critical variable of teacher buy-in, yoga teacher home practice, and yoga teacher value of yoga. Although we are waiting for the scientific evidence, seasoned yoga teachers know that their commitment to the preparation and discovery of the class yields quality classes. Recall the Mindful and Yogic Self as Effective Learner (MY-SEL) model in Chapter 3. Mindfulness and yoga are effective tools for helping students develop skills for self -regulation and to prepare them for effective engagement in class. These are good over-arching goals. Other good goals can be related to health and wellness, physical fitness, neuro-logical integrating, stress reduction, and so on. Within that context, be sure you have clearly defined goals and objectives just as you would for any other class (Childress & Harper, 2015). Scaffold your yoga lesson plans to build upon each other (Childress & Harper, 2015). You will want your lesson plans to encompass all the elements of school-based yoga (i.e., yoga poses, breathing exercises, relaxation, and meditation) as well as integration of content to meet the age, diversity, and specific needs of your students (Childress & Harper, 2015). As with all other lesson plans, include ways to assess your students' understanding in the moment (i.e., formative evaluation) and after class (i.e., summative evaluation; Childress & Harper, 2015).

Yoga programs align well with health and wellness, physical education, and some history and human biology/science standards. Herrington (2012) suggests aligning your yoga program goals and objectives with school physical education standards (see pp. 40–41 of Herrington [2012] for an alignment with the National Association for Sports and Physical Education Standards). Physical education standards often include the following: devel-opment of motor skills, understanding movement concepts, engaging in regular physical activity, maintaining health-enhancing levels of physical fitness, demonstrating interper-sonal respect during physical activities, and learning the value of physical activity for health and enjoyment (Herrington, 2012; www.shapeamerica.org/standards/pe/).

Your Presence Is the Most Powerful Teacher

A quote often attributed to Gandhi speaks volumes, "What we do speaks so loudly to chil-dren, that when we talk they cannot hear us." Your modeling of the practice will be one of the most powerful things you do. Center yourself before class (Flynn, 2013). As mentioned previously, your own mindfulness and yoga practice will serve you well as you do the work needed to stay steady and centered during instruction (Flynn, 2013; Harper, 2013). Intentions can involve consistency, responsiveness, awareness, and connection (Flynn, 2013). And have fun (Flynn, 2013). If you love the practices and are having fun, it is likely the students will as well. Create a session that you want to be present in.

If you are a school-based yoga teacher working with classroom teachers, encourage the classroom teachers to participate (Childress & Harper, 2015). There are a variety of benefits. Students take this as a cue that yoga is valued and valuable (Childress & Harper, 2015). Students may feel safer when their teacher is practicing with them (Childress &

Harper, 2015). This is a great time for teachers to engage in their own self-care and yoga practices (Childress & Harper, 2015). Last, as classroom teachers gain experience with yoga techniques, they can reinforce the principles and practices of school-based yoga throughout the school day (Childress & Harper, 2015).

DEVELOPMENTAL ISSUES

Consider the developmental appropriateness of the practice you are delivering (Childress & Harper, 2015). See Table 10.2 for recommendations of yoga teaching practices for each age group.

TABLE 10.2 Yoga Practice Recommendations by Age

AGE	YOGA PRACTICE TIPS
Grades K–2	• Yoga sessions 15–45 minutes (the younger and less experienced, the shorter the session) • Use clear and simple language • Use guided relaxation and meditation more than silence • Use props (breathing buddies; feathers; maximum one prop per session) • Use themes and stories (link to Language Arts and literature) • Use animal, elements of nature, and shapes to describe poses • Establish rituals and routines • Be consistent and predictable • Use preparation and predictability to establish a sense of safety • Make it fun, safe, and warm • Use play to support learning • Engage all senses in fun activities, move to stillness and inward focus • Don't explain everything; let them experience • Take time to spell out rules and expectations for participation • Remember that all behavior communicates a need, *listen* to how students behave and be responsive • Help them see cause and effect • Use music intentionally allowing for quiet time for reflection • Note that younger students can become overwhelmed or distracted by too much stimuli • Offer options for closing their eyes (e.g., choose a focus point) • Integrate the principles of embodied growth and learning
Grades 3–5	• Yoga sessions 20–40 minutes • Integrate yoga games and songs • Can spend more time in silent practices • Can increase depth of breathing and relaxation exercises • Use visualization techniques during relaxation exercises (e.g., images, stories). • Use yoga journals • Embodied games and practices are still important; engage through play • Routine still important • Can begin to move toward a more typical formal yoga class • Increase focus on alignment in poses

(continued)

TABLE 10.2 Yoga Practice Recommendations by Age (*continued*)

AGE	YOGA PRACTICE TIPS
	• Consider introducing more challenging poses • Introduce longer flowing sequences • Use partner work • Allow students to learn through experience rather than telling them • Give students opportunities to lead • Give them the rational reason for learning a lesson • Be mindful of placement of males behind females in class • Fully explore the principles of embodied growth and learning
Grades 6–8	• Yoga session 45–60 minutes • Silent and reflective practice can extend to 20 minutes • Encourage proper alignment in poses • Model proper alignment and suggest adjustments • Let students try poses together using photos and descriptions of poses • Integrate the internet in their exploration of new poses and techniques • Explain the benefits of exercises and poses, bringing in science and health curricula • Teach lessons along with explanations of their benefits • Connect yoga tools to developmental challenges (e.g., moodiness, achievement, social stress, emotional sensitivity) • Allow appropriate expressions of emotions • Keep a steady pace in sessions • Use variety in poses, discussions, relaxation, and meditations • Use sharing and partner work to allow time for peer support and bonding • Teach how lessons can be integrated into lives out of school • Emphasize emotional safety, creating a judgment-free space • Do not allow negative body talk directed toward self or others • Shift "I can't" statements to "I'll try" • Rotate class schedules to create implementation challenges and necessitate team work • Establish after-school yoga clubs, yoga-based interventions, and yoga integrated into wellness and physical education class to create accessibility • Be mindful of placement of males behind females in class • Offer time during and after class for clarifying questions and working through poses • Integrate the principles of embodied growth and learning, applying them to the students' current life experiences
Grades 9–12	• Yoga sessions from 60–90 minutes • Yoga sessions are more aligned with formal yoga class structure • Model proper alignment and suggest adjustments • Present new concepts, practice tools, and allow for dialogue and reactions • Use body-positive talk • Emphasize emotional safety, creating a judgment-free space • Foster a sense of belonging • Be discerning when doing partner work

(continued)

TABLE 10.2 Yoga Practice Recommendations by Age (*continued*)

Age	Yoga Practice Tips
	• Do not allow negative body talk directed toward self or others • Shift "I can't" statements to "I'll try" • Practices can be used before tests, athletic events, and other potential stressful experiences • Encourage proper alignment in poses • Consider integrating yoga teacher training programs into school curriculum • Rotating class schedules creates implementation challenges and necessitates team work • Establish after-school mindfulness clubs, yoga-based interventions, and yoga integrated into wellness and physical education class to create accessibility • Journals can be useful tools of self-reflection and growth • Integrate sharing and partner work • Support self-determination • Be mindful of placement of males behind females in class • Offer time during and after class for clarifying questions and working through poses • Integrate the principles of embodied growth and learning • Teach how lessons can be integrated into lives out of school • Encourage a self-directed practice

Note: See Chapter 5, Table 5.1 for Developmental Notes by Age.
Source: Childress & Harper, 2015; Flynn, 2013; Herrington, 2012.

CREATING A YOGA PROGRAM IN YOUR CLASSROOM OR SCHOOL

Getting ready for a yoga session in your classroom or school is completely manageable. One of my favorite aspects of yoga is it that requires very little, if any, equipment. When my research team went to Kenya in 2013 to study the Africa Yoga project, we were able to visit yoga classes in the most impoverished areas of Kenya. Students used tarps for yoga mats or simply practiced on the clay floors. There was complete joy in practice and no need for fancy mats, blocks, or yoga clothes. In this section, I cover class size, how to create a yoga space, special tips and tools, developmental notes, and an overview of the components of a yoga session. Note that Chapter 11 details the specific poses, breathing exercises, relaxation strategies, and meditations.

Creating a Yoga Space

Space depends on the number of students that you will be teaching. The average class size across the United States is between 20 and 25, although I have heard of classes as large as 35 students. When working with one yoga teacher without an assistant or classroom teacher in the room, the ideal yoga class size for younger students is between 8 and 14 (Cook-Cottone, et al., 2013; Herrington, 2012). For older students, you can have as many as 20 to 30. With larger groups, it is best to have the classroom teacher in the room practice with you or assist, co-teach with another trained yoga teacher, or work with a yoga assistant.

Any space can be a yoga space. You will need about 12 square feet for each 2 x 6 foot yoga mat with plenty of extra space. In terms of space needs, for 30 students, you will need 360 square feet (20 × 18 foot space in the middle of the room). Choose a space with safe and comfortable flooring (Flynn, 2013). Ideally, the floor should be a smooth wood floor or a low-pile carpet (Flynn, 2013). Carla Tantillo (2012), in her book *Cooling Down Your Classroom*, offers an elementary classroom floor plan (p. 24) that designates the areas to the left and right of desks for yoga (i.e., yoga spots). Over the years of providing yoga in school settings, I have found that classroom desks and tables can be easily moved (Childress & Harper, 2015). Placing tennis balls on the feet of tables and chairs reduces sound. At the university we invested in tables that collapse and that have wheels. We can transition from a lecture to a yoga space in about 5 to 10 minutes. Other spaces I have used for yoga spaces include the stage, gymnasium, and library. I found the music room and cafeteria can be challenging as you need to coordinate with cleaning staff to make sure the floor is clean.

Prepare the space you have. Declutter the room as much as possible and minimize distraction and stimuli (e.g., computers turned off; Flynn, 2013; Gillen & Gillen, 2007). Make sure the area is quiet (Flynn, 2013). Turn down school-wide announcement speakers, classroom phones, and place a sign on the door "Yoga in session" (Flynn, 2013). Use natural light or soften the room lights (Flynn, 2013; Gillen & Gillen, 2007). If the view is beautiful and natural, leave the blinds open (Harper, 2013); if the view is distracting or chaotic, consider closing the blinds (Harper, 2013). The ideal temperature is between 65 to 78 degrees (Flynn, 2013). Fresh air is nice. Open windows when you can (Flynn, 2013). Although it is wonderful to have a dedicated space, you do not need one to create the shift into yoga time. Use the removal of shoes, or changing into yoga clothes (which is optional) as a symbol of entering yoga time. See Chapter 5 of this text for more tips on creating a mindful space. For school-based yoga you should consider the following supplies:

- Hang posters and pictures of the yoga poses for reference (Herrington, 2012).
- Yoga mats or substitutes (e.g., beach towels, cut-to-size blankets; Flynn, 2013; Harper, 2013). Herrington (2012) recommends child-size mats; see The Little Yoga Mat Store at www.thelittleyogamat.com).
- Mat cleaner (use all-natural products; Flynn, 2013; Herrington, 2012).
- Blocks and straps (Flynn, 2013; especially for older students in more typical, formal yoga classes).
- Heavy cotton blankets (can be used as props and for relaxation work; Flynn, 2013; Harper, 2013).
- A chime or something to signal the end of meditation (Flynn, 2013; Harrington, 2012).
- A speaker and plug for yoga and relaxation music and scripts (Herrington, 2012).
- A white noise machine to muffle sounds outside of the classroom (Childress & Harper, 2015).
- Scarves for breath and movement work (Flynn, 2013).
- Tissues and feathers can be helpful in teaching breath work (Herrington, 2012; see also Chapter 6 for other tools for meditation; e.g., meditation pebble, breathing buddy).
- Pose cards (Flynn, 2013; good brands include Yoga Pretzels and Yoga 4 Classrooms®). Flynn (2013) also offers tips for making your own pose cards. It can be a fun activity for the class to do together.
- Breathing buddies (Flynn, 2013; see Chapter 5).

- Lamps to use for lower lighting if classroom lights cannot be softened (Harper, 2013).
- Journals (Harper, 2013).

  Do not use:

- A room with mirrors. If there are mirrors you can uses sheets or curtains to cover them (Cook-Cottone et al., 2013; Harper, 2013).
- Eye pillows due to contagion of pink eye and other infections (Herrington, 2012).
- Tibetan singing bowls may be viewed as reminiscent of Buddhist practices and therefore not secular (Cook-Cottone, Lemish, & Guyker, 2016).
- Hands in prayer (it's better to use a hand on the belly and a hand on the heart).
- Do not use music with Sanskrit words or references (Childress & Harper, 2015).
- Do not use the entire class time focusing on the props (only use one major prop a session; Flynn, 2013).

Structure of a Yoga Session

Yoga classes should have a structure and routine (Harper, 2013). Once you set the structure and routine, you should work for consistency (Harper, 2013). The length of a children's yoga class can be anywhere from 10 minutes (i.e., a yoga break), to an hour or more for adolescents (Harper, 2013; Herrington, 2012). Each step of getting through the class session should be modeled and broken into segments (Herrington, 2012). Tips for breaking down the yoga session into segments follow. The time spent on each segment will vary depending on the type of class you choose to teach that day (e.g., restorative, vigorous, contemplative). Note that a lesson planning sheet should include each of the sections listed with sections for the overall goal of the session, assessment of the goal, and materials needed (see Herrington, 2012, p. 147, for a sample planning sheet). I have integrated guidance from several experts on yoga in the schools, as well as tips based on my own experience for you in this section (i.e., Flynn, 2013; Harper, 2013; Herrington, 2012):

- PREPARE: Setting up the room (5 minutes)
- CONNECT: Tuning inward (3–5 minutes)
- ENGAGE: Warm-up (8–10 minutes)
- CHALLENGE: Challenging and vigorous poses (10–15 minutes)
- GROW: Learning and trying time (15–20 minutes)
- CENTER: Re-centering and grounding time (10–15 minutes)
- CALM: Relaxation (5–10 minutes)
- CLOSE: Check in and transition back to class (5 minutes)

PREPARE: Setting Up

Setting up time includes students removing and getting their shoes to the designated area (Herrington, 2012). Decide ahead of time if getting the mats and setting them up will be the students' work or your work (Herrington, 2012). For younger kids, I have found it helpful to add structure by having the mats set up with a block and strap for everyone. With more challenging groups, I have assigned mats by placing their journals (with their names on them) on individual mats before they arrive. Students often feel safer with the mats in a circle facing each other so no one is behind them. If there is no space for this, carefully consider who is in front of whom. Although research on gender and yoga in schools is only in its infancy, yoga conference discussions on best practices suggest that female students may feel vulnerable practicing in front of male students in mixed-gender classrooms. Experienced teachers have observed and reported that this occurs most often in middle and high school age groups. Have a feedback tool for students to talk about their comfort level and class set up. In our work, we used the journals as a tool for student feedback. Each week students had journal writing time. The yoga teachers read and responded to journals between sessions. Several times we were able to adjust our methods to increase student comfort. Finally, as part of set up, let the students know how you would like them to be ready on their mats when it is time for class (e.g., sitting with legs crossed, checking in with their journals). One way to mark the transition to class is to play music during the transition and then turn it off when you are ready to begin (Herrington, 2012).

CONNECT: Turning Inward

Begin with an opening routine (Harper, 2013). Herrington (2012) uses this time to bring everyone to focus. This is a time for connection (Harper, 2013). You want to choose exercises that bring awareness to the felt sense of self (i.e., feelings), breath, and/or physical presence (e.g., physical sensations, body scan). The first weeks of the program you can make a game out of learning the set up (e.g., seeing how fast they can get it done and be on their mats; Herrington, 2012). She asks the students to shift from the outward to the inward by sitting and getting quiet (Herrington, 2012). Herrington suggests asking the students, "How do you feel today?" (p. 68). From a scale of 1 to 10, the students "check in" as you write their responses on the board using a line or a graph. Herrington (2012) suggests checking back in after class and assessing change. They can also record this in their journals.

Once the class is set up and ready to go, you will want to bring students' attention to the current moment and to physical and mental presence. I think of it as two points of focus—time and space. These two points are highlighted in the principles of embodied growth and learning: principle 3, I am mindfully aware, and principle 2, I work toward presence in my physical body. In terms of time, or present moment awareness, ask the students to let go of what has happened before yoga class and what will happen after yoga class and be present right in this moment. Getting even more specific, you can ask them to let go of the pose before and the next pose and be exactly in this pose. In terms of space, I begin by asking them to bring their attention and focus from the school, to the room, to their mats, to their bodies, and then to their breath. In each pose, the specific point of focus may be different (e.g., the feet in Warrior I pose). However, the breath is always a good choice for focus and it works especially well for turning inward. You can also ask students to bring their awareness from all the people in their lives, to the people in the class, to themselves. I like to remind students of principle 1, I am worth the effort. That is, each of them is someone who is worth paying attention to. Poses that work in this section include: Supine Butterfly Pose, Child's Pose, Forward Fold, Downward Facing Dog, and Standing Pose (i.e., Tadasana or Mountain Pose; see Chapter 11 for review of poses).

ENGAGE: Warm-up

In the warm-up section of the session you want to move the students into their bodies, getting their breath and physical selves moving. Herrington (2012) uses breath work here (see Chapter 11). This is also the section of class when many teachers guide the students through sun salutations, a sequence of poses meant to warm your muscles up and get you breathing (Herrington, 2012; see Chapter 11). You can add in an extra challenge at the end that goes with the flow, such as flipping over a Downward Facing Dog to see if any of the students can move the pose into a backbend.

CHALLENGE: Vigorous and Challenging Poses

This section of the class often includes lunges, twisting lunges, chair poses, twisting chair poses, side angle poses, and arm balances, like the Crow pose (see Chapter 11 for pose descriptions). This section moves students into more intensity. As such, this section is a good teaching point for the principles (see Chapter 3): When things appear challenging, remind students that they are worth the effort (principle 1). Encourage the students to use their tools such as breath, awareness, and presence (principles 2, 3, and 4) and to allow their feelings to come through as they work (principle 5). Here, choice is important (principle 7). They can take a break if they need to or want to. However, they want to be in inquiry (principle 6) about what it takes to do the work (principle 8). When they are deciding about taking a break, ask them to consider the balance between effort and rest that is required for sustainability (principle 9). Will taking a break right now help you keep going?

As with all of the sections of the session, remind students to honor efforts toward growing (i.e., "Thank yourself for trying even if you don't get the pose"; principle 10). Remind them to be kind as they coach themselves through the poses ("Use kind words to yourself, 'Good work, Catherine,' 'I am proud of you for trying Catherine'"; principle 11). This section and the following section of the session (i.e., learning and trying time) are the sections in which they can find the most possibility in terms of lived experience (principle 12). As you close this section, balancing poses (i.e., Eagle, Extended Leg raise, Airplane Dancer, Half-Moon, Warrior III, Tree; see Chapter 11) are good for refocusing energy and creating a sense of equanimity.

GROW: Learning and Trying Time

Herrington (2012) suggests that you pick two or three poses to workshop each class. She suggests that you model the pose for the class pointing out key details and points of focus (Herrington, 2012). Next, have two or three students demonstrate the pose. Then, have all the students try the pose. Herrington (2012) suggests that you allow them to work together and encourage each other. You can use any pose here. The intention is really getting into the pose and understanding and practicing the specifics with body, breath, and intention. Herrington (2012) suggests putting the poses of the day up on the board before class. The experience should be positive overall. Make sure the students experience more successes than challenges (Harper, 2013).

CENTER: Grounding and Re-Centering

This part of the sequence should emphasize poses that require grounding and connection to the mat and internal awareness. Poses include Triangle; Warriors I, II, and Peaceful

Warrior; Side Angle; and Wide Legged Forward Fold (see Chapter 11 for pose descriptions and photos). Encourage breath awareness, and physical presence here (principles 2, 3, and 4). Adult classes sometimes include inversions here (e.g., headstand, handstand, forward balance). However, inversions are considered to be the riskiest of yoga poses and are not recommended for schools (Childress & Harper, 2015).

CALM and CLOSE: Relaxation and Closing

The goal of this section of the yoga session is to quiet the body and slow the breath. This section can begin with floor stretches (e.g., Supine Leg Twist, Figure Four). Move into relaxation techniques (Herrington, 2012). End with mindfulness meditations (see Chapters 6 and 11). Classes typically end in a seated position. Rather than placing hands in prayer, ask the students to place one hand on their bellies and one on their hearts as they tune in to their own breathing. Herrington (2012) suggests having students check back in (scale of 1–10) to bring an awareness to the shift that has occurred during yoga practice. Transition out of the session is just as important as transition into it (Childress & Harper, 2015). Have students complete the session by moving through the end of session sequence (e.g., mats put away, straps and blocks put away, shoes on, and desks back into place). The resetting of the room can be part of the mindful movement conducted in class.

BE SAFE AND INCLUSIVE

It is important for school-based yoga teachers to emphasize inclusion and safety (Childress & Harper, 2015). These are traditional school values. In addition, school-based yoga teachers should align programs as much as possible with school curriculum. Safety first. There are a few key practices. First, be very attentive when students are attempting poses (Flynn, 2013). Remind students that if something does not feel right, stop doing it (Harper, 2013). Harper (2013) reminds us that it is always okay in yoga to take a rest, slow down, or take a different form of the pose. It is also important to pace the class carefully, taking time to bring awareness to the qualities of a pose or activity (Harper, 2013). Teachers who focus on quantity over quality often lead a rushed class that misses the point of base awareness, engagement of the senses, and neurological integration. It is important to think of yoga this way: "There is nothing to accomplish here, only things to practice" (Harper, 2013, p. 31). You will want your yoga space to be free of clutter to avoid inadvertent injuries.

Inclusiveness is critical. In order to be inclusive, consult with your school physical therapist, occupational therapist, special education teachers, and school mental health professionals (i.e., school psychologist, school counselor, and school social worker). With their help you can better develop lessons plans with appropriate accommodations and supports. There are several wonderful books addressing yoga for children with special needs. For example, Lois Goldberg (2013) wrote a wonderful book titled *Yoga for Children With Autism and Special Needs* that serves as a how-to manual for yoga for kids in classrooms and therapeutic settings. As a second mention, Barbara Neiman (2015) has written a good resource for students with more emotional needs titled, *Mindfulness and Yoga Skills for Children and Adolescents: 115 Activities for Trauma, Self-Regulation Special Needs, and Anxiety.*

CONCLUSION

This chapter reviewed the key neurological and self-regulation processes that can be supported by yoga practices (i.e., yoga poses, breathing exercises, relaxation, and meditation). Addressing the shift in school-based and best-practices advice in yoga-based curriculum delivery, trauma and trauma-sensitive yoga practices were reviewed. Guidance for teaching to specific age groups was provided to enhance developmental sensitivity. An overall yoga session sequence and directions for setting up a yoga space were offered. In order to reduce redundancy, I did not repeat suggestions offered in Chapter 5 for creating a supportive environment of a mindful practice; please refer to this chapter for creating a smaller mindful space within the classroom (i.e., peace place; Herrington, 2012). Recall from Chapter 5 that the important supportive teaching practices are beginning with what you know; remembering that practices look and feel different from student to student; being mindful of how you teach mindfulness and yoga; using mindful words; explaining mindfulness and yoga practices to students; using imagination, metaphor, and story; connecting to the senses; planning and scheduling mindful and yoga practices; and teaching to developmental levels and age. The following chapters address formal and informal yoga practices and review the research on yoga in schools.

REFERENCES

Ahlers, k., Stanick, C., & Machek, G. R. (2016). Trauma-informed schools: Issues and possible benefits from a recent California lawsuit. *Communiqué, 44*, 1–25.

Barwick, D. D. (1983). *A treasury of days: 365 thoughts on the art of living*. Florence, AL: CR Gibson.

Childress, T., & Harper, J. C. (2015). *Best practices for yoga in schools*. Yoga Service Best Practices Guide Vol. 1 Atlanta, GA: YSC- Omega Publications.

Cook-Cottone, C. P. (2004). Childhood posttraumatic stress disorder: Diagnosis, treatment, and school reintegration. *School Psychology Review, 33*, 127–139.

Cook-Cottone, C. P. (2015). Mindfulness and yoga for self-regulation: A primer for mental health professionals. New York, NY: Springer Publishing.

Cook-Cottone, C. P., Kane, L., Keddie, E., & Haugli, S. (2013). *Girls growing in wellness and balance: Yoga and life skills to empower*. Stoddard, WI: Schoolhouse Educational Services, LLC.

Cook-Cottone, C. P., Lemish, E., & Guyker, W. (2016). Yoga is religion lawsuit: Phenomenological analysis of the Encinitas Union School District experience. Yoga in the Schools Symposium, March 2016, Kripalu, MA.

Douglass, L. (2011). Thinking through the body: The conceptualization of yoga as therapy for individuals with eating disorders. *Eating Disorders, 19*, 83–96.

Eknath, E., & Nagler, M. N. (2007). *The Upanishads*. Tomales, CA: Nilgiri Press.

Emerson, D. (2015). *Trauma-sensitive yoga In therapy: Bring the body into treatment*. New York, NY: W. W. Norton.

Emerson, D., & Hopper, E. (2011). *Overcoming trauma through yoga: Reclaiming your body*. Berkeley, CA: North Atlantic Books.

Field, T. (2011). Yoga clinical research review. *Contemporary Therapies in Clinical Practice, 17*, 1–18.

Flynn, L. (2013). *Yoga for children: 200+ yoga poses, breathing exercises, and meditation for healthier, happier, more resilient children*. Avon, MA: Adams Media.

Gillen, L., & Gillen, J. (2007). *Yoga calm for children: Educating heart, mind, and body*. Portland, OR: Three Pebble Press.

Goldberg, L. (2013). *Yoga for children with autism and special needs.* New York, NY: W. W. Norton.

Harper, J. C. (2013). *Little flower yoga for kids: A yoga and mindfulness programs to help your children improve attention and emotional balance.* Oakland, CA: New Harbinger Publications.

Herrington, S. (2012). *Om schooled: A guide to teaching kids yoga in real-world schools.* San Marcos, CA: Addriya.

Iyengar, B. K. S. (1966). *Light on yoga.* New York, NY: Schocken Books.

Levine, P. L. (2010). *In an unspoken voice: How the body releases trauma and restores goodness.* Berkeley, CA: North Atlantic Books.

McCall, T. (2007). *Yoga as medicine: The yogic prescription for health and healing.* New York, NY: Bantam Dell, Random House, Inc.

Nakazawa, D. J. (2015). *Childhood disrupted: How your biology becomes your biology and how you can heal.* New York, NY: Atria Books.

Neiman, B. (2015). *Mindfulness and yoga skills for children and adolescents: 115 activities for trauma, self-regulation special needs, and anxiety.* Eau Claire, WI: PESI Publishing & Media.

Olson, K. (2014). *The invisible classroom: Relationships, neuroscience, and mindfulness in school.* New York, NY: W. W. Norton & Company.

Porges, S. W. (2011). *The polyvagal theory: Neurophysiological foundations of emotions, attachment, communication, and self-regulation.* New York, NY: W. W. Norton.

Shanker, S. (2016). Self reg: How to help your children (and you) breath the stress cycle and successfully engage with life. Tononto, ON: Penguin Press.

Siegel, D. J. (2010). *The mindful therapist. A clinician's guide to mindsight and neurological integration.* New York, NY: W. W. Norton.

Siegel, D. J. (2012). *Pocket guide to interpersonal neurobiology: An integrative handbook of the mind.* New York, NY: W. W. Norton.

Tantillo, C. (2012). *Cooling down your classroom: Using yoga, relaxation, and breathing strategies to help students learn to keep their cool.* Oak Park, IL: Mindful Practices.

Telles, S., Singh, N., & Balkrishna, A. (2012). Managing mental health disorders resulting from trauma through yoga: A review. *Depression Research and Treatment, 9,* doi:10.1155/2012/401513

CHAPTER 11

ON THE MAT: FORMAL YOGA PRACTICES FOR SELF-REGULATION AND ENGAGEMENT

The Anchor Spot:
Please put your hand mindfully
on your anchor spot,
your heart or your belly,
breathing in, breathing out.

(Kellie Love, Aliza's Yoga Teacher)

It's like having a safe haven in your pocket.

(Zarida, Aliza's Mom; *Aliza and the Mind Jar*, Bronx, New York; Love, 2015)

Yoga means connection. You are truly practicing yoga when you connect with your self. The anchor spot is a term used in children's yoga to guide students in finding a point of inner connection. To *anchor* is to find a connection that keeps you from drifting. With boats it's a heavy metal object. In yoga, it's a place within. The *anchor spot* is your heart or your belly. By placing your hands on your heart or your belly, you add an external feedback loop (i.e., your hands to your body) to your internal feedback (i.e., the internal sensation of breath and heartbeat). Closing your eyes, you can bring your awareness to the internal and external sensory experience for your breath and heartbeat. It is a wonderful self-soothing technique. In this way, the ability to calm and soothe comes from your own settling down and turning inward. Students feel empowered as they are the source of their own self-regulation. Like Zarida, Aliza's mom said in the video "Aliza and the Mind Jar," having an anchor spot or the ability to turn inward for calm, "It's like having a safe haven in your pocket" (Love, 2015; see vimeo.com/119439978). This is the connection of yoga.

I find it fascinating to see how hard it is for us humans to stay connected and present. Baptiste (2016) suggests that being fully present can be scary for us. The trauma specialists agree that for some of us, it can be downright terrifying to be fully present (Levine, 2010). As a default we disconnect. As adults we model checking out, reacting, and losing our connection to the students. The students, faced with stress and challenge, emulate what they see. The result is a disconnected, hard-to-manage classroom that feels very stressful to be in for everyone—teachers and students alike. The answer for the class-room lies in the answer for all of us: connection, breath, self-soothing, and engagement. As this is not easy to do, we must practice over and over and over again. As we do, we model and teach the students how to reconnect, over and over and over again. Note, a solid informal practice (i.e., the integration of mindfulness and yoga techniques into our daily lives) is rooted in a steady formal practice. This chapter reviews yoga poses (asana), breathing exercises, relaxation techniques, and meditation. These are the on-your-mat, formal practices of school-based yoga.

YOGA POSES: ASANAS

Yoga postures (asanas) have many benefits such as increased flexibility, strengthened mus-cles, enhanced balance, improved immune system, better posture, enhanced lung function, slower and deeper breathing, enhanced oxygenation of tissues, and relaxation of the ner-vous system (Anderson & Sovik, 2000; Cook-Cottone, 2015; McCall, 2007; Stephens, 2010). In his book, *Yoga as Medicine*, McCall (2007) lists and details over 40 benefits. The yoga pos-tures, or asanas, stretch and tone muscles, help keep the tissues and joints flexible, and may, in some poses, massage internal organs and glands (Cook-Cottone, 2015; Field, 2011). Poses are typically done in concert with deep, diaphragmatic breath (Field, 2011). Connection in yoga is found in the alignment of breath, attention, and intention as you move through and stay in the yoga poses (Cook-Cottone, 2015).

Yoga poses let us, and students, be empowered in the present moment (Willard, 2016). Willard (2016) cites an emerging line of research that suggests that how you hold your body can shape who you are. If you have not seen it yet, watch Amy Cuddy's (2012) TED Talk, "Your body language shapes who you are." In brief, there is evidence that holding a power pose has neuroendocrine, behavioral, and social benefits. Power poses have the following qualities: expansiveness (i.e., taking up more space) and openness (i.e., keeping limbs open or closed; Carney, Cuddy, & Yap, 2010). The results of Carney et al. (2010) study found that posing in high-power displays (i.e., open and expansive) when compared to low-power displays (i.e., closed and restricted) caused psychological and behavioral changes consistent with literature on those that hold social power. That is, high-power displays yielded elevation of testosterone, reduction in the stress hor-mone cortisol, and increased behaviorally demonstrated risk tolerance and feelings of power (Carney et al., 2010). More research is needed, especially research specific to yoga. However, the implications are compelling as we look more into the empowering role of embodying Warrior Pose, Mountain Pose, and powerful Lunge Pose.

In Chapter 10, the overall structure of the yoga class was presented. Here I cover the various poses within the section that they might fit: setting up the room (Prepare), turning inward (Connect), warm-up (Engage), challenging and vigorous poses (Challenge), learn-ing and trying time (Grow), centering time and grounding (Center), relaxation (Calm), and closing (Close). As reviewed in Chapter 10, preparing, or setting up the room involves the transition from classwork time to yoga time. It may include moving furniture, removing shoes and changing (although specific yoga clothes are not needed), setting up mats, and getting out yoga props (e.g., blocks and straps).

Each of the other sections of the overall yoga class layout are associated with a series of poses that are believed to serve the overall intention of that section of the sequence (e.g., sun salutations help students engage their bodies and warm up). Short descriptions of the poses, the key instructional points, and a photograph are offered for poses in each section. The twelve Principles of Embodied Growth and Learning can be offered as themes for the week and re-enforced during the class (see Chapter 3 for a review of the principles; worth (1), breath (2), awareness (3), presence (4), feeling (5), inquiry (6), choice (7), self-determination (8), sustainability (9), compassion (10), kindness (11), and possibility (12). There are about 36 weeks in a school year. A classroom teacher could rotate through the themes three times a year.

Tips for Teaching Poses

There are a few things to remember when teaching poses to students. First, no book or video can replace a quality teacher-training program. This text is meant as a resource to reinforce knowledge or introduce you to new ideas. It is not meant to replace a teacher-training program (see Chapter 3 for notes on training). The following are tips from some of the best school- and youth-based teacher trainers and some things I have learned over the years in my own yoga teaching.

- Establish foundational poses first (Flynn, 2013). These are (a) Easy Seated Cross-Legged Pose, (b) Mountain Pose, and (c) Resting Pose (Flynn, 2013). According to Flynn (2013) these foundational poses provide a home base to return to between other poses. Further, Mountain Pose is considered to be *the* foundational pose from which all other poses are generated. The alignment in Mountain Pose is a framework for alignment in yoga.
- Build each pose from the ground up and center outward. When teaching alignment, begin with the ground as a root or base for the pose. Then instruct the students to notice the connection of their hands and/or feet with the floor. Ask them to ground, press, or engage here. Move your instruction up the legs and/or arms, to the core, and to the crown of the head (or whatever body part is closest to the ceiling). As you do this, instruct the pose from the center outward. Even in expansive poses (e.g., Half Moon), the student is more stable and can experience more success and expansion from a grounded and integrated starting point.
- Speak to action, body part, direction, and anchor (Stephens, 2010). That is, when giving refinements for a pose, first tell the students the action you would like them to take (e.g., press, move, step, engage, draw, reach). Next, tell them to which body part you are referring (e.g., your foot, hand, body, eyes, tops of femurs). Next, tell them the direction (e.g., inward, toward, into, away from, back, forward, up, down). Last, provide an anchor point for the action and direction (e.g., spine, back of room, ceiling, floor). All together it sounds like this, "Draw your naval toward your spine," "Reach your hands up toward the ceiling," "Press your foot into the mat."
- Prioritize breath awareness (Flynn, 2013). For critical outcomes like decreased stress and increased self-regulation the breath is central (Cook-Cottone, 2015). This is why after the

principle on self-worth, the second principle of the Principles of Embodied Growth and Learning refers to breath (i.e., my breath is my most powerful tool). As you teach, continuously bring awareness back to breath, instruct to breathe, and remind students to breathe. If there is no breath work, there is no yoga.

- Emphasize mindful awareness (principle 3, I am mindfully aware). As you instruct poses encourage mindful awareness by bringing the students' awareness to their bodies (Flynn, 2013). Ask them to notice where they are feeling the stretch, to notice the feeling of the mat under their feet, attend to the sensation of their ribs as they breathe in and out, and the tension in their muscles as they soften or work hard. Ask them to notice their thoughts and information coming in through their senses (e.g., sights, smells, sounds).

- Establish an anchor spot or focal point (Flynn, 2013). I like to establish the root of a pose to dig into. For example in Half Moon, it is the grounded foot and then the belly. From there, establish a point upon which students can anchor their gaze. Suggestions are provided for each pose. As always, the breath should be part of any yoga focus.

- Be clear about the distinction between challenge (and the discomfort of challenge) and pain that means risk for injury. It's okay to feel work and effort in the belly of muscles. If a student feels sharp pain or pain at a joint or near the ends of muscles, this is a sign of risk and an internal message telling the student to ease off the pose. Although we do want students to feel the work of a pose, sharp pain is to be avoided and should not be part of the experience of yoga.

- Prioritize connection over correction. Teach with an intention to help students connect. When we teach from an intention to correct poses, breath, and behavior as the priority, we lose opportunities to teach connection. Approach your class and students from connection first, then help them with alignment, breath work, and behavior. It is not one or the other; it is connection first. From Harvard Business School researchers and colleagues, Cuddy, Kohut, and Neffinger (2013), "A growing body of research suggests that the way to influence—and to lead—is to begin with warmth" (p. 56).

- Use second-person, personal, possessive, and reflexive pronouns to describe body parts and accessories (i.e., you, yours, and yourself). We live in a world that objectifies bodies. Often students feel little personal ownership of their own bodies. To say, "Press *that* foot into *the* mat," depersonalizes the body and distances students from the process. Better is "Press *your* foot into *your* mat." The practice is their practice. Their bodies are their bodies. With our words we want to work toward encouraging personal empowerment and a sense of ownership over their bodies. In the same way, unless you are intentionally working to create group unity, defer to second-person pronouns above first-person plural pronouns (e.g., we, us, ours, and ourselves).

- Honor diversity and cultivate connection. Yoga means union and connection. Connection, by definition is the joining of distinct entities. To join and connect does not mean the loss of what makes us unique—our cultures, ethnicities, body size and shape, race, and personal histories. It means that we can hold onto all that is who we are and practice connection with ourselves and others.

- Be ready to modify and work with special populations as addressed in Chapter 10. Work with physical therapy, occupational therapy, and mental health professionals in your school to problem solve modifications specific to each student who would benefit from them. I have noted a few modifications for each pose. Research deeper; there is much more to be learned. (See Gillen and Gillen [2007] for a quality list of modifications for a variety of poses; see also texts, blogs, and research on chair yoga and yoga for kids with special needs.)

CONNECT: Turning Inward

The CONNECT portion of class is intended to bring the students toward a connection with their breath and bodies (see Chapter 10; Harper, 2013). You want to choose exercises that bring awareness to the felt sense of self (i.e., feelings), breath, and/or physical presence (e.g., physical sensations, body scan). Have students check in (Herrington, 2012). Remind students to be present in their own bodies and in the present moment. Emphasize the Principle of Embodied Learning and Growth for the week (see Chapter 3). Of note, the first five principles (i.e., Mindful Embodiment; Worth [1], Breath [2], Awareness [3], Presence [4], and Feeling [5]) capture the goal of this portion of the sequence.

Easy Seated Cross-Legged Pose

This pose can also be called Criss-Cross-Applesauce, Easy Pose, or the Pretzel (Herrington, 2012; Walsh, 2008). Here you see Kayla with her hands on her anchor spots (i.e., belly and heart; she is breathing and turning inward). Easy Pose calms and balances, strengthens the back and spine, and stretches the legs, ankles, and feet (Flynn, 2013).

POSE 11.1 EASY SEATED CROSS-LEGGED POSE (ANCHOR SPOTS)

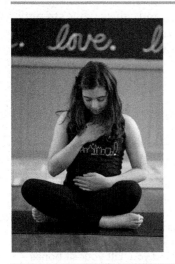

Pose	Easy Seated Cross-Legged Pose
Instruct	Sit on the floor. Knees bent, cross your ankles. Soften your gaze. Place one hand on your belly and one hand on your heart. You can bow your head or lengthen through your spine and lift from your sit bones, through the crown of your head.
Anchor Point	Heart and belly. Eyes are closed, focal point is internal to breath.
Breath Work	Slow, deep, steady breaths. This is a good pose for seated meditations and discussions.

Photograph by Madison Weber; model Kayla Tiedemann.
Source: Curran, 2013; Flynn, 2013; Gillen & Gillen, 2007; Harper, 2013; Herrington, 2012; Walsh, 2008.

Child's Pose

Child's Pose is a good go-to pose when the class feels overwhelmed and students need to take a break. Remind students that it is always okay to take Child's Pose (Harper, 2013). The pose reduces sensory input and is very soothing. It is considered to be a stress reliever and serves as a resting pose (Flynn, 2013). Child's Pose stretches the thighs, hips, ankles, and knees and is believed to relieve back strain (Flynn, 2013).

POSE 11.2 CHILD'S POSE

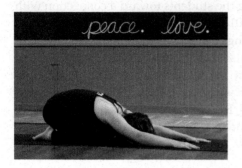

Pose	Child's Pose
Instruct	Come down to your mat on your knees. Extend your toes and make your knees wider than your hips. Fold forward resting your forehead on the mat or a block. Place your hands along your side, palms facing up, or reach them toward the front end of your mat, palms down.
Anchor Point	Breath and internal awareness with eyes closed.
Breath Work	Slow, relaxed, natural breathing.

Photograph by Madison Weber; model Kayla Tiedemann.
Source: Curran, 2013; Flynn, 2013; Gillen & Gillen, 2007; Harper, 2013; Herrington, 2012; Walsh, 2008.

Downward Facing Dog

Downward Facing Dog stretches the shoulders, arms, hamstrings, and calves while strengthening the arms, shoulders, and back (Flynn, 2013). To modify, students can drop their knees as in Table Pose, then draw their sit bones toward the back of the room and stretch their arms forward.

POSE 11.3 DOWNWARD FACING DOG

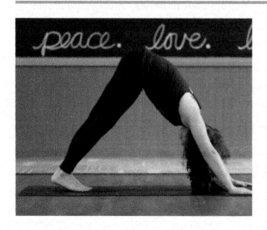

Pose	Downward Facing Dog
Instruct	From Table Pose or Child's Pose, press your hands, especially your thumbs and first fingers, into your mat. Press your feet into your mat, reaching your heels toward the floor behind you. Lift your sit bones toward the ceiling, pressing your chest toward your thighs and your heels even more toward the floor. Soften through your neck.
Anchor Point	Hands and feet. The focal point is a few feet behind the legs on the floor.
Breath Work	Deep, steady, intentional breath.

Photograph by Madison Weber; model Kayla Tiedemann.
Source: Flynn, 2013; Harper, 2013; Herrington, 2012; Neiman, 2015; Walsh, 2008.

Table, Cat, and Cow Poses

Table, Cat, and Cow Poses all begin with the same basic framework of Table Pose (Herrington, 2012). Table Pose helps with core strengthening and stabilization. Cat and Cow Poses improve physical coordination and coordination with breath (Flynn, 2013). Table Pose is presented here with a reaching variation. For Cow Pose, begin from Table Pose and drop your belly, lifting your chest and sit bones on an inhalation (see Flynn, 2013, pp. 120–121). For Cat Pose, arch your spine toward the ceiling, drop your head, and pull your naval to your spine on an exhale (see Flynn, 2013, pp. 120–121). Cycle between Cat Pose and Cow Pose with each inhalation and exhalation (Herrington, 2012).

POSE 11.4 TABLE WITH EXTENSION

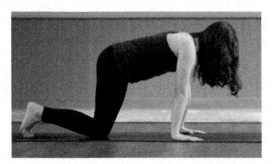 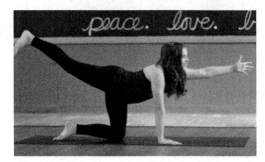

Pose	Table With Extension
Instruct	Come to the floor on your hands and knees with toes tucked under. Press down on your mat, through your thumbs and first fingers. Spread your fingers. Pull your naval up and in toward your spine. Lengthen from your tailbone through the crown of your head. To extend, look slightly forward, reach your left hand forward and your right leg back. Press into the floor and engage your belly. Release and come back to Table Pose. Continue on other side.
Anchor Point	Hands, knees, and belly. Focal point the floor and front wall.
Breath Work	Breathe steadily. Take deep breaths. Inhale for reaches and exhale for releases.

Photograph by Madison Weber; model Kayla Tiedemann.
Source: Curran, 2013; Flynn, 2013; Gillen & Gillen, 2007; Harper, 2013; Walsh, 2008.

Forward Fold

Forward Fold is also called Rag Doll if you weave opposite hand to opposite elbow with arms bent and let your arms hang heavy (Herrington, 2012). It is considered a calming and soothing pose (Flynn, 2013). Forward Fold stretches the back side of the body including the hamstrings, spine, and neck (Flynn, 2013). To modify the pose, encourage students to press their hands on the front of their shins and soften their knees slightly.

POSE 11.5 FORWARD FOLD

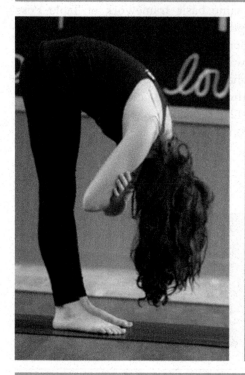

Pose	Forward Fold (Rag Doll)
Instruct	From Mountain Pose, heel–toe your feet to hip-distance apart, engage your belly, and fold at the hips. Allow the very tops of your femurs to move forward while pressing your shins back. Continue to pull your naval in toward your spine. Allow your head to hang heavy with a soft neck.
Anchor Point	The naval pulling in and up toward the spine. The focal point is internal awareness if eyes are closed or a spot directly behind you if eyes are open.
Breath Work	Breath should be steady, even, and natural.

Photograph by Madison Weber; model Kayla Tiedemann.
Source: Curran, 2013; Flynn, 2013; Gillen & Gillen, 2007; Herrington, 2012; Walsh, 2008.

ENGAGE: Warm-up

The ENGAGE section of class warms the students up and gets them ready for more vigorous and challenging poses. The main components of this section are Sun Salutations A (Sun A) and Sun Salutations B (Sun B). A Sun Salutation is a sequence of poses that takes you from standing down to the floor and then back to standing. Some school-based yoga teachers like to call them Warm-up Sequence A and B, as a more secular option, discerning them from more traditional titles. Sun A is the basic core sequence and Sun B builds on Sun A adding Chair and Warrior Poses (Herrington, 2012). See Table 11.1 for the sequences for Sun A and Sun B. I have also added suggestions for breath (i.e., in = inhale, out = exhale). All of the poses are described in the following section with the exception of Half-Lift. In Half Lift, students' feet are on the floor, legs straight, their spines are extended so that they are parallel with the floor, and the crowns of their heads are reaching toward the front of the room. Hands can be placed on the floor or shins. The core muscles should be used to support the back.

During the ENGAGE section, continue to reinforce the breath, connection, and intention. You want to bring a deep engagement into the physical experience (principle 4, I work toward the possibility of presence in my physical body).

TABLE 11.1 Sun Salutation A and B Sequences

Sᴜɴ Sᴀʟᴜᴛᴀᴛɪᴏɴ A Sᴇǫᴜᴇɴᴄᴇ (Bʀᴇᴀᴛʜs)	Sᴜɴ Sᴀʟᴜᴛᴀᴛɪᴏɴ B Sᴇǫᴜᴇɴᴄᴇ (Bʀᴇᴀᴛʜs)
Mountain Pose—Hands High (in)	Chair Pose (in)
Forward Fold (out)	Forward Fold (out)
Half-Lift (in)	Half-Lift (in)
High Plank to Low Plank (out)	High Plank, Low Plank (out)
Upward Facing Dog (in)	Upward Facing Dog (in)
Downward Facing Dog (out)	Downward Facing Dog (out)
Step or Hop Forward (in)	Warrior I—Right Side (in)
Forward Fold (out)	Warrior II—Right Side (optional)
Half Lift (in)	High Plank, Low Plank (out)
Forward Fold (out)	Upward Facing Dog (in)
Mountain Pose—Hands High (in)	Downward Facing Dog (out)
	Repeat Warriors—Left Side
	High Plank, Low Plank (out)
	Upward Facing Dog (in)
	Downward Facing Dog (out)
	Step or Hop Forward (in)
	Forward Fold (out)
	Half Lift (in)
	Forward Fold (out)
	Chair Pose (in)

Source: Herrington, 2012.

Mountain Pose

This is considered to be the base, or foundation, for all poses (Flynn, 2013; Harper, 2013; Herrington, 2012). It can be a good way to check in with your body during the school day (Harper, 2013). It is a centering pose that promotes a healthy spine and good posture (Flynn, 2013).

POSE 11.6 MOUNTAIN POSE (STANDING POSE)

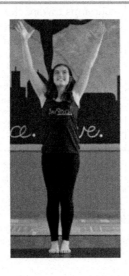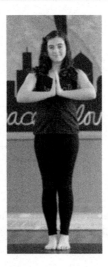

Pose	Mountain Pose
Instruct	Standing with your big toes touching and your heels directly behind your second and third toes, press your feet into the mat. Be aware of all four corners of your feet. Emphasize the inner rims of your feet as you press down. Engage your legs, contracting the muscles while you soften slightly at your knees. Draw your tailbone toward the floor as you lift your naval up and in and toward your spine. Lift through your chest, while you draw your lower ribs into your body. Soften at the shoulders and reach the crown of your head toward the ceiling; your chin is neutral.
Anchor Point	Your feet and belly. The focal point is straight ahead.
Breath Work	Breath is steady and natural.

Photograph by Madison Weber; model Kayla Tiedemann.
Source: Curran, 2013; Flynn, 2013; Harper, 2013; Gillen & Gillen, 2007; Herrington, 2012; Neiman, 2015; Walsh, 2008.

Chair Pose

Chair Pose strengthens feet, ankles, calves, core, and thighs (Flynn, 2013). It also strengthens and stretches shoulders, arms, and upper back (Flynn, 2013). It is a signature component of Sun B.

POSE 11.7 CHAIR POSE

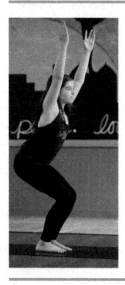

Pose	Chair Pose
Instruct	From Mountain Pose, press into your feet, settle much of your weight into your heels. Lift your arms toward the ceiling. Look forward and up slightly. Bending at your knees, sink your sit bones toward the back of the room and down. Draw your naval in toward your spine and your lower front ribs down. To come out, press into your feet, engage your belly and come to Mountain Pose.
Anchor Point	Feet and belly. Focal point is forward and slightly up.
Breath Work	Breath should be steady and deep. Exhale to sink into the pose, inhale to come out.

Photograph by Madison Weber; model Kayla Tiedemann.
Source: Flynn, 2013; Gillen & Gillen, 2007; Walsh, 2008.

Plank Pose

Plank Pose strengthens arms, shoulders, wrists, ankles, legs, and core (Flynn, 2013). It is believed to promote a healthy spine and good posture (Flynn, 2013). To accommodate students in the pose, encourage them to drop their knees for support as shown. Half Plank Pose, pictured in the following, is achieved by drawing the elbows toward the back of the room and lowering to elbow height, keeping the chest open and shoulders integrated into the body. The feet, hands, and core stay activated. For an added challenge, you can ask students to press into Plank Pose, squeeze their feet and legs together, roll their heels to the right as they ground into the right hand and take Side Plank Pose (Harper, 2013). This pose engages the oblique core, leg, and arm muscles.

POSE 11.8 HIGH PLANK (WITH MODIFICATION AND HALF PLANK)

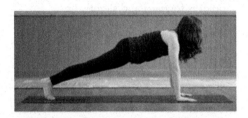
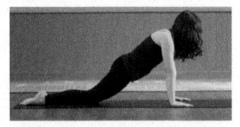
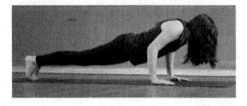

Pose	Plank Pose
Instruct	From Downward Facing Dog, or half-lift, engage your belly pulling your naval to your spine. Press your hands, especially the thumbs and first fingers into the floor. Press the balls of your feet into the floor. Drop your hips so that your whole body becomes parallel to the floor with your hips between your ankles and your shoulders. Draw your triceps toward the back of the room, look slightly forward, and open across the chest.
Anchor Point	Feet, hands, and belly. The focal point is slightly forward.
Breath Work	The breath should be deep, intentional, and steady.

Photograph by Madison Weber; model Kayla Tiedemann.
Source: Gillen & Gillen, 2007; Walsh, 2008.

Upward Facing Dog Pose

Upward Facing Dog is a chest opening pose that strengthens the lower back, spine, and gluteus muscles (Flynn, 2013). To modify, students can do Cobra Pose in which the legs and hips remain engaged with the mat and the chest is lifted only slightly, gaze is forward and up (see Flynn, 2013, p. 124).

POSE 11.9 UPWARD FACING DOG

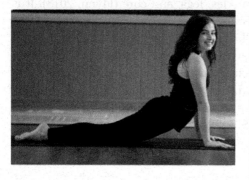

Pose	Upward Facing Dog
Instruct	From lying on the floor face down, place your hands underneath your shoulders and press down into your mat through the thumb and first fingers. Lift your chest up, pull your belly in and draw your shoulder blades back and down. Pressing the tops of your feet into the mat, lift your hips and reach through the crown of your head. Look forward and slightly up.
Anchor Point	Tops of feet, hands, and belly. Focal point is forward and slightly up.
Breath Work	Breath is steady, intentional, and deep.

Photograph by Madison Weber; model Kayla Tiedemann.
Source: Gillen & Gillen, 2007; Walsh, 2008.

Warrior I Pose

Warrior I is considered a strengthening pose (Flynn, 2013; Harper, 2013). It improves balance, and promotes focus (Flynn, 2013; Herrington, 2012). To modify for students in Warrior, I, give them a chair to help them stabilize.

POSE 11.10 WARRIOR I POSE

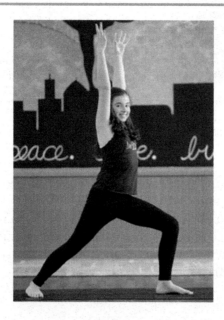

Pose	Warrior I
Instruct	From Downward Facing Dog, step your left foot between your hands, press down your right foot, engage your legs and your belly and lift up to standing. Press the outer rim of your back foot into your mat. Turn your back foot slightly outward. Stabilize the pose by pressing all four corners of your left foot into the mat. Engage both legs by pressing your feet into the mat and pulling them toward center. Draw your naval into your spine. Lift through your chest and crown of your head and reach your hands up to the ceiling.
Anchor Point	Your feet, belly, heart and hands, from the floor up. The focal point is between your hands.
Breath Work	Your breath should be deep and steady.

Photograph by Madison Weber; model Kayla Tiedemann.
Source: Flynn, 2013; Gillen & Gillen, 2007; Harper, 2013; Herrington, 2012; Neiman, 2015; Walsh, 2008.

Warrior II Pose

Warrior II is also considered a strengthening pose (Flynn, 2013; Harper, 2013). A chair is a good support here for students who have yet to develop good balance.

POSE 11.11 WARRIOR II POSE

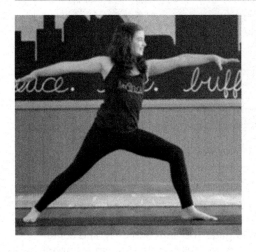

Pose	Warrior II
Instruct	From Warrior I (leftside), turn your back foot so that it is perpendicular to your front foot and spine at the hips. Reach your right hand behind you and your left hand forward, looking over the second and third fingers of your left hand.
Anchor Point	Your feet, belly, heart, and hands, from the floor up. The focal point is beyond your left second and third fingers.
Breath Work	Your breath should be deep and steady.

Photograph by Madison Weber; model Kayla Tiedemann.
Source: Flynn, 2013; Gillen & Gillen, 2007; Harper, 2013; Herrington, 2012; Neiman, 2015; Walsh, 2008.

CHALLENGE: Challenging and Vigorous Poses

This section of the class moves students into more intensity. As a teacher you want to be a positive, compassionate, and kind coach as you help students work hard. As such, this section is a good teaching point for the principles (see Chapter 3). This section of the class often includes lunges, twisting lunges, chair poses, twisting chair poses, side angle poses, and arm balances, like Crow Pose. See Chapter 10 for a review of this section and an integration with the principles.

Lunge Pose

The Lunge Pose is a strengthening pose (Harper, 2013). It helps build strength in the legs, core, and arms. This pose also stretches the hip flexor of the extended leg. It requires substantial effort and can trigger resistance for students who struggle with feeling uncomfortable in challenge. This pose can be modified by dropping the back knee to the floor or stabilizing with a chair at the front of the mat. To add challenge, ask the students to reach through the crown of their heads and twist, opposite elbow to opposite knee (shown with a dropped knee). For more of a challenge and a balance, ask the students to try Warrior III (Harper, 2013). They can find Warrior III from Lunge Pose by pressing into the forward foot and lifting the back leg up parallel to the floor. Hands can meet at the chest palms together, or reach forward, gaze forward.

POSE 11.12 LUNGE POSE

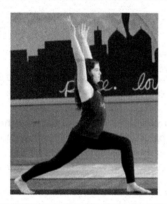 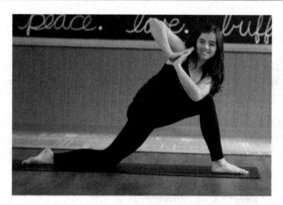

Pose	Lunge
Instruct	From Downward Facing Dog, step your left foot forward in between your hands. Step onto the ball of your back foot, press both feet into your mat, engage your legs and belly, and come to standing, reaching toward the ceiling with your arms. Engage your entire body from your feet, to legs, to core, to arms, to fingers. Press down into your mat, pull into your belly, to reach and look up.
Anchor Point	Your feet, belly, and hands. The focal point is upward between your hands.
Breath Work	Breath should be steady, deep, and intentional.

Photograph by Madison Weber; model Kayla Tiedemann.
Source: Gillen & Gillen, 2007; Harper, 2013; Walsh, 2008.

Boat Pose

Boat Pose is a core strengthening pose and uses the entire body (Flynn, 2013; Harper, 2013). It also stretches and challenges the hamstrings and integrates balance (Flynn, 2013; Herrington, 2012). Many people find it to be one of the most difficult yoga poses. To modify this pose, ask students to support the pose by holding their hands underneath the knees or by keeping their toes touching the floor. For a challenge, ask the students to bend their knees, take their knees wide, touch their feet together, weave their hands under their knees, and place their palms up, holding the balance (Harper, 2013). This is Flower Pose (Harper, 2013; Herrington, 2012).

POSE 11.13 BOAT POSE

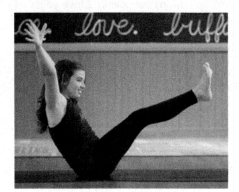

Pose	Boat Pose
Instruct	From sitting on the floor, knees bent, chest lifted, engage your core. Press your sit bones toward the floor, lift your chest, holding your hands on the backs of your knees as you lift your feet. Extending your hands forward, lifting through your chest, pull your belly toward your spine and press your heels out and up toward the upper edge of the wall. Release back to seated, knees bent, and feet on the floor. Pull your chest toward your knees and breathe.
Anchor Point	The sit bones to belly, focal point forward and slightly up (Kayla could look up here and be more comfortable).
Breath Work	Breath should be deep and steady.

Photograph by Madison Weber; model Kayla Tiedemann.
Source: Flynn, 2013; Harper, 2013; Herrington, 2012; Walsh, 2008)

Bridge Pose

Bridge Pose strengthens the legs, back, and gluteus muscles and opens the chest and lungs (Flynn, 2013). This can also be called Baby Wheel Pose (Herrington, 2012). It is considered a back-bending pose and a chest opener. Modifications include placing a block under the student's sit bones for support.

POSE 11.14 BRIDGE POSE

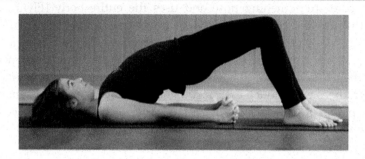

Pose	Bridge Pose
Instruct	From lying on your back, knees bent, and feet on the floor, press your feet into the floor, engage your belly and press your hips up toward the ceiling. Move your upper arms toward each other and under you, interlacing your fingers and pressing your palms together (if that feels okay). Press down into your arms and feet to lift up. Slowly release your arms and then your hips and shift your knees from side to side to rest.
Anchor Point	Feet and upper arms. Focal point is the ceiling.
Breath Work	Breath should be deep and steady.

Photograph by Madison Weber; model Kayla Tiedemann.
Source: Gillen & Gillen, 2007; Herrington, 2012; Walsh, 2008.

Wheel Pose

Wheel Pose is a challenging pose. It improves the flexibility of the spine and builds and strengthens muscles throughout the body (Flynn, 2013).

POSE 11.15 WHEEL POSE

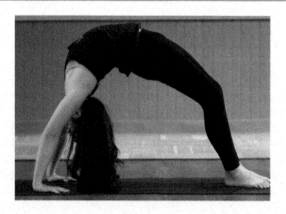

Pose	Wheel Pose
Instruct	From lying on your back, bend your knees and place the soles of your feet on your mat. Bring your hands by your ears and place the palms of your hands up over your head, then place your hands, palms down on, the mat next to your ears. Press down into your hands and feet at the same time, lifting your core up toward the ceiling. Push into your hands, straighten your arms, and press down into the inner rims of your feet to lift up even higher. Expand through your chest as you pull your naval in toward your spine.
Anchor Point	Your feet, hands, and belly. The focal point is directly behind you.
Breath Work	Your breath should be deep, steady, and intentional.

Photograph by Madison Weber; model Kayla Tiedemann.
Source: Walsh, 2008.

GROW: Learning and Trying Time

The GROW portion of the yoga session is the time to learn. Herrington (2012) suggests that you pick two or three poses to workshop each class. Model the pose for the class pointing out key details and points of focus (Herrington, 2012). Next, have two or three students demonstrate the pose. Then, have the students try the pose. The intention is really getting into the pose and understanding and practicing the specifics with body, breath, and intention. Herrington (2012) suggests putting the poses of the day up on the board before class. The experience should be positive overall. Make sure the students experience more successes than challenges (Harper, 2013). There are many fun poses you can try here. I have included a few suggestions. The principles of inquiry (6), choice (7), self-determination (8), sustainability (9), compassion (10), kindness (11), and possibility (12) can all be powerfully used here (see Chapter 3).

Dancer Pose

Dancer Pose is considered a balancing and integrating pose (Flynn, 2013). Dancer Pose develops balance and focus, stretches the shoulders and chest, and strengthens the ankles

POSE 11.16 DANCER POSE

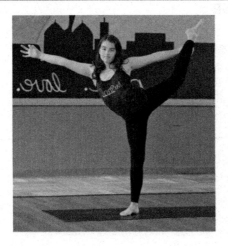

Pose	Dancer Pose
Instruct	From Mountain Pose, press your right foot into your mat, bringing your awareness to the center line of your right foot. Lift your left foot, bend at the knee, and take your ankle or sole of your foot into the palm of your left hand. Present your chest forward and up, look forward, pull your naval to your spine, lift the crown of your head up, and kick into your hand, opening your hip flexor. Press down into your mat with your foot and reach even higher with your chest and head.
Anchor Point	The inner rim of your grounded foot, your belly, and the connection of your hand and lifted foot. The local point is forward and up.
Breath Work	Slow deep intentional breaths. Watch for holding breath during balance poses.

Photograph by Madison Weber; model Kayla Tiedemann.
Source: Flynn, 2013; Herrington, 2012; Walsh, 2008.

and legs (Flynn, 2013). Kayla is facing the camera for the photo. When practicing, ask students to face forward and present their chests forward. Direct them to kick their back legs directly behind them. To modify, you can support students by giving them a strap to help reach their lifted foot (students with tight hips have trouble here).

Crow Pose

Crow Pose is an arm balance that strengthens the arms and the core. It requires strength and persistence (see principle 8, I do the work). It can be helpful to put your hands on blocks to create access for those with tighter hips. Also, when practicing, place a blanket or pillow in front of the hands to break the landing if the student falls forward. A modification is to encourage a student to sit in a deep squat, or do a series of squats, and work on stretching and strengthening through the hips.

POSE 11.17 CROW POSE

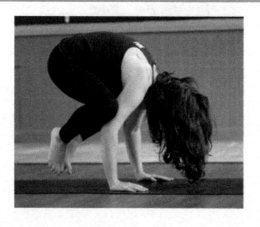

Pose	Crow
Instruct	With your feet hip-distance apart, squat so that your hips are near your ankles. Take your knees to the tops of your triceps (the backs of your upper arms) and press your knees into your arms. Press your hands into your mat, shoulder distance apart. Pressing your knees into your bent arms, come to balance on your arms, pulling your belly in and squeezing your knees and feet toward the center line of your body. Once steady, work to straighten arms and look up.
Anchor Point	Your hands, core, and feet. Your focal point is slightly in front of your hands.
Breath Work	Slow deep intentional breaths. Watch for holding breath during balance poses.

Photograph by Madison Weber; model Kayla Tiedemann.
Source: Walsh, 2008)

Camel Pose

Camel Pose stretches the shoulders, thighs, and hips and opens the throat, chest, and lungs (Flynn, 2013). It is considered a chest-opening pose. Modifications include students placing their hands behind them, as if placing their hands in their back pockets, rather than dropping all the way back to their feet.

POSE 11.18 CAMEL POSE

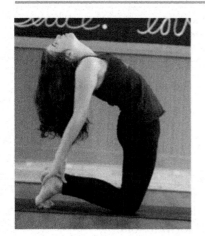

Pose	Camel Pose
Instruct	From a kneeling position, tuck your toes under, bring your hands to your lower back as if you were placing your hands into your back pockets. Next, engage your belly pulling your naval toward your spine and open across your chest. Try reaching back with one hand at a time to reach your heels. Press your hips forward toward the front wall as you look up toward the ceiling, opening even further across your chest. Slowly bring one hand and then the other back to your back pockets, engage your belly, and come back to kneeling.
Anchor Point	Feet, knees, belly, and chest. Focus point is the ceiling.
Breath Work	Deep steady breathing.

Photograph by Madison Weber; model Kayla Tiedemann.
Source: Flynn, 2013; Walsh, 2008.

Standing Extended Toe Pose

Standing Extended Toe is an advanced balance pose. As such, it builds balance and integration. The pose builds strength in the supporting leg and core. It can be modified by bending the lifted leg and taking the bent knee out to the side or using a strap to help extend the leg.

POSE 11.19 STANDING EXTENDED TOE POSE

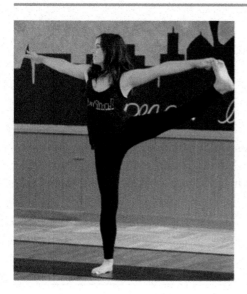

Pose	Standing Extended Toe
Instruct	From Mountain Pose, lift your left knee to your belly and squeeze into your belly with both hands. Take your left hand to the outside of your left foot and extend your left leg forward, pushing your right foot into the floor and your left heel toward the front wall. Pressing into the inner rim of your right foot, reach your left leg out to the left. Look right.
Anchor Point	Your right foot, inner rim, and core. The focal point is forward and then right.
Breath Work	Slow deep intentional breaths. Watch for holding breath during balance poses.

Photograph by Madison Weber; model Kayla Tiedemann.
Source: Walsh, 2008.

CENTER: Centering and Grounding

The CENTER part of the sequence emphasizes poses that require balancing, grounding, and connection to the mat and internal awareness. Poses include balance poses, triangle; warriors I, II, and peaceful warrior; side angle; and wide legged forward fold.

Eagle Pose

Eagle Pose is considered a balancing and integrating pose. It is believed to help develop balance and coordination (Flynn, 2013). Eagle Pose stretches the shoulders and upper back while strengthening legs, knees, and ankles (Flynn, 2013). To modify this pose, place the ball of the foot of the crossed-leg on the floor for balance, and with elbows bent, cross your arms at your chest and place the opposite hand on the opposite shoulder (Flynn, 2013)

POSE 11.20 EAGLE POSE

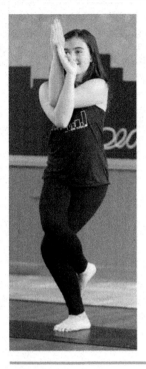

Pose	Eagle Pose
Instruct	From standing, bring your arms to goal-post arms, upper arms extended and parallel to the floor, elbows bent, hands pointing up. Press your left foot into your mat and begin to bend at the knee as you bring your right leg up and over your left leg, crossing at the thighs. Some like to hook their right foot around the back of the left calf. Sink your hips toward the floor as you lift the crown of your head toward the ceiling. Cross your right arm under your left and then wrap your forearms together, clasping your hands at the centerline of your body or placing hands back to back.
Anchor Point	The grounded foot and center-line of your body. Focal point is forward.
Breath Work	Slow deep intentional breaths. Watch for holding breath during balance poses.

Photograph by Madison Weber; model Kayla Tiedemann.
Source: Flynn, 2013; Gillen & Gillen, 2007; Herrington, 2012; Walsh, 2008.

Airplane Pose

Airplane Pose is considered a balancing pose. It can help improve balance and coordination (Flynn, 2013). Airplane Pose strengthens and stretches the hamstrings, back, and arms (Flynn, 2013).

POSE 11.21 AIRPLANE POSE

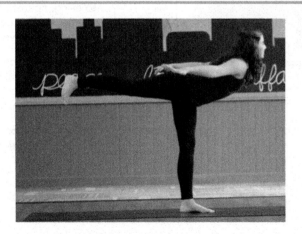

Pose	Airplane
Instruct	From Mountain Pose (or Lunge/Warrior I), find a focal point. Press down into to your left foot, feeling all four corners of your foot. Engage your left leg, pulling your muscles toward your bones. Engage your belly; pressing into your left foot lift your right leg behind you. Your hands extend toward the back of the room, palms facing down. To release, soften the grounded leg, engage your belly, and gently bring feet together into Mountain Pose.
Anchor Point	Grounded foot and belly, focal point a few feet forward, and breathe.
Breath Work	Slow deep intentional breaths. Watch for holding breath during balance poses.

Photograph by Madison Weber; model Kayla Tiedemann.
Source: Flynn, 2013; Herrington, 2012; Walsh, 2008.

Half Moon Pose

Half Moon Pose is considered a balancing and integrating pose (Flynn, 2013). Harper (2013) suggests that this pose may be the most challenging pose students will practice. It strengthens the core, legs, and spine (Flynn, 2013). Use a block or two to help the students reach the floor with their bottom hand. To modify, have students practice with a chair or against a wall for support.

POSE 11.22 HALF MOON POSE

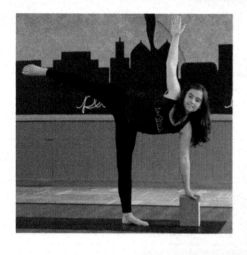

Pose	Half Moon
Instruct	From Warrior II, make sure your left foot is at 12:00 on a clock (pointing toward the front of the room). Pull your belly in toward your spine, engage your leg and arm muscles, and press into your left foot, lifting your right leg, stacking your hips. Drop your left hand to a block and reach your right hand up toward the ceiling, opening across the chest. Activating your gluteus muscles, point your right toes toward the ceiling.
Anchor Point	The inner rim of the grounded foot and belly. The focal point begins at the floor and gradually moves toward the ceiling or to reaching hand.
Breath Work	Slow deep intentional breaths. Watch for holding breath during balance poses.

Photograph by Madison Weber; model Kayla Tiedemann.
Source: Flynn, 2013; Herrington, 2012; Walsh, 2008.

Tree Pose

Tree Pose is a balancing and integrating pose (Flynn, 2013; Harper, 2013; Herrington, 2012). It helps students develop focus, improves balance, and stretches and strengthens the legs, especially the inner thigh (Flynn, 2013). To adapt the pose, have students place the ball of the lifted leg on the floor. To modify, place a stable chair next to the student to support balance.

POSE 11.23 TREE POSE

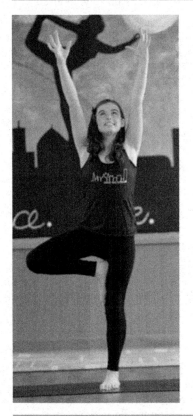

Pose	Tree
Instruct	From Mountain Pose, bend your right knee and bring your right foot to the inside of your left calf or inner thigh. Press your left foot into the mat, especially the inner rim of the foot. Engage your left leg and press the sole of your right foot into your left thigh. Engage your belly and place your palms together at your chest. Pressing down into your left foot, integrate your right leg by pressing your foot into the left leg, pull your belly in. From here, lift your arms up to the ceiling.
Anchor Point	The foot and belly. The focal point is forward and up.
Breath Work	Slow deep intentional breaths. Watch for holding breath during balance poses.

Photograph by Madison Weber; model Kayla Tiedemann.
Source: Flynn, 2013; Harper, 2013; Herrington, 2012; Walsh, 2008.

Triangle Pose

Triangle Pose stretches and strengthens the legs, arms, back, and core, elongates the spine, and opens the chest (Flynn, 2013). To modify, use a block or two to help the students reach the floor.

POSE 11.24 TRIANGLE POSE

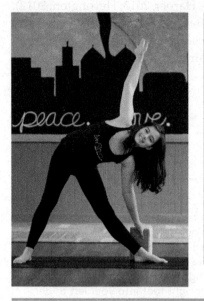

Pose	Triangle
Instruct	From Warrior II (left side), reach forward with your left hand to elongate your spine. Bending sideways, press your feet into your mat, soften your knees slightly, and use your core muscles to stack your lungs on top of each other. Reach your left hand down to a block and reach your right hand up to the ceiling. Keeping your chin neutral, look up to your lifted hand.
Anchor Point	Your feet and core. The focal point is to the lifted hand.
Breath Work	Breath should be deep, intentional, and steady,

Photograph by Madison Weber; model Kayla Tiedemann.
Source: Flynn, 2013; Gillen & Gillen, 2007; Harper, 2013; Herrington, 2012; Neiman, 2015; Walsh, 2008.

Wide-Legged Forward Fold Pose

Wide-Legged Forward Fold is considered a calming pose (Flynn, 2013). To modify, students can use blocks to help them reach the floor more easily.

POSE 11.25 WIDE-LEGGED FORWARD FOLD POSE

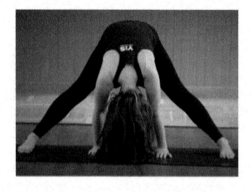

Pose	Wide-Legged Forward Fold
Instruct	Step or hop your feet wide apart. Place your hands on your hips, soften your knees, and fold at the hips. Place your hands on the floor, draw your naval toward your spine, and hang your head heavy and allow yourself to lean forward, making sure your heels stay connected to the floor.
Anchor Point	The feet and belly. The breath is always an anchor point.
Breath Work	Allow your breath to be smooth, even, and natural.

Photograph by Madison Weber; model Kayla Tiedemann.
Source: Flynn, 2013; Neiman, 2015; Walsh, 2008)

CALM: Relaxation

The goal of this section of the yoga session is to quiet the body, slow the breath, and bring the students to an awareness of the effects of their practice. This section begins with floor stretches (e.g., Supine Leg Twist, Happy Baby) and moves into relaxation techniques (Herrington, 2012). In traditional studio classes, this section may also include inversions. However, many inversions are considered to include too much physical risk to be integrated into school-based yoga (e.g., headstands and handstands; Childress & Harper, 2015). If you do want to include an inversion, consider the Modified Candle Pose (see Flynn, 2013, pp. 118–119). In this pose, ask the student to place a block underneath his or her sacrum (i.e., the triangular bone at the base of the spine) and let the feet float up toward the ceiling. This gives the sensation and benefits of an inversion without the risk. Follow with resting pose. Yoga classes typically end with students in a seated position with one hand on their bellies and one on their hearts as they tune into their own breathing. It is a good time to practice mindfulness meditations (see Chapter 6 and the mediation section of this chapter).

Happy Baby Pose

Happy Baby Pose stretches the hips, gluteus muscles, and the groin as it soothes the lower back (Flynn, 2013). To modify, students can hold the back of their knees instead of the outsides of their feet.

POSE 11.26 HAPPY BABY POSE

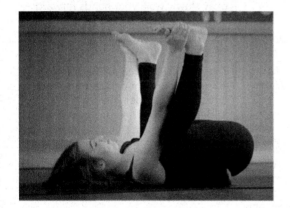

Pose	Happy Baby Pose
Instruct	Lying on your back, bend your knees taking your thighs to the sides of your body. The soles of your feet face the ceiling. Grab the outer edges of your feet with your hands and draw your thighs more deeply toward the floor and the outsides of your body. You can gently rock from side to side here or straighten your legs and push through your heels.
Anchor Point	Your back on the floor. The focal point is the ceiling or internal awareness with eyes closed.
Breath Work	Breath should be smooth and natural.

Photograph by Madison Weber; model Kayla Tiedemann.
Source: Flynn, 2013; Walsh, 2008)

Pigeon Pose

Pigeon Pose is considered a hip stretching pose (Flynn, 2013). It stretches the gluteus muscles, groin, and hamstrings, while elongating the back (Flynn, 2013). It can be done as Half Pigeon Pose, with one leg directly behind the student. Or as Double Pigeon Pose with both legs stacked on top of each other, ankle on knee on each side. To modify the Half Pigeon Pose, place a block under the thigh of the bent leg to give more support for the hips. To modify Double Pigeon Pose, place a block under the external side of each thigh for support

POSE 11.27 HALF PIGEON POSE

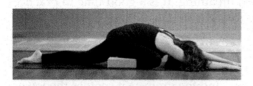
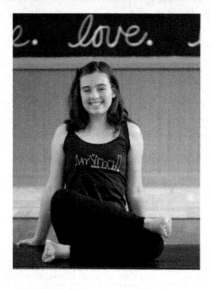

Pose	Half Pigeon Pose
Instruct	From Downward Facing Dog, step your right foot forward and heel-toe your foot over to the left side. Drop your knee to the right so your shin is parallel to the front edge of your mat. Place a block under your right thigh. Press into your hands to square your hips, drawing your left leg directly behind you, pressing the top of your foot into your mat and then release it to the floor. If it feels okay slowly walk your hands forward coming to a fold over your right leg, or use a block to support your elbows.
Anchor Point	Your hips. The focal point is forward if arms are straight and chest is lifted, directly to your mat and down if folded forward, or eyes closed with internal awareness.
Breath Work	Work for gentle, natural breathing.

Photograph by Madison Weber; model Kayla Tiedemann.
Source: Walsh, 2008.

Seated Forward Fold Pose

Seated Forward Fold is a calming pose (Flynn, 2013; Harper, 2013). It is also called Sandwich Pose (Herrington, 2012). This pose stretches the back side of the body from the heels to the neck (Flynn, 2013). To modify the pose, provide the students with a strap. Place the strap around the feet and hold the strap with both hands. One-Legged Forward Fold can be more accessible for those with tight hamstrings.

POSE 11.28 ONE-LEGGED FORWARD FOLD POSE

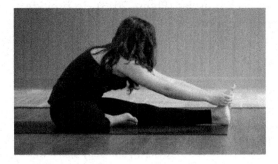

Pose	One-Legged Forward Fold
Instruct	From a seated position, straighten your legs out in front of you on the mat. Bending your right knee place the sole of your right foot on your left inner thigh. Engaging your belly, reach your chest toward your left big toe, elongate your spine. Place your hands on either side of your left shin or hold your left foot.
Anchor Point	Your sit bones and belly. The focal point is forward.
Breath Work	Work toward steady, natural, relaxed breath.

Photograph by Madison Weber; model Kayla Tiedemann.
Source: Flynn, 2013; Harper, 2013; Herrington, 2012; Walsh, 2008.

Reclined Butterfly Pose

Reclined Butterfly Pose is a restoration pose. It creates a stretch through the hips and groin, while calming the nervous system. Some students feel vulnerable here or have very tight hips and can't stay in this pose in comfort for more than a few breaths. To modify, have students take their feet to the edge of their mats and let their knees fall together.

POSE 11.29 RECLINED BUTTERFLY POSE

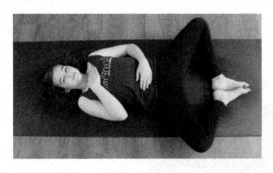

Pose	Reclined Butterfly Pose
Instruct	Lying on your back, bring the soles of your feet together. Let your knees fall wide open. Place one hand on your belly and one hand on your heart.
Anchor Point	Your belly and your heart. The focal point is internal or a soft gaze if eyes are open.
Breath Work	Breath should be calm, easy, and natural.

Photograph by Madison Weber; model Kayla Tiedemann.
Source: Walsh, 2008.

Reclining Twist Pose

Reclining Twist stretches the back, gluteus, and neck muscles (Flynn, 2013). To provide a modification, place a block under the bent knee for support.

POSE 11.30 RECLINING TWIST POSE

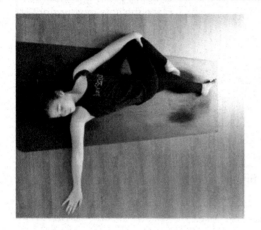

Pose	Reclining Twist
Instruct	Lying on your back, draw your right knee in toward your belly and hug it in using both hands. Take your left hand to the outside of your right knee, draw your knee over to your left side. Extend your right arm and turn your head to gaze at or beyond your right hand.
Anchor Point	Your back and outer part of the hip of your bent leg. The focal point is beyond your extended hand.
Breath Work	Your breath should be natural and relaxed.

Photograph by Madison Weber; model Kayla Tiedemann.
Source: Gillen & Gillen, 2007; Walsh, 2008.

Resting Pose

Resting Pose relaxes the body and is considered a restorative pose (Flynn, 2013; Harper, 2013). Some students feel safer seated with their backs against the wall and eyes slightly open. Other students like a heavy blanket to help calm them.

POSE 11.31 RESTING POSE

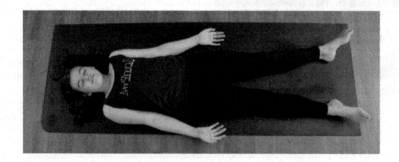

Pose	Resting Pose
Instruct	Lie down on your back and extend your legs. Place your arms along the sides of your body and face your palms up toward the ceiling. Soften and release from your feet to the crown of your head. Soften or close your eyes.
Anchor Point	The anchor point is the belly and heart. With your eyes closed, or softened gaze, your focal point is internal awareness.
Breath Work	Allow the breath to be steady, soft, and natural.

Photograph by Madison Weber; model Kayla Tiedemann.
Source: Curran, 2013; Flynn, 2013; Harper, 2013; Walsh, 2008)

CLOSE: Closing

Herrington (2012) suggests having students check back in (scale of 1 to 10) to bring an awareness to the shift that has occurred during yoga practice. Transition out of the session is as important as transition into it (Childress & Harper, 2015). Have students complete the session by moving through the end-of-session sequence (e.g., mats put away, straps and blocks put away, shoes on, and desks back into place). The re-setting of the room can be part of the mindful movement conducted in class.

There are many, many more poses: Frog Pose, Side Plank, Starfish, Gate, Shark Pose, Fish, Mermaid Pose, Splits, Plow Pose, Hero Pose, Rabbit Pose, and more (see Flynn, 2013). Accordingly, there are many guides for instruction in asana practice for adults and children. These include texts and videos (see Anderson & Sovik, 2000; Cook-Cottone, Kane, Keddie, & Haugli, 2013; Flynn, 2013; Gillen & Gillen, 2007; Harper, 2013; Herrington, 2012; McCall, 2007; Stephens, 2010; Walsh, 2008). *Yoga Journal* (www.yogajournal.com) offers free access to detailed descriptions of nearly all known yoga poses, instruction for sequencing a class, sample classes, and boundless information on yoga. Yoga journals' pose descriptions offer instruction on yoga poses including step-by-step instructions, tips, and contraindications for each pose. See also these texts for more yoga poses for students: Flynn (2013) *Yoga for Children: 200+ Yoga Poses, Breathing Exercises, and Meditations for Healthier, Happier, More Resilient Children* (pp. 104 to 201), and Harper (2013), *Little Flower Yoga for Kids: A Yoga and Mindfulness Program to Help Your Child Improve Attention and Emotional Balance* (pp. 84 to 119).

BREATH WORK

"Without awareness of breathing, there is no yoga" (Sovik, 2005, p. 11). Flynn (2013) says it this way, "Breathing is arguably the single most important aspect of yoga" (p. 80). In yoga breathing, the breath is used to calm and strengthen the nervous system and enhance concentration (Anderson & Sovik, 2000; Cook-Cottone, 2015; Flynn, 2013; Gillen & Gillen, 2007). The typical tempo of breath is slow, averaging about 16 breaths a minute (Anderson & Sovik, 2000). The rate of breathing varies throughout the day in service of your autonomic nervous system, as well as your intentional direction of the breath

(Anderson & Sovik, 2000; Flynn, 2013). It is the only function of the autonomic nervous system that can be accessed in an intentional manner (Anderson & Sovik, 2000). The breath is a barometer for the nervous system, changing as the nervous system experiences stress and imbalance (Cook-Cottone, 2015). The breath and the nervous system create an internal feedback loop. Changes in breathing can indicate internal distress (Anderson & Sovik, 2000; Flynn, 2013). Conversely, relaxed, deep, diaphragmatic breathing can restore the nervous system to a coordinated, integrated functioning (Anderson & Sovik, 2000; Flynn, 2013). Equalizing the length of inhalation and exhalation can help students bring their minds and bodies into balance (Flynn, 2013).

In yoga, there are various types of breath exercises to help students work with breath to create calm and active engagement. Flynn (2013) suggests bringing at least one breathing activity into each yoga session. When teaching students breathing exercises, it is important to key them into how working with the breath affects their bodies and feelings (Flynn, 2013). Gillen and Gillen (2007) remind teachers to include the following healthy breathing principles in breath work instruction: mindful awareness, breathing through the nose to allow the moisturizing and warming functions of the nose, relaxation to allow efficient use of the diaphragm, and slow and deep breath.

Diaphragmatic Breathing

Due to the importance of yogic breath in self-regulation, many beginner yoga sessions start with instruction in diaphragmatic breathing (Anderson & Sovik, 2000). Teaching students about diaphragmatic breathing is crucial to supporting their efforts at embodied self-regulation. Diaphragmatic breathing involves breathing deep into the belly. The lungs are not made of muscle fibers and depend on the muscles of respiration (e.g., diaphragm, intercostal muscles, pectoralis minor and major, sternocleidomastoid, serratus interior and superior, and transcersospinal, scalene, and abdominal muscles; Anderson & Sovik, Cook-Cottone, 2015; 2000: Stephens, 2010). Stress and the development of bad breathing habits can result in shallow, restricted breathing (Anderson & Sovik, 2000; Stephens, 2010). In healthy, diaphragmatic breathing the abdomen expands as one inhales (Anderson & Sovik, 2000; McCall, 2007). This expansion signifies the compression of the organs in the abdomen as the diaphragm presses down making space for the expansion of the lungs (McCall, 2007). On exhalations, your diaphragm releases moving back up toward the lungs, leaving more room for the organs (McCall, 2007). The Practice Script 11.1 can be used to guide students through diaphragmatic breathing.

PRACTICE SCRIPT 11.1: DIAPHRAGMATIC BREATHING

(Approximate timing: 5 minutes for practice)

Begin by getting comfortable in your seat. Place one hand on your chest and one hand on your belly. Bring your awareness to your breath. Soften your belly so that it is free to move. Rest the muscles connected to your rib cage. Slowly begin to breathe deeply extending your inhalation by one count and your exhalations by one count. Continue to breathe deeply as you use your breath. Notice your

(continued)

PRACTICE SCRIPT 11.1 (*continued*)

hands, your chest, and your belly. Notice your hands rise and fall with your breath. Notice, does the hand on your rib cage move more or less than the hand on your belly? To bring your breath toward deep, diaphragmatic breath, inhale so deeply that the hand on your belly lifts as the belly expands. See if you can breathe so that the hand on your chest is moving only slightly as your rib cage expands and the hand on your belly is rising and falling noticeably with each breath. Be sure to keep your breath slow, deep, smooth, and even. If you notice that you are getting lightheaded, pause at the end of each inhalation and exhalation and count to four before cycling to the next part of your breath. Continue breathing with your hands on your chest and your belly, breathing deeply into the hands on your belly for 10 more breath cycles.

Source: Cook-Cottone, 2015; informed by Anderson & Sovik, 2000; McCall, 2007; Stephens, 2010.

Victory Breathing

Victory breathing involves breathing through the nose, mouth closed with a slightly constricted throat (Cook-Cottone, 2015; Herrington, 2012; Neiman, 2015; Stephens, 2010). It is a breath that sounds like the ocean (Herrington, 2012). Some teach victory breath by asking practitioners to first make the "ha" sound as if fogging a mirror with their mouth open. Next, they ask the practitioner to make the same "ha" sound with the mouth closed and the breath moving through the nose (McCall, 2007). Creation of the same sound and sensation while inhaling and exhaling is encouraged (Stephens, 2010). This type of breath is believed to provide additional physiological and sensory feedback regarding the breath. It has the effects of both energizing the body and bringing focus to the mind (Cook-Cottone, 2015; McCall, 2007; Neiman, 2015; Stephens, 2010; Weintraub, 2004).

Whole Body Breathing

Whole body breathing uses your whole body in the inhalation and exhalation of breath. Begin by asking students to stand in Mountain Pose. Have them scan their bodies and notice any tensions and see if they can begin to soften tension with their breath. Begin with shoulder shrugs. As they inhale through their noses, ask them to bring their shoulders all the way up to their ears, squeezing tightly. As they exhale, have them drop their shoulders and exhale the breath through their mouths. Repeat this for 5 or 6 cycles of breath, gradually lengthening the breaths each time until you get to a count of three for the inhale and four for the exhale. Next, in the inhale, ask students to reach their hands all the way up toward the ceiling and look up as they take a long, deep inhalation. Next, on the exhalation have them drop their hands and fold all the way over until their head is reaching toward the floor and their hands go all the way to the floor. Repeat five or six times until they are standing up on their tip toes as they inhale and folding forward so that their hands go between their legs behind them. Close the activity by centering the students in Mountain Pose with their hands on their anchor spot (i.e., belly or heart). Have them check back into their bodies noticing any last bit of tension that they can let go.

Calming Breath Countdown

The calming breath is a great breath exercise for students and school personnel. The time to use this breath is when students are presenting as over-stimulated, anxious, wound-up, or upset (Flynn, 2013; Harper, 2013). It is just as important for students to have a felt sense of when they are over-stimulated and wound-up as knowing what it feels like to be calm (Harper, 2013). As most students (and people) today spend a lot of time in a heightened, anxious state, this can feel normal. Teaching students what calm feels like is a good way to start teaching them what the over-stimulated states feels like. When a student is feeling upset, agitated, frustrated, or anxious (any one of these heighted states), ask the student to check in. Have the student notice any tension, breath rate, and his or her thoughts as an observer. Coach the student through the experience with guided questions checking into the body, feelings, and thoughts.

By slowing and deepening the breath, our bodies will slow down and relax (Flynn, 2013; Harper, 2013). After checking in and becoming the observer, have the student sit up or stand up tall, lengthening throughout the spine (Flynn, 2013). Ask the student to breathe in and lift one finger at a time and count to five (Flynn, 2013). Then ask the students to exhale and count backward from five to one (Flynn, 2013). To effectively down-regulate the nervous system, cycle through the breaths about three to five times (Flynn, 2013).

Balloon Breath

The Balloon Breath is a very simple practice that integrates a repetitive movement in the body with breathing (Harper, 2013). Harper (2013) suggests that this breath exercise can be helpful for students who struggle with breath control. As an added benefit, it helps with opening across the chest, stretching the upper body and arms, and mobility in the mid and upper spine. Begin by sitting in Easy Sitting Pose with ankles crossed. It can help with comfort to put a small pillow or yoga block under your sit bones. Imagine that your body is a balloon. Each time you inhale your body fills with air and each time you exhale your body empties and deflates. Begin with an inhale and as you inhale press down through your legs and sit bones, engage your belly and breathe in lifting your arms. Continue inhaling filling your belly and your chest with air. As you breathe in the very last of your inhalation, your arms are spread wide and your hands are reaching up and you are looking up. Now, begin the exhalation from there. Slowly let the air out from your belly, then your chest. Your arms slowly move downward toward your body as you let the air out. During the very last moment of your exhale, wrap your arms around you, drop your head and bring your gaze down. From here inhale and begin the process again (Harper, 2013).

S.E.L.F. Breath (Slow, Even, Long, Full Breath)

Tantillo (2012) created this easy-to-remember breathing exercise. She suggests using this exercise to calm students after a hard day of testing. Ask students to lie on their bellies or sit at their desks and make a pillow with their hands by placing one hand on top of the other (Tantillo, 2012). Ask them to rest their right cheek on their hands and relax their bodies (Tantillo, 2012). Have them observe their breath in each inhale and exhale, making each breath slower, and become more observant as they breathe. Bring their awareness to the feeling of their breath in their bodies, belly, back, ribs, and whole torso (Tantillo, 2012). Encourage them to make their breath smooth like a stream flowing in and out. At this point, ask them to create a S.E.L.F breath—Slow, Even, Long, and Full breath in and a Slow, Even, Long, and Full Breath out (Tantillo, 2012). Remind students that deep, even breathing helps them nourish and take care of who they are, "Know that each breath you take, you are nourishing and taking care of yourself. With each breath you take, you feel good about who you are" (Tantillo, p. 79).

RELAXATION

Relaxation exercises create a bridge from the more active, external practices of yoga to the internal, meditative practices (Anderson & Sovik, 2000; Stephens, 2010). Relaxation and meditation are part of a continuous process of deepening and stilling the mind and moving toward self-awareness (Stephens, 2010). Once there, the meditation process in yoga is much like meditation in mindfulness.

Self-Massage

School-based yoga is focused on empowering students to be the regulators of their own bodies, minds, and behaviors. Self-massage is a great tool for showing students how much they can help their bodies relax. Recall that is it very difficult to have an anxious mind in a calm body. This is a simple self-massage technique described by Flynn (2013). The students should be in a seated pose either on the floor with ankles crossed or at their desks. Read Practice Script 11.2, adapted from Flynn (2013, pp. 62–63).

PRACTICE SCRIPT 11.2: SELF-MASSAGE
(Approximate timing: 10 minutes for practice)

Become aware of your body, beginning with your feet and the connection of your sit bones on your chair or floor. Notice any tension you are holding in your body and breathe into the tension spots, reminding yourself to soften. Breathe. Place your hands together and rub them gently, feeling the warmth you create as you rub them together. Now place your second and third fingers on your temples and gently press and begin massaging in small circles on your temples. Keeping the small massaging circles going, move the massage into your scalp and hair; move across the sides of your head, slowly moving your massage toward the back of your head. Next, bring your second and third fingers to your forehead and make the same small, massaging circles. Massage slowly and use all of your fingers, taking the massaging circles into your hair and scalp all the way to the back of your head. Now take your second and third fingers back to your temples and massage in small circles. This time take all of your fingers into your hair and massage your scalp as you move just over your ears and down into your neck as you massage toward the back of your head and neck.

(continued)

PRACTICE SCRIPT 11.2 (*continued*)

Next, using all of your fingers massage your neck in small circles finding any place you feel you are holding stress and tension. Massage and breathe. Move your hands to the top of your shoulders. Massaging any tensions there. Now, bring your hands to the front of your shoulders to the spot just beneath your collar bone on each side. You can use all of your fingers to massage any tension there. Take a deep breath in and a big exhale out. Give yourself a big squeeze wrapping your arms over your chest. Squeeze tight, lift your shoulders, and squeeze more, until you feel like you can't squeeze anymore, then release your shoulders and your arms. Interlace your fingers, bring your palms together and make figure-8s with your clasped hands releasing any tension in your wrists. Then, take one hand in the other and find the soft spot between the thumb and first finger and massage there. Move your massage to the center of your hand and then to each finger starting with the pinky finger and then ending with your thumb. Now, do the same for the other hand: soft spot, center, pinky finger to thumb. Rest your hands on your desk or your legs. Notice your body again from your feet and sitting bones to the crown of your head. Take a deep breath in and breathe out. Slowly open your eyes and consider a half-smile.

Source: Adapted from Flynn, 2013.

Systematic Relaxation

In systematic relaxation, your awareness moves across the length of your body from the head to the toes and back to the crown of the head (Anderson & Sovik, 2000; Flynn, 2013; Gillen & Gillen, 2007). At each area at which attention is focused, maintain a deep, diaphragmatic breath while bringing a release and relaxation to the muscle (Anderson & Sovik, 2000; Flynn, 2013; Gillen & Gillen, 2007). Systematic relaxation is like the body scan (see Chapter 6). However, in the body scan, awareness is brought to each area of the body and in systematic relaxation, deep relaxation is brought to each area of the body. Once awareness, breath, and relaxation have been brought to the body, focus is returned to the breath for 10 breath cycles (Anderson & Sovik, 2000). Associated principles for Embodied Growth and Learning include: principle 2, my breath is my most powerful tool; principle 3, I am mindfully aware; and principle 4, I work toward presence in my physical body.

PRACTICE SCRIPT 11.3: SYSTEMATIC RELAXATION
(*Approximate timing: 20 minutes for practice*)

Lie down or get in a very comfortable, supported seated position. Bring your awareness to your breath becoming aware of its qualities. Is it smooth and even? Are you moving from inhalation to exhalation without pause? Slowly deepen your breath to diaphragmatic breathing. Feel your belly expand with each inhalation and release with each exhalation. Breathe here for three deep cycles of breath.

(*continued*)

PRACTICE SCRIPT 11.3 (*continued*)

Now, bring your awareness to the crown of your head. Breathe as if you could breathe into the crown of your head. Notice if you feel any tension in your muscles. Breathe into the tension and bring a softness, a letting go, into the muscles. With each inhalation, bring awareness and with each exhalation, bring relaxation and softness. As you relax the crown of the head and the muscles of your scalp, be aware of your breathing and bring attention back to deep, diaphragmatic breathing when necessary. Breathe here and relax (pause).

[Continue this same process through the rest of your body pausing to relax at each of these points: crown of the head, forehead, temples, eye area, nose, cheeks, jaw, mouth, chin, throat, neck, shoulders, arms, hands, fingers, palms of the hands, back up the arms, shoulders, chest, rib cage, spine, heart, belly, sides, lower back, hips, gluteus region, thighs, knees, calves, feet, toes, and the soles of the feet. Pause at the feet and reverse the order going all the way back through the body to the crown of the head.]

Bring your awareness to your whole body. Breathe as if you can breathe into your whole body for three cycles of deep, diaphragmatic breath. Allow your breath to return to normal. Continue with 10 breath cycles. Slowly bring your awareness back to the room, bend your elbows and your knees. Roll to your right side, the softest side for your heart. Slowly come to a seated position. Cross your ankles and bring your hands to touch in front of your heart. Slowly open your eyes.

Source: Cook-Cottone, 2015; informed by Anderson & Sovik, 2000; Flynn, 2013; Gillen & Gillen, 2007; Walsh, 2008).

Guided Visualization

Guided visualization is imagery to create calm and relaxation (Harper, 2013). Take the students on a journey to a relaxing place with lots of smells, sounds, and sights to imagine. I have a guided relaxation I use called the Worry Tree. It helps students let their worries go for exams, school, work, or performances. Gillen and Gillen (2007) suggest the following topics for guided relaxation: student riding on a magic carpet, a teacher doing something silly or funny, a boat with cozy pillows floating down a river, riding a dolphin in the ocean, and a garden with giant-sized flowers (Gillen & Gillen, 2007;).

PRACTICE SCRIPT 11. 4: THE WORRY TREE
(*Approximate timing: 20 minutes for practice*)

There is a tree called The Worry Tree. The Worry Tree is strong. It grows strong from the honor of holding people's worries. People go to The Worry Tree and leave their worries for safekeeping. You want to go see The Worry Tree and leave some of your worries there for her to hold.

To get there you must walk through the fields of sunflowers and corn. You must hike into the forest over rocks and down a lightly traveled path. As you walk, you see densely grown trees. You see waist-high ferns and foliage all around. There are beautiful colors including all shades of

(continued)

PRACTICE SCRIPT 11.4 *(continued)*

greens and browns. Your feet crunch on the pine needles and you hear birds chirping. As you walk, you see little meadows that open up to sunshine and wildflowers. The flowers are in all colors, mostly your favorite color. You hear water and look to find it. You see a big river to your right just over a hill. Funny, you still hear water. You look and there is another river to your left. You keep hiking onward looking for The Worry Tree. You see it, up ahead, where the two rivers join, The Worry Tree.

Its bark is old and strong, a deep dark, brown. The bark seems as if it was the holder and protector of strength. Its branches are bigger than anything you have ever seen. Moss is growing all over the tree and the tree's roots descend deep into the earth. You notice that the The Worry Tree is alive. Its branches move like arms.

You have heard the stories about The Worry Tree. You have heard how you can give her your worries and she holds them for you as long as you need her to. You decide you would like to give the Worry Tree some of your worries to hold. You think carefully and pick a few really heavy worries. You take your worries in your hands and reach your hands up to the tree. The tree's branches extend toward your outreached hands. You stand on your toes and stretch your worries toward the tree's branches. The tree's leaves open and wrap around your worries and pulled them in tight. The Worry Tree draws the worries into her grand branches with tiny branches and thick, strong leaves wrapping around your worries tightly sealing them in, safe and sound. You feel a little less weight on your shoulders and in your heart.

There is a sign there that says you can leave your worry with the tree as long as you want to. You decide to leave them there for now, until you are ready to get them back. It feels good to know your worries are safe. You do not need to hold them all of the time. You walk back through the flowers, the ferns, the forest, the meadows, and the fields. You come all the way back to the present moment. You begin to bring yourself to awareness of your breath. You notice the feeling of your feet on the floor and your body in your chair. Take a big, deep breath in and a big exhalation out. One more time, breathe in, and breathe out. Slowly open your eyes as you count to five.

Source: Adapted from Cook-Cottone, The Worry Tree, www.thyogabag.blogspot.com.

MEDITATION

Meditation is an integral part of yoga. In Chapter 6 the formal practice of meditation has been covered in detail including: the process of meditation, finding insight through meditation, getting seated, visualizations, basic meditation practices, the meditating pebble practice, breath awareness, breathing buddies, body scan, the calming mind jar, the sensory sloth practice, mindful eating, walking meditations, and the loving kindness meditation. Chapter 6 also includes meditation work for older students including: the seeking in the wrong places reflection; the space between meditation; and the soften, soothe allow meditation. Finally, Chapter 6 provides tips for home practice and how to write your own home practice script. In this section, I have added a few techniques described in yoga books for children and youth that were not covered in Chapter 6.

Thought River Meditation

The Thought River Meditation helps students be more mindfully aware and discerning about their thoughts. Begin by asking the students to notice if they have many thoughts in their heads (Harper, 2013). Explain to the students that the brain is like a thought-generating machine (Harper, 2013). It makes lots and lots of thoughts. Thoughts come from stories that you have heard, movies you have watched, or things that people have told you. Some thoughts are important and true. Others are not. Tell the students that it is their job to decide which of the thoughts they want to keep and believe (Harper, 2013). To guide the meditation, tell the students this. "As you sit quietly, imagine that as your mind makes thoughts, it drops the thoughts into the river. You can watch the thoughts float by in the river. As your thoughts begin to come to mind they fall into the river. You do not need to pick them up; simply watch them flow by. Notice them. Are they true? Memories? Stories? Are they linked together? Are they about people? Worries? Plans? Notice as much as you can about them so that you can describe to your peers what you saw floating down the river." After 3 to 5 minutes, play a chime to let them know the time is up (Harper, 2013). Ask the students to journal the types of thoughts that they saw. Provide time for the students to discuss what they observed. Ask them how they might decide which thoughts to keep and which to let go.

Flow Meditation

This meditation is an embodied flow using flowy scarves (Flynn, 2013). It works for students of all ages especially younger students. Each student receives a scarf or two to hold (Flynn, 2013). The scarves can become waves, breath, seaweed, wind, or the ocean (Flynn, 2013). This flow meditation can be paired with music, a poem, a guided meditation, or silence. The goal is the promotion of mindful movement and it is believed to encourage body awareness and mindfulness (Flynn, 2013). Encourage the students to hold the scarf. Play the music, read a poem, or begin a script (Flynn, 2013). Encourage them to follow the words or sounds (Flynn, 2013). To integrate the practice with breath, ask the students to sit in a circle. Hold a corner of the scarf in each hand. Breathe in, lifting the scarf up and breath out, letting the scarf fall. Breathe together, synchronizing the breath and the movement of the scarves.

Anchor Breath

The anchor breath is considered a core concept of mindfulness and yoga (Rechtschaffen, 2014). It is a focusing exercise in which students notice the way their breathing feels in their bellies (Rechtschaffen, 2014). When there is a lot of chaos and stress in students' lives, the anchor breath can bring them back to a calm and relaxed state (Rechtschaffen, 2014). Ask the students to sit comfortably in their seats. Ask them to place one hand on their hearts and one hand on their bellies and to breathe deeply. Explain to them that the deepest breathing, the most effective breathing, goes right to their bellies and will help the hand on their bellies rise and fall. Remind them that they can always find their anchor breath there. Ask them to imagine that there are times that all of the stuff they need to do starts pulling their attention all over, and, like a boat getting tossed around in a rough sea, they need an anchor. Remind them that as the waves of emotions, fear, anxiety, and sadness come and go, the anchor breath will keep them steady (Rechtschaffen, 2014). Have them feel how the deep breath in the belly is calming the waves and holding them in place. Ask them to notice how the tension is leaving their bodies as they soften into the deep belly breathing of the anchor breath. After about 10 cycles of breath, have them check in with their bodies and get back to work, steady and at ease.

Mirroring: Moving Mindful Meditation

Mirroring is an activity done in pairs (Curran, 2013; Neiman, 2015). According to Neiman (2015) it is an opportunity to practice connecting and sensing oneself, as well as connecting to and sensing another person. Because there is no touching, it is an emotionally and especially physically safe way to work in partners in the school setting (Curran, 2013). To do this, place the students in pairs. Have the students stand or sit facing each other (Curran, 2013; Neiman, 2015). The activity begins with the partners placing their palms facing each other (fingertips to the ceiling; Curran, 2013; Neiman, 2014). There is no set leader. The practice is to be a mirror to your partner's movements (Curran, 2013; Neiman, 2015). Ask the students to move slowly and mindfully (Curran, 2013; Neiman, 2015). Remind the students to use all of their senses, to see and feel what is happening. You can also have the students take turns being leader and mirror. Ask them to process what they noticed. Did it matter if there was a leader? What was it like to not have a leader? What helped them be mirrors?

CONCLUSION

Yoga is embodied learning. During each yoga practice, our students are learning how to be with and for themselves and others. This chapter reviewed the four key practices of school-based yoga: yoga poses, breathing exercises, relaxation, and meditation. Consider this your starting point. I have been on my yoga journey for nearly 20 years now. As an ongoing practice, it is never finished. There are many wonderful yoga-based resources to bring into your classroom or school as formal practices. For a broad overview of poses see Flynn (2013) *Yoga for Children: 200+ Yoga Poses, Breathing Exercises, and Meditations for Healthier, Happier, More Resilient Children.* For a review of conceptually cohesive yoga practices with children, see Harper (2013), *Little Flower Yoga for Kids: A Yoga and Mindfulness Program to Help Your Child Improve Attention and Emotional Balance.* For a set of classroom yoga-based practices that are in a teacher-friendly lesson plan and worksheet format, see Tantillo (2012), *Cooling Down Your Classroom: Using Yoga, Relaxation, and Breathing Strategies to Help Students Learn to Keep Their Cool.* Gillen and Gillen (2007), in their book *Yoga Calm for Children: Educating Heart, Mind, and Body,* do a wonderful job providing modifications for yoga poses, as does Lois Goldberg (2013) in her book, *Yoga for Children With Autism and Special Needs.* Finally, for a good how-to for students who have experienced trauma, see Neiman (2015), *Mindfulness and Yoga Skills for Children and Adolescents: 115 Activities for Trauma, Self-Regulation, and Special Needs.* There is still more to learn in this book. Specifically, Chapter 12 will review the informal applications of school-based yoga and Chapter 13 will review programs and research.

REFERENCES

Anderson, S., & Sovik, R. (2000). *Yoga mastering the basics.* Honesdale, PA: The Himalayan Institute.

Baptiste, B. (2016). *Perfectly imperfect: The art and soul of yoga practice.* Carlsbad, CA: Hay House.

Carney, D. R., Cuddy, A. J., & Yap, A. J. (2010). Power posing: Brief nonverbal displays affect neuroendocrine levels and risk tolerance. *Psychological Science, 21,* 1363–1368.

Childress, T., & Harper, J. (2015). *Best practices for yoga in the schools.* Rhinebeck, NY: Omega Institute, Yoga Service Council.

Cook-Cottone, C. P. (2015). *Mindfulness and yoga for self-regulation: A primer for mental health professionals.* New York, NY: Springer Publishing.

Cook-Cottone, C. P., Kane, L. S., Keddie, E., & Haugli, S. (2013). *Girls growing in wellness and balance: Yoga and life skills to empower.* Stoddard, WI: Schoolhouse Educational Services.

Cuddy, A. (2012). *Your body language shapes who you are.* San Francisco, CA: TEDGlobal.

Cuddy, A. J. C., Kohut, M., & Neffinger, J. (2013). Connect, then lead: To exert influence, you must balance competence with warmth. *Harvard Business Review,* July-August, 55–61.

Curran, L. (2013). *101 trauma-informed interventions: Activities, exercises and assignments to move the client and therapy forward.* Eau Claire, WI: PESI Publishing & Media.

Field, T. (2011). Yoga clinical research review. *Complementary Therapies in Clinical Practice, 17,* 1–8.

Flynn, L. (2013). *Yoga for children: 200+ yoga poses, breathing exercises, and meditations for healthier, happier, more resilient children.* Avon, MA: Adams Media.

Gillen, L., & Gillen, J. (2007). *Yoga calm for children: Educating heart, mind, and body.* Portland, OR: Three Pebble Press.

Goldberg, L. (2013). *Yoga therapy for children with autism and special needs.* New York, NY: W.W. Norton.

Harper, J. C. (2013). *Little flower yoga for kids: A yoga and mindfulness programs to help your children improve attention and emotional balance.* Oakland, CA: New Harbinger Publications.

Herrington, S. (2012). Om schooled: a guide to teaching kids yoga in real-world schools. San Marcos, CA: Addriya.

Levine, P. L. (2010). *In an unspoken voice: How the body releases trauma and restores goodness.* Berkeley, CA: North Atlantic Books.

Love, K. (2015). Aliza and the mind jar: How a school in New York City teaches mindfulness to kids. *Elephant Journal,* www.elephantjournal.com/2015/03/aliza-the-mind-jar-hoa-a-school-in-NYC-teaches-mindfulnessto-kids-short-film/

McCall, T. (2007). *Yoga as medicine: The yogic prescription for health and healing.* New York, NY: Bantam Dell, Random House, Inc.

Neiman, B. (2015). *Mindfulness and yoga skills for children and adolescents: 115 activities for trauma, self-regulation, special needs.* Eau Claire, WI: PESI Publishing & Media.

Rechtschaffen, D. (2014). *The way of mindful education: Cultivating well-being in teachers and students.* New York, NY: W. W. Norton.

Stephens, M. (2010). *Teaching yoga: Essential foundations and techniques.* Berkeley, CA: North Atlantic Books.

Tantillo, C. (2012). *Cooling down your classroom: Using yoga, relaxation, and breathing strategies to help students learn to keep their cool.* Oak Park, IL: Mindful Practices.

Walsh, G. B. (2008). *Yoga in the Classroom: A step-by-step manual for K-12 school teachers.* New City, NY: Yoga Mountain Press.

Weintraub, A. (2004). *Yoga for depression: A compassionate guide to relieve suffering through yoga.* New York, NY: Broadway Books.

Willard, C. (2016). *Growing up mindful: Essential practices to help children, teens, and families find balance, cam, and resilience.* Boulder, CO: Sounds True.

CHAPTER 12

YOGA PRACTICE TO CULTIVATE THE SELF OFF THE MAT: MANAGING FEELINGS AND BROADENING COMPETENCIES

We are what we repeatedly do

—Aristotle

Love, compassion, joy, and equanimity are the very nature of an enlightened person. They are the four aspects of true love within ourselves and within everyone and everything.

—Thich Nhat Hanh (1999, p. 170)

As Aristotle says, "We are what we repeatedly do." A yoga-friendly way of saying that is we are what we repeatedly embody. Traditional yoga is an eight-limbed practice with a broad array of tools designed to help you manage your body, feelings, and relationships (Cook-Cottone, 2015). Off-the-mat practices provide ways to be in yoga, in connection throughout the day. From an integrated place, we all can be better versions of ourselves (see Chapter 1: Mindful and Yogic Self as Effective Learner [MY-SEL] model). As illustrated in the MY-SEL model, yoga practice involves a positive relationship with one's body, emotions, and thoughts that facilitates a healthy engagement in relationships, schoolwork, and community. The informal practice of yoga extends far beyond the mat and includes the building of basic self-care skills to create stability in the physical body and emotions, the cultivation of positive emotions (e.g., joy, loving-kindness), a skill set for managing negative or difficult emotions, and the ability to weave the four formal school-based yoga practices into the typical school day (i.e., yoga poses, breathing exercises, relaxation, and meditation; see Figure 12.1).

This chapter reviews the ways to teach and practice yoga off-the-mat and in your life. To do this, the broad-and-build theory as a rationale for engagement in informal yoga practice is reviewed. This chapter also reviews the role of emotions in our lives from a yoga perspective. Next, the four immeasurables (i.e., joy, equanimity, compassion, and loving-kindness) are reviewed within the context of the discussion on broadening and building positive feelings and experiencing for our students. Last, ways to integrate yoga into your school day in a more formal way are reviewed.

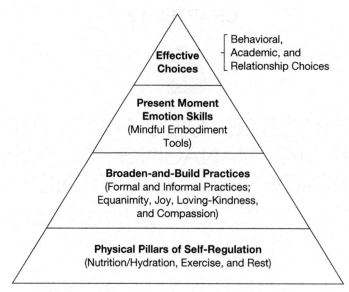

FIGURE 12.1 Building behavioral, academic, and relational competence.

BROADEN AND BUILD THE POSITIVE

Positive emotions are the basis for the motivation to learn, the development of a sense of security and the sense of community needed to build a rich and effective learning community (Jennings, 2015). Jennings (2015) explains that negative emotions (e.g., fear, sadness, anger) can inhibit the learning process and do little to cultivate community. Mastering emotions and learning to cultivate the emotions that serve learning and connections will allow you to orchestrate the promotion of positive engagement and academic success (Jennings, 2015).

The broaden-and-build theory (Fredrickson, 2013) aligns nicely with the MY-SEL model, suggesting that positive attunement and integration support students' self-regulation and intentional reflective engagement (see Chapter 1). It is built on the premise that individuals must begin with cultivating positive emotions, via intentional experiences, to trigger a positive growth trajectory (Fredrickson, 2013). It can be explained this way: First, research suggests that negative emotions narrow the scope of people's attention and thinking and support the enactment of specific *action urges* associated with the human survival instinct (e.g., fight, flight, freeze, experience disgust; Garland et al., 2010). An action urge is the automatic urge that we feel when we are experiencing an emotion. When an individual experiences negative emotions, the action urges are constricted by the negative mood state to urges that do not tend to potentiate active problem solving and connection (e.g., wanting to give someone a piece of your mind, e-mailing angry thoughts and accusations, becoming stuck and not able to move or act, an urge to quit or leave a project, or a feeling of disgust).

Conversely, research suggests that positive emotions broaden individuals' thought-action repertoires (Fredrickson, 2009, 2013; Garland et al., 2010). From a positive emotional state, individuals can draw flexibly on higher-level cognitive connections and wider-than-usual ranges of perceptions, ideas, and action urges. This positive emotion-cognition-behavioral influence is called an *upward spiral* (Fredrickson, 2009, 2013). Garland et al. (2010) explain that positive emotions and consequent broadened cognition create a base for behavioral flexibility that, over time, builds personal resources (e.g., mindfulness, resilience, social intimacy, physical health). It is theorized that positive emotions drive an incremental accrual of cognitive, psychological, social, and physical resources (Garland et al., 2010). The accumulation of these resources may have provided human ancestors with an evolutionary advantage by increasing their subsequent chances of survival (Garland et al., 2010). The critical point to note is that, while emotions are transient, coming and going, the resources created as a result of positive mood states are durable (Garland et al., 2010).

In a review of the literature, Garland et al. (2010) integrate Fredrickson's broaden-and-build theory of positive emotions (see Fredrickson, 2009, 2013) with advances in affective neuroscience and plasticity in the neural circuitry of emotions. Specifically, researchers describe a body of research that supports the notion that: (a) positive emotions broaden cognition and behavioral repertoires, and (b) positive emotions lead to the building of long-lasting personal resources that support coping and flourishing mental health (Garland et al., 2010). Note that interventions listed in the literature that help support the upward spiral process include mindfulness and yoga practices (i.e., loving-kindness meditation; Garland et al., 2010). See Fredrickson (2009) for an in-depth review of the broaden-and-build theory.

Yoga From the Bottom Up: Being With and For the Body

How do we even begin to broaden and build? The process begins with engagement in behaviors that help create a positive mood state. It is a *bottom-up* process (i.e., behavior to emotion to cognition process; see Figure 12.1 for a framework). Western psychology has focused on changing individual behavior from the *top-down* for many years (e.g., from brain to body; Cook-Cottone, 2015). These top-down approaches have taken many forms ideologically. For example, there is the notion that one must understand a person's trauma or past history before being able to help that person change (e.g., psychoanalysis), or that re-framing a way of thinking about something can shift behavior (e.g., cognitive behavioral approaches; Cook-Cottone, 2015). Classic behavior management for children and youth is not much different. Here, the top-down approach is not cognitive control; rather, it is behavioral control based on external contingencies managed by adults. The behavioral regulation comes from the outside in and not the inside out and does not adequately address the role of emotion and mood. It is important to acknowledge that for some students these approaches are effective. However, for others a focus on actionable methodologies or tools (e.g., yoga and mindfulness) moves them more effectively toward positive self-regulating behaviors that are contingency free and self-sustaining (Cook-Cottone, 2015).

Linehan (1993), whose work focuses on behavioral self-regulation among patients with borderline personality disorder, was among the first to suggest focus must begin with the provision of skills to negotiate experiences. There are two main conceptual components of the physiological foundations: (a) a calm and relaxed body fosters a calm and relaxed mind, and (b) taking reliable, steady care of your body fosters a reliable, steady state of mind (Cook-Cottone, 2015).

Calm Body, Calm Mind

Many teachers and older students are often fairly well versed in positive affirmations, the power of positive thinking, and the ability to look at the positive side of things (Cook-Cottone, 2015). However, I have noticed that they rarely consider the body as a potential source of soothing (Cook-Cottone, 2015). Citing the effectiveness of progressive muscle relaxation and breathing techniques, Bourne (2010), in his top-selling anxiety workbook, suggests that it is quite difficult for one to have an anxious mind within a relaxed body. In both private practice and in yoga classes, I provide guidance and support in ways to access the body as a source of soothing, groundedness, and calm during stressful situations. Of course, going for a walk, attending a relaxation-based yoga class (i.e., a yin class), or a traditional yoga class can all be ways to calm the body and relax the mind (Cook-Cottone, 2015). However, it is often in daily life, when there is no yoga mat to be found, that we need access to calming tools (Cook-Cottone, 2015). Effective strategies include: physical self-care, diaphragmatic breathing (see Chapter 11), sensate focus, and the stop refocus breath (SRB). See Bourne's (2010) *The Anxiety and Phobia Workbook*, Fifth Edition, for a variety of breathing, relaxation, and meditation techniques for calming the mind. Two effective techniques are explicated here.

Taking Good Care of the Body: The Physical Pillars of Emotional Regulation

Emotional regulation is inextricably connected to physical stability and homeostasis (Cook-Cottone, 2015; Cook-Cottone, Tribole, & Tylka, 2013). The more regulated the body, the more regulated and steady the mind (Cook-Cottone, 2015). Daily maintenance of the body provides a physiological steadiness, reducing cravings and sensitivity to triggers and supporting health-positive behavioral choices (Anderson & Sovik, 2000). In Linehan's (1993) manual for dialectic behavioral therapy (DBT), sleep, nutrition, and exercise are key components of the emotional regulation facet of treatment.

Each of the pillars plays a role in creating a solid physiological baseline for students. First, nutrition and hydration matter. For example, nutrition is known to play a role in mood, sleep, cognitive efficiency, and emotional stability (e.g., Anderson & Sovik, 2000; Cook-Cottone et al., 2013; Kennedy, Jones, Haskell, & Benton, 2011). Further, even mild dehydration has been linked to alterations in mood (e.g., Armstrong et al., 2012). When not understood and minded, nutrition- and hydration-based drops in energy can quickly become triggers for difficulties with self-regulation (Cook-Cottone, 2015).

Next, exercise helps with self-regulation. In 2013, Lees and Hopkins (2013) conducted a systematic review of randomized controlled trials of the effect of exercise on cognition and psychosocial function in children and found a positive association. Although more research is needed, there is some evidence that suggests that daily exercise plays a role in preventing, delaying the onset, and enhancing treatment outcomes in mental disorder (e.g., Zschucke,

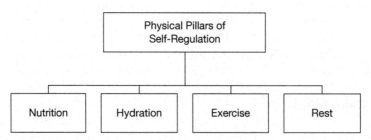

FIGURE 12. 2 The physical pillars of self-regulation.
Source: Adapted from Cook-Cottone (2015); Cook-Cottone et al. (2013).

Gaudlitz & Ströhle, 2013). Linehan (1993) encourages at least 20 minutes of vigorous exercise every day. I encourage students to target 30 to 60 minutes a day depending on the exercise. This would translate to a yoga class, a hike, a walk with a friend, or a pick-up soccer game. Researchers suspect that the mechanisms of action include changes in neurotransmitters such as serotonin and endorphins, which relate to mood and positive effects on stress reactivity (e.g., the hypothalamus-pituitary-adrenal axis; Zschucke et al., 2013). Potential psychological mechanisms of action may include changes in body-related and health-based attitudes and behaviors, social reinforcement, experience of mastery, shift of an external to a more internal locus of control, and improved coping strategies (Zschucke et al., 2013).

Getting adequate rest matters (Anderson & Sovik, 2000). Sleep deprivation can place students at risk (Cook-Cottone, 2015). In 2012, Astill, Van der Heijden, Van Ijzendoorn, and Van Scomeren conducted a meta-analysis on sleep, cognition, and behavioral problems among school-age children analyzing 86 studies. The authors reported that in practical terms, the findings suggest that insufficient sleep in children is associated with deficits in higher-order and complex cognitive functions and an increase in behavioral problems (Astill et al., 2012). In their review of research, Gujar, Yoo, Hu, and Walker (2011) concluded that sleep deprivation is associated with enhanced reactivity toward negative stimuli, amplified reward-relevant reactivity toward pleasure-evoking stimuli, and increased emotional reactivity. Simple rest, the allowing of yourself to do nothing, is also an important aspect of creating a stable base for self-regulation (Cook-Cottone, 2015; Stahl & Goldstein, 2010). Doing nothing and resting can take many forms: lying on a hammock, going to a green space with friends, cooking with grandma, sitting on the deck or stoop, and putting the cell phone and the computer away (Cook-Cottone, 2015; Stahl & Goldstein, 2010).

As the research suggests, it does not make a lot of sense to talk about managing student behavior without supporting nutrition, hydration, exercise, and rest. See Cook-Cottone et al. (2013) to read more about changing your school environment to help support healthy physical self-care. Associated Principles of Embodied Growth and Learning include: 1, I am worth the effort; 2, my breath is my most powerful tool; 3, I am mindfully aware; 4 I work toward presence in my physical body; 6, I ask questions about my physical experiences, feelings, and thoughts; 7, I choose my focus and actions; 8, I do the work; and 12, I work toward the possibility of effectiveness and growth in my life (see Chapter 3).

Turning the Mind Toward the Body: Sensate Focus

In Linehan's (1993) DBT, self-soothing, as a bottom-up approach, takes the form of sensate focus (Siegel, 2010). Sensate focus refers to bringing mindful awareness to the sensory input from each of the senses. For example, sensate focus using the eyes refers to the intentional awareness of what you are seeing. Perhaps you bring your attention to each and every detail of a rose. You study the curve of the petal, the sturdiness of the stem, each leaf, and how all the different parts of the flower come together creating the whole flower. You notice the shadows and places where the light reflects. Sensate focus can be done with each of the senses: vision, hearing, smell, taste, and touch. By bringing your awareness back to your sensations, you allow your mental processes to clear, becoming immersed in sensations rather than thoughts (Siegel, 2010). This can lead to a new way of considering things, free from confining or habit reinforcing conceptualizations. Associated Principles of Embodied Growth and Learning include: 2, my breath is my most powerful tool; 3, I am mindfully aware; 4, I work toward presence in my physical body; 6, I ask questions about my physical experiences, feelings, and thoughts; 7, I choose my focus and actions; 8, I do the work; and 12, I work toward the possibility of effectiveness and growth in my life (see Chapter 3).

Turning the Mind Toward the Breath: SRB

Mindful breathing techniques are helpful in self-regulation (e.g., Cook-Cottone, 2015; Garland, Schwarz, Kelly, Whitt, & Howard, 2012; Stahl & Goldstein, 2010). SRB is a simple breathing technique that can be applied as needed or used prophylactically to down-regulate the physical and emotional systems (see Practice Script 12.1). I explain to students in my yoga classes that the brain can be like a toddler fascinated with an electrical outlet. The toddler, curious and persistent, will continually return to the outlet unless you give the toddler something else on which to focus (Cook-Cottone, 2015). Worse is if you say, "Do not touch that outlet," "Do not touch that outlet," and repeat, "Do not touch that outlet," you have repeatedly reinforced, "… touch that outlet" several times. Imagine we were saying, "Do not eat that cheesecake." My brain hears the cheesecake. More effectively, you tell the toddler, "No!" and then you say to the toddler, "Hey buddy, look over here," as you point to something that will catch the toddler's interest. Students can use SRB in this same way to refocus the brain. The *outlet* is a metaphor for anything that might be anxiety provoking and the *toddler* is a metaphor for the easily guided brain (Cook-Cottone, 2015). In SRB, the brain is redirected to the breath as a point of concentration. In order to maintain focus, a breath in three parts can be practiced (i.e., inhale for a count of four, hold for a count of four, and exhale for a count of four). Repeat the breath cycle four times. Associated Principles of Embodied Growth and Learning include: 1, I am worth the effort; 2, my breath is my most powerful tool; 3, I am mindfully aware; 6, I ask questions about my physical experiences, feelings, and thoughts; 7, I choose my focus and actions; 8, I do the work; and 12, I work toward the possibility of effectiveness and growth in my life.

PRACTICE SCRIPT 12.1: SRB
Approximate timing: 3 minutes for practice

Stop: Either in response to an internal or external stressor or as a systematic practice scheduled throughout the day, tell your brain to "STOP" thinking. This might be a gentle reminder or a firm directive.

Refocus: Tell your brain "REFOCUS" as a gentle reminder or a firm directive. Direct your brain to your breath.

Breathe: Complete a mindful breath in three parts. Hold your attention on the breath. Breathe in and count to four—1, 2, 3, 4. Now hold the breath for a count of four—1, 2, 3, 4. Next, exhale for a count of four—1, 2, 3, 4. Repeat this cycle three more times.

Source: Cook-Cottone (2015).

EMBODYING AND REGULATING FEELINGS

Yoga practice provides opportunities to experience your feelings as embodied (Cook-Cottone et al., 2013). Understanding what is happening in your body and how it affects your behavior are critical to self-regulation and active engagement. Our emotions matter. It is believed that our emotions evolved to help us survive (Jennings, 2015). Emotions coordinate behavior and physiological states during survival, salient events, and pleasurable interactions (Jennings, 2015; Nummenmaa, Glerean, Hari, & Hietanen, 2014). Rooted in survival, our emotions are intricately linked to everything we do. Emotions are wired to keep us safe and connected. Our sense of right and wrong, intrinsic reward for learning and getting things right, and happiness when we feel connected to the others in our lives, all stem from the deep influences of our emotional selves. In this way, school is also inherently emotional as it involves learning and relationships, two key human survival processes.

Mindfulness and yoga skills can help our students manage emotions. We now understand that the process of feeling emotions is intricate, is rooted in the body, and involves key regions across and within the brain (Cook-Cottone, 2015). In a functional MRI study of emotions, Oosterwijk et al. (2012) reported that body cues are a critical component of emotional mental life. Nummenmaa et al. (2014) agree. Emotions are felt in the body. Further, somatosensory feedback may trigger conscious emotional experiences. In order to map the location of emotions in the body, Nummenmaa et al. (2014) used a unique topographical self-report method. In a set of five experiments, participants ($n = 701$) were shown two silhouettes of bodies alongside emotional words, stories, movies, or facial expressions. Nummenmaa et al. (2014) asked participants to color the bodily regions where they felt activity increasing or decreasing while viewing each stimulus. After analysis, the researchers found that different emotions were consistently associated with statistically discernable bodily sensation maps (see Figure 12.3, which

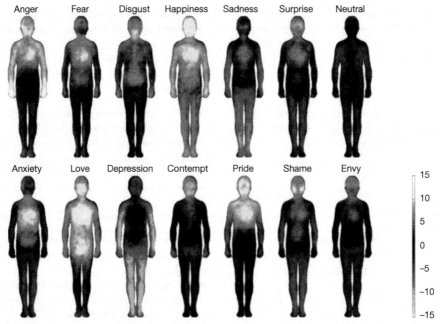

FIGURE 12.3 Topographical map of emotions in the body. (See inside back cover for a color version of this figure.)

Source: Nummenmaa et al., 2014.

appears in color on the inside back cover of this book). The authors concluded that emotions are represented in the somatosensory system as categorical somatotopic maps and perception of emotion-triggered bodily changes may play a key role in generating consciously felt emotions.

Allowing the sensations and experience of feelings, without action, is critical for self-regulation. Feelings often come with a felt sense of an imperative to act. Students, especially young students, are not aware of this process. They simply feel and do. The sensation, that one must act on, or escape from, a feeling is a disrupter of self-regulation. To enhance self-regulation, students can work with getting comfortable with their feelings (see Practice Script 12.2).

The mindful and yogic approach to emotional regulation is explicated in Table 12.1. The table aligns this approach to Koole, Van Dillen, and Sheppes's (2011) model of emotional regulation. In yogic approaches, regular practice of yoga poses, breathing exercises, relaxation, and meditation cultivate neurological integration and reduced reactivity over time (Cook-Cottone, 2015). Further, these practices are down-regulating, decreasing the

TABLE 12.1 Mindful and Yogic Processing of Feelings

STAGE	EMOTIONAL REGULATION (KOOLE ET AL., 2011)	MINDFULNESS AND YOGA PROCESS (ASSOCIATED PRINCIPLE, SEE CHAPTER 3)
Stage One	Situational triggers encountered (e.g., situational selection, situational modification)	*Situational shifts over time:* • Yoga practice (poses, breathing exercises, relaxation, and meditation) shift neurological reactivity to triggers over time. *In present time:* • External challenges and triggers; thoughts and memories.
Stage Two	Attention/inattention to emotionally relevant features (e.g., attentional deployment)	• Mindful awareness (Awareness, 3) • Selection of: attachment, avoidance, or allowing (Choice, 7). • Physical Presence (Presence, 4). • Honoring breath and physical experience (Breath, 2; Presence, 4).
Stage Three	Cognitive appraisal of the situation (e.g., cognitive change)	• Remembering that you are worth the effort no matter the challenge (Worth, 1). • Understanding of how and why brains and bodies feel the way they do (Inquiry, 6). • Awareness of impermanence, not-self, nonjudgment, and allowing (Awareness, 3; Choice, 7). • Maintaining equanimity (Sustainability, 9).
Stage Four	Emotions expressed in behaviors (e.g., response modulation)	• Expression of authentic self (*through intentional choice of movement or voice*; self-determination, 8). • Doing the work (Self-determination, 8). • Cultivating compassion and kindness (Compassion, 10; Kindness, 11). • Working toward new possibilities (Possibility, 12).

Source: Adapted from Cook-Cottone (2015); informed by Jackson (2013); Koole et al. (2011).

triggering potential of both distracting thoughts and memories and external challenges and frustrations (Cook-Cottone, 2015). Stages Two through Four in Table 12.1 reflect the mindful and yogic approach to negotiating emotionally salient information and behavioral choices. Ultimately, this process cultivates embodied self-regulation that honors the present moment experience, creates balanced and sustainable self-mastery, and allows attunement within self and with others (Cook-Cottone, 2015).

The practice script that follows is designed to bring awareness to feelings and the locations of feelings in the body. This activity can be especially helpful for those students who have very little awareness of emotions and the embodied experience of emotions.

Consider doing this activity in consultation with a school-based mental health professional in case you are in need of further referral or support. For students who have trauma histories or little experience with emotions this may be a challenging activity. When working with students with trauma in my role as a psychologist, I present the idea and allow the students to choose when we do it (e.g., "Let me know when you would like to try this activity in a session"). I also develop a cue or signal with which they can notify me that they need a break or would like to stop for the day. I also encourage students to schedule a quiet afternoon or evening with supportive family or friends if the session has been particularly challenging. Good candidates for doing this activity independently with a mental health professional are students who struggle with negative affect, show a tendency to try to escape from uncomfortable situations or emotional experiences, have deficits in the awareness of bodily states, show difficulty detecting triggers or cues in their bodies, self-objectify, and have experienced invalidating or abusive environments.

For most students, this is a fun activity that allows them to become more aware of their feelings. Before you begin, invite students to participate, explaining the process and the reasons for the process. I like to tell students that we are being *feeling detectives*. That is, we will be investigating exactly what feelings feel like in our bodies. Let them know that you will be asking them to elicit four feelings—safety and happiness, sadness, anger, and anxiety. Following the activity, it is important to engage in breath work and supportive communication in order to help the students return to baseline physiological activation.

PRACTICE SCRIPT 12.2: FEEL YOUR FEELINGS
(Approximate timing: 2 minutes for the introduction; 30 minutes for practice)

[To prepare, have four photocopied sheets of a gender-neutral outline of a human figure for each child and a box of colored pencils or crayons.]

Sit in a comfortable position. Be sure that you feel grounded, your feet on the floor and solid support under your sit bones and behind your back. Close your eyes and become aware of your breath. Breathe in and out noticing the air as it enters your body and as you exhale. Feel the sensation of your chest, rib cage, and belly as they expand to take in air and contract to release air. Allow your breathing to be steady and natural.

Now, bring your awareness to a time when you were feeling very safe and happy. Picture yourself in this moment. Have a sense of where you were, maybe even what you were wearing. Were you inside or outside? Recall who was around you. Bring to mind any sights, sounds, and smells. Now, bring your awareness to your body. Feel the feelings of safety and happiness. Explore where you feel these feelings in

(continued)

PRACTICE SCRIPT 12.2 (*continued*)

your body. Scan your body from your feet to the crown of your head. Feel your arms and legs. Breathe into the areas of your body where you are feeling. It might help to place one or both of your hands on the place that you are feeling something. Breathe as you watch the feeling arise and slowly pass away. Notice that feelings have a point at which you become aware of them, a peak, and then a gradual lessening. Breathe and notice. Take as much time as you need [pause]. When you are ready, slowly open your eyes. Reflect on your experience and draw what you were feeling in your body on the figure here. Choose whatever colors you'd like to reflect what you were feeling and where you were feeling it. Use color to show intensity and how the feeling may have felt different in various parts of your body. Let me know when you are done.

When you are ready, sit back and return your focus to your breath. Next, think of a time when you were feeling sad. Maybe you were disappointed or you lost a toy or favorite object. As before, cultivate a sense of your surroundings, the people, the sounds, sights, and smells of the environment. As you remember, see what you see and feel what you feel. Now, bring your awareness to your body. Locate the sadness in your body. Breathe and notice. Breathe into the areas of your body where you are feeling sadness. It might help to place one or both of your hands on the place(s) that you are feeling sadness. Breathe as you watch the feeling arise and slowly pass away. Notice if the emotions seem to peak. Breathe and notice. Take as much time as you need [pause]. When you are ready, open your eyes. Color on this sheet where you were feeling sadness in your body. Choose whatever colors you'd like in order to best reflect what you were feeling and where you were feeling it.

When you are ready, sit back and bring your focus to your breath. Close your eyes. Bring to mind a time when you were angry. Do you remember why you were angry? Maybe a friend borrowed something and did not give it back. Maybe someone did not play a game fairly. Think about the anger. Who was present when you were feeling angry? Where were you? Do you recall what you were wearing, or any sights, sounds, and smells? Bring the feeling of anger to your awareness. Now, bring your attention to your body. Where do you feel the anger in your body? Scan your body from the crown of your head to your feet. Feel your arms, your torso, and your legs. Feel what you feel. Breathe into the areas of your body where you are feeling the anger. It might help to place one or both of your hands on the place that you are feeling anger. Breathe as you watch the feeling arise and slowly pass way. Breathe and notice the feeling. Take as much time as you need [pause]. When you are ready, open your eyes. Color on a new sheet where you were feeling anger in your body. Indicate with colors where you were feeling anger in your body. Choose whatever colors you'd like to reflect what you were feeling and where you were feeling it.

When you are ready, return to a comfortable position and close your eyes. Bring your awareness to your breathing. This is the final emotion we will be working on today. Bring to mind a time when you were anxious. Maybe it was before a test or you were waiting to get a grade back. Think of something like that. Recall the circumstances, the location, and the people that were there. Recall if it was day or night and the location. Try to recall any sights, sounds, and smells. Now, turn your attention to your body. Where do you feel the anxiety in your body? Take time to scan your body, from your center out to your hands and feet, to the crown of your head. Feel what you feel. Breathe into the areas of your body where you are feeling anxiety. It might help to place one or both of your hands on the area that you are feeling the anxiety. Breathe as you watch the feeling arise and slowly pass way. Take as much time as you need [pause]. When you are ready, open your eyes. Color on this sheet where you were feeling anxiety in your body. Choose whatever colors you'd like to reflect what you were feeling and where you were feeling it.

[Label each of the drawings: safe and happy, sad, angry, and anxiety. Place them one next to the other on the table. Have your students describe the pictures to you, how the feelings showed

(continued)

PRACTICE SCRIPT 12.2 (continued)

up in their bodies, and how the feelings were similar and different. Ask the students to reflect on the process of feeling and drawing feelings. Some students will have many details and experiences to share with you and others will have few. There is no right or wrong, just what was experienced or not. Be sure to note that some people might not feel anything and that is okay. Once they are done describing, comparing, and reflecting, return your students to the breath].

Find your comfortable seat. Bring your awareness to your breath. Notice your breath as you inhale and notice your breath as you exhale. Each time you inhale, have a sense of gratitude for your willingness to explore, experience, and allow your feelings. Each time you exhale silently say the words, "Let go" and release any tensions that you may be experiencing. Do this for five breaths, inhaling gratitude and exhaling release. When you are ready, slowly open your eyes.

Source: Adapted from Cook-Cottone (2015).

This activity can be done once or in a series. As your students become increasingly aware of their felt sense, the drawings will change. I have found it very instructional to review the drawings that have been created over time and reflect on growth and challenges. Ultimately, feelings need to be felt, experienced, breathed through, and sometimes expressed. Associated Principles of Embodied Growth and Learning include: 3, I am mindfully aware; 4, I work toward presence in my physical body; 6, I ask questions about my physical experiences, feelings, and thoughts; 8, I do the work; and 12, I work toward the possibility of effectiveness and growth in my life (see Chapter 3).

Integrating the Thinking and Feeling Brain

The next step in working with feelings is learning to integrate the thinking part of the brain with the feeling part of the brain (Linehan, 1993). In Linehan's DBT, she refers to the joining of the emotional and cognitive aspects of self as *wise mind* (p. 109). The goal is to be present and to process the felt experience fully, including the physical, emotional, and cognitive aspects, without falling into reaction (Linehan, 1993). When working with students, I find it effective to draw a picture of the brain and explain that there are parts of the brain generally responsible for thinking and other parts of the brain that are primarily responsible for feeling (see Cook-Cottone, Kane, Keddie, & Haugli, 2013). When we defer to either thoughts or emotions, we run the risk of missing critical information that we need for making a decision. Despite the inherent challenge, I explain to students that we make the best decisions when we process all of the information available, integrating the thinking and the feeling brain (Cook-Cottone et al., 2013; see Figure 12.4).

Self-Regulation in the Palm of Your Hand: I Feel, I Think, I Say, I Do

In Girls Growing in Wellness and Balance: Life Skills and Yoga to Empower, our yoga-based eating disorder prevention program, we taught the girls how to do emotional problem solving using the palms of their hands (Cook-Cottone et al., 2013). We remind students that the source of wisdom is the integration of thoughts and feelings (see Figure 12.5). The teaching script follows.

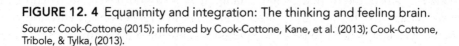

FIGURE 12. 4 Equanimity and integration: The thinking and feeling brain.

Source: Cook-Cottone (2015); informed by Cook-Cottone, Kane, et al. (2013); Cook-Cottone, Tribole, & Tylka, (2013).

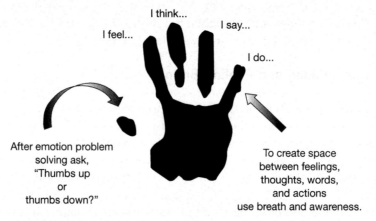

FIGURE 12.5 Emotional problem solving in the palm of your hand.

Source: Adapted from Cook-Cottone et al. (2013).

PRACTICE SCRIPT 12.3: YOU CAN SOLVE YOUR PROBLEMS WITH YOUR OWN HANDS

(Approximate timing: 2 minutes for the introduction; 30 minutes for practice)

One of the best ways to get the thinking and feeling parts of our brain to work together is by breathing. Breathing in and out with long, deep, smooth breaths helps the feeling part of the brain relax and gets the thinking part of your brain to pay attention to how the body is feeling. When breathing, put one

(continued)

PRACTICE SCRIPT 12.3 (*continued*)

hand on your belly. This not only allows you to feel your deep breaths in and out, but also shows that you have control over your breathing. When you have control of your breath, there is a good chance you will be able to manage how your brain reacts when it is trying to solve a problem or make a decision. We are all better able to feel and think with our brains when we are relaxed. When we are relaxed, both the thinking and the feeling parts of the brain have enough room and energy to work their best! Now, the feeling and thinking parts of the brain are ready to work together. You can help them work together by imagining just how they would do so.

Another way to think about how our brain works is by using the Hot Soup model. Imagine a freshly poured bowl of steaming hot soup. The soup spoon is right next to it, waiting to be lifted. You might sprinkle some crackers or cheese into the soup, or eat it just how it is. It smells delicious, and you can feel your mouth start to water at the sight of this delicious meal in front of you. The soup, however, cannot be eaten just yet; it is piping hot. When we are upset, frustrated, anxious, or hurt and are facing a problem to solve, our brain is just like hot soup: It is too hot and needs to be cooled before we can eat it (or use it in the case of our brains). Nothing is wrong with the soup; it is still going to be delicious and good for us, it just needs to cool down. Like the soup, when our brain is "too hot," or we are having strong feelings, it needs to be "cooled down" before acting or making decisions.

How can we cool our soup?

Our parents often tell us to "Wait a few minutes and it will cool off," or "Blow on it." The soup needs TIME and AIR. This is exactly what the brain needs when it is wound up and ready to react: TIME and AIR. Just like your soup, it is perfect, just too hot. So, we wait and we breathe. This way the thinking and the feeling parts of our brain can work effectively together to help us make a good choice.

There is a strategy that you can use that will help you make better choices in these types of situations. If you focus on your breath, just as we do when we practice our yoga or relaxation, you will calm yourself and allow yourself time and space to make better decisions. You can work on letting what you feel, what you think, what you say, and what you do be in harmony. That means that when you start to feel a particular way, you are able to think about what may be causing the feeling and the most effective way to react. Thinking about our feelings before acting is important, because if we act only on feelings we are missing out on a lot of extra information that can come from our thoughts. We want our actions to be because of the choices we make and not because we acted too fast without thinking first. It might even be helpful to think about it in terms of yoga:

I FEEL: "Frustrated!"
You might begin to feel frustrated because a particular asana or posture is difficult for you.

I THINK: "I can't do this. I am not good at anything. Everyone is better than me."
It is easy to feel angry and give up or have negative thoughts about yourself and your body.

I SAY (to myself or even out loud): "This is stupid. I can't do this."
At this point what you are thinking is shifting into things you are saying about yourself. You might even say things out loud. In this way, your feelings and thoughts are guiding your behavior.

I DO: You quit trying and start fidgeting and trying to distract your friend.

(*continued*)

PRACTICE SCRIPT 12.3 (*continued*)

However, if we breathe and then really think about it, we know we are each trying to do our own personal best. It is ok if we struggle with a yoga posture. It is important to understand that other people will be good at some postures that are difficult for us, and that we will be good at postures that other people struggle with. It is also important to remember that postures that were easy one day may be difficult another because we are tense or too distracted to focus on our breathing (or many other reasons); this feeling of frustration over a yoga move is actually giving us information about other areas of our lives, too. In order to make good choices, we need to know as much information as we can, so that we can be informed.

I FEEL: "Frustrated!" I BREATHE.
You might begin to feel frustrated because a particular asana or posture is difficult for you.

I THINK: "I can't do this. It seems like everyone is better than me." I BREATHE. "I can tell by my frustration and my thoughts that this is a real challenge for me. I need to BREATHE and choose what I am going to say and do.

You notice your thoughts ("I can't do this"). You notice that it seems as if everyone is doing better than you. Your feelings and thoughts are so important to notice and observe. Once you do this for a while you'll start to notice that when you are upset and the feeling part of your brain is really working, things SEEM different. Notice this as often as you can. Then, breathe and see if how you see things, or how they SEEM, changes. You are then ready to make a choice about what to say and/or do.

I SAY (to myself or even out loud): "This is hard to do. I know it only matters if I try." I know I am worth the effort.
At this point what you are thinking is shifting into things you are saying about yourself. You might even say things out loud. In this way, your feelings and thoughts are guiding your behavior.

I DO: You try.

Remember, between each of your fingers is time and air, which the brain needs in order to make good choices!

Source: Adapted from Cook-Cottone et al. (2013).

While taking the students through a yoga sequence, you can ask them to stop and go through the process (i.e., I feel, I think, I say, and I do). As an informal practice, whenever students appear to be struggling, have them use their hands to think through the process. If they think the process led them to a good behavioral choice—thumbs up—or if they decide they need to think it through again—thumbs down. You can also use this as a journaling assignment. Here are some questions to start with:

- Have you ever said or done something because you were feeling really angry, stressed, nervous, excited, or confused, and then regretted it later?
- Why do you think you acted that way when it was not something you would have done if you would have really thought about it?
- What could you have done to make the situation have a better ending? Break it down using I feel, I think, I say, and I do.

Associated Principles of Embodied Growth and Learning include: 1, I am worth the effort; 2, my breath is my most powerful tool; 3, I am mindfully aware; 4, I work toward presence in my physical body; 6, I ask questions about my physical experiences, feelings, and thoughts; 7, I choose my focus and actions; 8, I do the work; and 12, I work toward the possibility of effectiveness and growth in my life (see Chapter 3).

You and Me and Our Feelings Space

The felt sense of your emotions and someone else's emotions can be difficult to discern in your own body. Helping students have an awareness and sense of their own feelings and personal space and their peers' feelings and personal space can help them with emotion regulation. The simple personal space activity listed first can be done with students of elementary school age and older. The emotional space activity, described next, is best for middle and high school students. You will need a ruler, chalk, and chalkboard.

First, have two students come to the front of the room and stand about 10 to 12 feet apart, facing each other (Gillen & Gillen, 2007). Guide them through a quick body scan and ask them to pay close attention to their feelings and the sensations in their bodies. They are not to talk and should keep a neutral face and body posture while doing this activity. Ask Student A to begin walking slowly toward Student B (Gillen & Gillen, 2007). As Student A nears Student B, ask Student B to raise his or her hands to show when it feels like Student A has entered his or her personal space (Gillen & Gillen, 2007). Have the students measure the distance from Student B's feet and the edge of his or her personal space. Note the measurement in feet and inches on the chalkboard. Next, ask the students to switch roles and repeat. Have all of the students do this in pairs. Calculate the average of the distances and the range. Have the original Student A and B come up the front of the class and demonstrate the range of answers and the average. Lead a discussion about how the students knew the edge of their personal space zones and how they felt the personal space limits in their bodies.

Now, take half of the class (the Student As) to the side and ask them to think of something that they have been mad about in the past. Ask them to let the mad feelings be present in their bodies. Ask them to do the same activity, thinking about the mad thoughts and with face and body neutral. Have Student As walk slowly toward Student Bs. Ask Student Bs to indicate their personal space again; measure and post on the board. Repeat this again asking the Students As to cultivate gratitude, thinking of something for which they feel thankful. Ask them to take a moment to feel the sense of being thankful in their bodies. Have Student As walk toward Student Bs and measure and post again. Calculate the averages and ranges for mad and grateful. Ask the Student Bs to explain how they felt these each time. Were there differences in how their bodies felt? What did they notice? Reveal to the Student Bs the emotional primes given to the Student As. Now, ask Student Bs how they knew what Student As were feeling? Where did they have a felt sense that things were different? In day-to-day life, how can we be more sensitive to and aware of what others are feeling? Close the activity with a journal entry writing what they felt and what they may have learned in the activity. Associated Principles of Embodied Growth and Learning include: 1, I am worth the effort; 2, my breath is my most powerful tool; 3, I am mindfully aware; 4, I work toward presence in my physical body; 6, I ask questions about my physical experiences, feelings, and thoughts; and 7, I choose my focus and actions (see Chapter 3).

THE FOUR IMMEASURABLES

The four immeasurables are addressed both in mindful and yogic traditions reflecting the intertwining of the roots of these practices. The four immeasureables are equanimity, joy, loving-kindness, and compassion (Hanh, 1999). They are understood to be parallel to a set of negative states (McCown, Reibel, & Micozzi, 2010). It is believed that cultivating equanimity makes it more difficult for anxiety, attachment, and aversion to grow; loving-kindness can be developed to soften anger; joy for others combats jealousy; and compassion is a counterbalance for cruelty to self and others (McCown et al., 2010).

Equanimity

Equanimity is the quality of balance within the context of challenge or change (Stahl & Goldstein, 2010). McCown et al. (2010) describe equanimity as the most difficult of all of the immeasurables as it means to embrace and integrate all that arises—the feeling, thinking, good, bad, pleasant, and unpleasant. In yoga practice, true balance in a posture happens when the body has become neurologically integrated. That is, the various areas of the brain involved in maintaining a posture are working together. The same is true in our emotional lives. Balance comes from a balance of effort and rest, the use of the thinking part of our brains with the feeling part of our brains, or from the balance of independent and shared work. When we let ourselves fall too far to one side or another in a variety of contexts, we run the risk of losing our emotional balance.

Equanimity is often explored using the story of the farmer, his horse, and his son. During a storm his horse was lost (see Practice Script 12.4). Throughout the story, the farmer stayed steady as his neighbor watched in reaction to the tragedy and fortune as it moved in and out like the tide. Sometimes adolescent and college-age students are concerned that equanimity, or balance in reaction, seems more like dissociation, not connecting, or not caring. Equanimity is not the same as dissociating, not caring, or completely disconnecting. It is a process of staying centered and integrated during times of seemingly great fortune and times of seemingly great challenge. The story of the farmer and

PRACTICE SCRIPT 12.4: THE FARMER AND HIS HORSE

(Approximate timing: 2 minutes for the introduction; 1 minute for practice)

A long time ago there was a farmer. He and his family owned a fine horse. Late at night, during a terrible storm, the horse broke free and left the farm. Upon hearing of the farmer's loss, his neighbor said, "You must be so unhappy. This is horrible."

"Maybe," said the farmer. The next day, the horse returned bringing many wild horses with him. The neighbor said, "You must be so happy. This is wonderful."

"Maybe," said the farmer. The next day, the farmer's son rode the horse, fell, and broke his leg. The neighbor said, "You must be so unhappy. This is horrible."

"Maybe," Said the farmer. This accident ultimately saved the farmer's son from being recruited for active duty in the war. The farmer stayed steady as the neighbor reacted.

---

the horse does not tell us of the feelings and thoughts the farmer experienced. I am sure the farmer worried about his horse and was saddened when his son was hurt. Yet, the farmer stayed centered. I am sure he was happy when many horses returned with his horse, as well as when his son was spared from battle. The farmer likely used his breath, awareness, presence, and allowed his feelings rather than reacting to them. His yoga skills likely served him well as these skills can help all of us when fortunate and unfortunate things happen. The process of cultivating equanimity into daily life involves acceptance, nonjudgment, and a focus on speaking and behaving in service of effectiveness and *not* in service of reaction (Linehan, 1993).

Cultivating equanimity can bring a sense of peace and contentment into the lives of our students (Hanson & Mendius, 2009). Stahl and Goldstein (2010) suggest that equanimity allows for a deep understanding of the nature of change and how to be with change. As the practice of equanimity dampens the stress-response system, we need not overthink or get lost in our emotional reaction (Hanson & Mendius, 2009). When faced with emotional challenge, we want integration. We do not want to respond with constricted emotional control or abandonment of reason (see Figure 12.6). We are looking for the center path. When experiencing the integration and presence that can be found in the center (see Figure 12.6), Siegel (2010) suggests that these five qualities are present: flexibility, adaptability, coherence, energy, and stability (i.e., FACES). That is, your students will be able to show more (F) flexibility in response to challenge, they will be (A) adaptive to new situations, their response will reflect a central (C) coherence and organization, they will have (E) energy, and they will show more (S) stability over time (Siegel, 2010).

You can use your Language Arts curriculum to process this concept (e.g., *Romeo and Juliet*). Work with Figure 12.6 as you walk your students through a literature story. Ask them to identify times when the character abandoned reason and let emotions take over, and times when he or she shut down the emotional self and allowed reason to run the show. Ask students to consider what could happen if the character used both sources of wisdom to guide action during times of change.

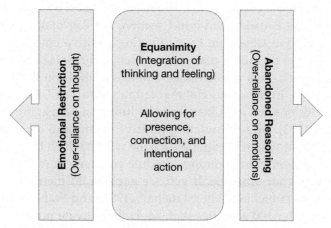

FIGURE 12.6 Equanimity within challenge.
Source: Cook-Cottone (2015).

The Associated Principles of Embodied Growth and Learning aligned with equanimity practices include: 1, I am worth the effort; 2, my breath is my most powerful tool; 3, I am mindfully aware; 4, I work toward presence in my physical body; 6, I ask questions about my physical experiences, feelings, and thoughts; 7, I choose my focus and actions; 8, I do the work; and 12, I work toward the possibility of effectiveness and growth in my life (see Chapter 3).

Loving-Kindness and Joy

Joy and loving-kindness are positive emotional states associated with our feelings toward ourselves and others. Cultivation of positive feelings states have been found to be an important component in programs that effectively address self-regulation (e.g., Hanson & Mendius, 2009; Jennings, 2015; Linehan, 1993; Shapiro & Carlson, 2009). Hanson and Mendius (2009) remind us that the brain preferentially scans for negative and potentially threatening information. Our negative implicit memory system grows faster than our positive implicit memory system (Hanson & Mendius, 2009). It is critical to purposely cultivate positive emotions such as joy and loving-kindness. In her book on mindfulness for teachers, Jennings (2015) dedicates two chapters in support of the development of positive emotions: Chapter 3, "Understanding Your Negative Emotions" (pp. 51–82) and "The Power of Positivity" (pp. 84–109).

In mindfulness and yoga teaching, sympathetic joy goes a step beyond simply cultivating joy. Sympathetic joy involves the cultivation of joyful feelings when we see others doing well (Cook-Cottone, 2015). The practice of sympathetic joy pairs well with loving-kindness practices. Consistent with these teachings, Linehan (1993) instructs patients to change current emotions by active opposition to the current emotion. The loving-kindness meditation (see Chapter 6 for a practice script) is useful for cultivating feelings of loving-kindness and warmth toward yourself, people that you care about in your life, as well as people who might get on your nerves (Stahl & Goldstein, 2010). Siegel (2010) believes that practice of the loving-kindness meditation helps activate the social and self-engagement systems of the brain. Stahl and Goldstein (2010) recommend that you practice the loving-kindness meditation in the face of resistance, "perhaps there is no greater healing than to learn to love yourself and others with an open heart" (p. 150).

As described in the broaden-and-build section, we can make great strides in creating a warm, productive classroom by cultivating positive emotions such as loving-kindness and joy. We can do this by planning and scheduling pleasant events throughout the school day and week. This research-based practice builds on the early DBT work of Marsha Linehan (1993). In the emotional regulation module of DBT, patients are taught to build positive emotions and joyfulness by scheduling and engaging in pleasant events each day (Linehan, 1993). By accumulating positive events and corresponding positive emotional states, patients begin to experience a life within which they want to be present (Linehan, 1993). Look over your planning schedule and make sure there are positive, fun experiences built into your schedule. If you see gaps, build them in (e.g., yoga breaks, mini dance parties, or stretching time). Linehan (1993) and Stahl and Goldstein (2010) both provide lists of over 100 activities that can help cultivate positive experiences. See also Jennings (2015) for ideas for your classroom. Associated Principles of Embodied Growth and Learning include: 1, I am worth the effort; 2, my breath is my most powerful tool; 3, I am mindfully aware; 4, I work toward presence in my physical body; 6, I ask questions about my physical experiences, feelings, and thoughts; 7, I choose my focus and actions; 8, I do the work; and 12, I work toward the possibility of effectiveness and growth in my life (see Chapter 3).

Compassion for Self and Others

Compassion means to wish for the suffering in others to be removed (McCown et al., 2010). The roots of the word compassion are shared with the word kindness (Wallace, 2010). When you experience compassion, you are fully present with the struggle within the other person or yourself. There is no avoidance, denial, or dissociation. Compassion for self and others also includes the awareness that struggling is part of being human. I remind my students and yoga students that it is not about the winning, getting it right, or being perfect. It is about the trying. Further, in the trying there will be some instances of getting right, landing the part in the play, and nailing the test or performance or maybe even the pose. However, there will also be times when they get it wrong, fall, lose a sense of purpose, and experience what the world sees as failure. Self-compassion is loving yourself through all of it. Compassion is the kindness you show to others as they succeed, fail, try, and forget how to try. For a tool to assess compassion, see Pommier (2011), which is accessible at www.self-compassion/self-compassion-sales-for-researchers.

Research suggests that self-compassion may promote the successful self-regulation of health-related behaviors (Terry & Leary, 2011). It is believed that improved self-regulation is possible due to a lowering of defensiveness, negative emotional states, and self-blame. Additionally, it is theorized that people high in self-compassion may be less depleted. Being less depleted, they cope better because they have greater self-regulatory resources to devote to self-care (Terry & Leary, 2011). To assess self-compassion see Raes, Pommier, Neff, and Van Gucht (2011). The scale is accessible at www.self-compassion/self-compassion-sales-for-researchers. Associated Principles of Embodied Growth and Learning include: 1, I am worth the effort; 2, my breath is my most powerful tool; 3, I am mindfully aware; 4, I work toward presence in my physical body; 6, I ask questions about my physical experiences, feelings, and thoughts; 7, I choose my focus and actions; 8, I do the work; 10, I honor efforts to grow and learn; 11, I am kind to myself and others; and 12, I work toward the possibility of effectiveness and growth in my life (see Chapter 3).

YOGA THROUGHOUT THE SCHOOL DAY

Childress and Harper (2015) contend that in order to have the greatest impact and create access for the most students, yoga programs should be integrated into the school day. This can be done with a mix of formal and informal practices woven into the classroom experience, as well as by offering stand-alone yoga classes and/or after school programs. It is important to note that efforts to provide access should be balanced with a commitment to creating an invitational environment (Childress & Harper, 2015). This chapter, from beginning to end, is intended to inspire and empower you to integrate informal yoga concepts and practices into your school day. Weaving in the informal practices can begin with the broader work of emphasizing and practicing the physical pillars of self-regulation (i.e., nutrition, hydration, exercise, and rest). Next, create a framework for a positive and problem-solving approach to emotions. Last, with a wider view on a broaden-and-build approach for your classroom and school, intersperse positive embodied activities with challenging academic tasks. The following provides a few more ideas for integrating yoga in the classroom.

Yoga Breaks

A yoga break is a 5 to 10 minute break to stretch between academic tasks, allowing students time to assimilate knowledge, build a positive mood state, and support physical health (Asencia, 2006). This can be done first thing in the morning, during class times when you notice that their attention and focus are waning, between tasks, while students are waiting in line, before or after lunch, after recess, before a test or exam, when student appear tense or tired, and at the end of the day (Asencia, 2006). Types of breaks include breathing breaks in which you guide students through one of the breathing exercises (Asencia, 2006), taking a few moments to coordinate breath with movement (i.e., raising arms up and down, opening and closing arms, stretching side to side, or folding forward and standing up). Asencia (2006) suggests stretching the inhale and the exhale out longer than the movement. For an entire book on yoga breaks, see Goldberg (2016).

Quick Yoga Games

When working with students of all ages but especially younger students, bringing a sense of play into practice can help engage the students. Most books on children's yoga include a section on yoga games (e.g., Tantillo, 2012). Choose a game that meets the needs of the class. Offer what is missing in the room. If the class has been working hard on seated work, do a quick active yoga game. If students are wound up and are struggling to settle, have them do a reflective game. You want to avoid relying on yoga games for yoga practice. The choice of the game should be done with an eye on attunement to their needs, and should build on more formal yoga practice that builds inner connection and basic yoga skills.

There are lots of ideas for yoga games online and in most yoga for kids books. Many of these games integrate yoga into traditional games. For example, Red Light, Green Light is played with the traditional or familiar rules adding a yoga pose when the students freeze. Yoga Freeze is a simple game of skipping and dancing around the room, freezing and doing a yoga pose, when the music stops, and moving again when the music starts (Tantillo, 2012). Musical Cards works like musical chairs, except the students dance around yoga pose cards. When the music stops they quickly take the pose on the card (Tantillo, 2012). Last, Pass the Cup involves sitting in a circle and passing a half cup of water in silence, noticing sounds and sensations (Greenland, 2010). Pass it in one direction and then the other. Next, pass the cup with eyes closed. Process with the students by asking students what it felt like to use their eyes and then to rely on other senses to pass the cup. Similarly, you can play pass the breath using a Hober-man sphere (i.e., expanding ball toy) with each person taking a breath (Willard, 2016). See Herrington (2012), Flynn (2013), and Harper (2013) for ideas for yoga games, activities, and yoga-based art.

Mindful Body Awareness

Body awareness is an integral aspect of yoga. It is awareness of your body, body sensations inside and out, and a sense of your body in space. Body awareness includes an awareness of the nonverbal messages in communication and the way they feel in our bodies (David, 2009). Body awareness lets us know when we are tired, hungry, in need of exercise or when we need to stop and rest (Cook-Cottone et al., 2013). David (2009) suggests that there are many informal ways to apply mindful awareness to physical sensations and movement of the body. David (2009) encourages you to start with a body scan (see Chapter 6). Next, you can use the body scan experience to bring awareness to the body when the class is walking. When walking somewhere as a class you can guide them to walk silently as if everyone is watching them, as if they are very tired, as if they want to pass unnoticed, or as if they are paying attention to each step (David, 2009). Throughout the day, you can ask the class to check in with their bodies, notice any tightness, and breathe into the tightness and relax. David encourages "mini mindfulness movement techniques" (2009, pp. 123–126). These include a check-in with legs and feet while students are walking, dialing into the energy level of the body at any point in the day, noticing physical sensations while working on the computer, and digging into a felt-awareness during a mini stretch break.

CONCLUSION

Going back to where we started this chapter, Aristotle says, "We are what we repeatedly do." Educational research tells us that spaced practice creates durable learning (e.g., Kang, 2016). Formal practice is important and adding in informal practice throughout the day, along with yoga breaks and yoga games, can enhance outcomes. This chapter reviewed the ways to teach and practice yoga off-the-mat, in your classroom, and in your life. The broad-and-build theory was offered as a conceptual framework for informal practice and for work with emotions. The role and management of emotions was explicated from a yoga perspective. Next, the four immeasurables (i.e., joy, equanimity, compassion, and loving-kindness) were discussed within the context of broadening and building positive feelings and experiences for your students. Last, quick and easy ways to integrate yoga into your school day were reviewed (e.g., yoga breaks and games). Note that, although the theory is compelling and some informal practices have been found to be beneficial (i.e., loving-kindness meditation), more research is needed to explore the role of yoga poses, breathing exercises, and the broader role of a variety of relaxation and mindfulness techniques and how they can help students broaden and build their coping repertoire and set of resources. To add to your resource library consider these texts:

- For lots of ways to integrate social-emotional learning to your school day, see Philbert (2016a), *Everyday SEL in Elementary School: Integrating Social-Emotional Learning and Mindfulness Into Your Classroom*, and Philbert (2016b), *Everyday SEL in Middle School: Integrating Social-Emotional Learning and Mindfulness Into Your Classroom*.
- For yoga games, see Tantillo (2012), *Cooling Down Your Classroom: Using Yoga Relaxation and Breathing Strategies to Help Students Learn to Keep Their Cool*.
- For yoga breaks, see Golberg (2016), *Classroom Yoga Breaks: Brief Exercises to Create Calm*.

REFERENCES

Anderson, S., & Sovik, R. (2000). *Yoga mastering the basics*. Honsedale, PA: The Himalayan Institute.

Armstrong, L. E., Ganio, M. S., Casa, D. J., Lee, E. C., McDermott, B. P., Klau, J. F., ... & Lieberman, H. R. (2012). Mild dehydration affects mood in healthy young women. *The Journal of nutrition, 142*(2), 382–388.

Asencia, T. (2006). *Yoga in your school: Exercises for classroom, gym and playground*. Highstown, NJ: Princeton.

Astill, R. G., Van der Heijden, K. B., Van IJzendoorn, M. H., & Van Someren, E. J. (2012). Sleep, cognition, and behavioral problems in school-age children: A century of research meta-analyzed. *Psychological Bulletin, 138,* 1109–1138.

Bourne, E. J. (2010). *The anxiety and phobia workbook, fifth edition.* Oakland, CA: New Harbinger Publications.

Childress, T., & Harper, J. C. (2015). *Best practices for yoga in the schools.* Best Practices Guide Vol. 1. Atlanta, GA: YEC Omega Publications.

Cook-Cottone, C. P. (2015). *Mindfulness and yoga for self-regulation: A primer for mental health professionals.* New York, NY: Springer Publishing.

Cook-Cottone, C. P. Kane, L. S., Keddie, E., Haugli, S. (2013). *Girls growing in wellness and balance: Yoga and life skills to empower.* Stoddard, WI: Schoolhouse Educational Services, LLC

Cook-Cottone, C. P., Tribole, E., & Tylka, T. L. (2013). *Healthy eating in schools: Evidence-based interventions to help kids thrive.* Washington, DC. American Psychological Association.

David, D. S. (2009). *Mindful Teaching and teaching mindfulness: A guide for anyone who teaches anything.* Boston, MA: Wisdom Publications.

Flynn, L. (2013). *Yoga for children: 200+ yoga poses, breathing exercises, and meditations for healthier, happier, more resilient children.* Avon, MA: Adams Media.

Fredrickson, B. L. (2009). *Positivity: Groundbreaking research reveals how to embrace the hidden strength of positive emotions, overcome negativity, and thrive.* New York, NY: Crown Publishing Group.

Fredrickson, B. L. (2013). Positive emotions broaden and build. *Advances in Experimental Social Psychology, 47,* 53.

Garland, E. L., Fredrickson, B., Kring, A. M., Johnson, D. P., Meyer, P. S., & Penn, D. L. (2010). Upward spirals of positive emotions counter downward spirals of negativity: Insights from the broaden-and-build theory and affective neuroscience on the treatment of emotion dysfunctions and deficits in psychopathology. *Clinical Psychology Review, 30,* 849–864.

Garland, E. L., Schwarz, N. R., Kelly, A., Whitt, A., & Howard, M. O. (2012). Mindfulness-oriented recovery enhancement for alcohol dependence: Therapeutic mechanisms and intervention acceptability. *Journal of social work practice in the addictions, 12*(3), 242–263.

Gillen, L., & Gillen, J. (2007). *Yoga calm for children: Educating heart, mind, and body.* Portland, OR: Three Pebble Press.

Golberg, L. (2016). *Classroom yoga breaks: Brief exercise to create calm.* New York, NY: W. W. Norton.

Greenland, S. K. (2010). *The mindful child: How to help your kids manage stress and become happier, kinder, and more compassionate.* New York, NY: Atria.

Gujar, N., Yoo, S. S., Hu, P., & Walker, M. P. (2011). Sleep deprivation amplifies reactivity of brain reward networks, biasing the appraisal of positive emotional experiences. *The Journal of Neuroscience, 31,* 4466–4474.

Hanh, T. N. (1999). *The heart of Buddha's teachings: Transforming suffering into peace, joy, and liberation.* New York, NY: Broadway Books.

Hanson, R., & Mendius, R. (2009). *Buddha's brain: The practical neuroscience of happiness, love, and wisdom.* Oakland, CA: New Harbinger Publications.

Harper, J. C. (2013). *Little flower yoga for kids: A yoga and mindfulness programs to help your children improve attention and emotional balance.* Oakland, CA: New Harbinger Publications.

Herrington, S. (2012). *Om schooled: A guide to teaching kids yoga in real-world schools.* San Marcos, CA: Addriya.

Jennings, P. A. (2015). *Mindfulness for teachers: Simple skills for peace and productivity in the classroom.* New York, NY: W. W. Norton.

Kang, S. H. (2016). Spaced repetition promotes efficient and effective learning policy implications for instruction. *Policy Insights from the Behavioral and Brain Sciences, 3,* 12–19.

Kennedy, D., Jones, E., Haskell, C., & Benton, D. (2011). Vitamin status, cognition and mood in cognitively intact adults. *Lifetime nutritional influences on cognition, behaviour and psychiatric illness, 16,* 194–250.

Koole, S. L., van Dillen, L. F., & Sheppes, G. (2011). The self-regulation of emotion. In K. D. Vohs & R. F. Baumeister (Eds.), *Handbook of self-regulation, second edition:Research, theory and applications* (pp. 22–40). New York, NY: The Guilford Press.

Lees, C., & Hopkins, J. (2013). Effect of aerobic exercise on cognition, academic achievement, and psychosocial function in children: A systematic review of randomized control trials. *Preventing Chronic Disease, 10*(10). doi:10.5888/pcd10.130010.

Linehan, M. (1993). *Cognitive-behavioral treatment of borderline personality disorder.* New York, NY: Guilford Press.

McCown, D., Reibel, D., & Micozzi, M. S. (2010). *Teaching mindfulness: A practical guide for clinicians and educators.* New York, NY: Springer.

Nummenmaa, L., Glerean, E., Hari, R., & Hietanen, J. K. (2014). Bodily maps of emotions. *Proceedings of the National Academy of Sciences, 111,* 646–651.

Oosterwijk, S., Lindquist, K. A., Anderson, E., Dautoff, R., Moriguchi, Y., & Barrett, L. F. (2012). States of mind: Emotions, body feelings, and thoughts share distributed neural networks. *NeuroImage, 62,* 2110–2128.

Philbert, C. T. (2016a). *Everyday SEL in elementary school: Integrating social-emotional learning and mindfulness into your classroom.* New York, NY: Routledge.

Philbert, C. T. (2016b). *Everyday SEL in middle school: Integrating social-emotional learning and mindfulness into your classroom.* New York, NY: Routledge.

Pommier, E. A. (2011). The compassion scale. *Dissertation Abstracts International Section A: Humanities and Social Sciences, 72,* 1174.

Raes, F., Pommier, E., Neff, K. D., & Van Gucht, D. (2011). Construction and factorial validation of a short form of the Self-Compassion Scale. *Clinical Psychology & Psychotherapy, 18,* 250–255.

Siegel, D. J. (2010). *The mindful therapist: A clinician's guide to mindsight and neural integration.* New York, NY: W. W. Norton.

Stahl, B., & Goldstein, E. (2010). *A mindfulness-based stress reduction workbook.* Oakland, CA: New Harbinger Publications.

Tantillo, C. (2012). *Cooling down your classroom: Using yoga relaxation and breathing strategies to help students learn to keep their cool.* Chicago, IL: Mindful Practices.

Terry, M. L., & Leary, M. R. (2011). Self-compassion, self-regulation, and health. *Self and Identity, 10,* 352–362.

Wallace, A. (2010). *The four immeasurables: Practices to open the heart.* Boulder, CO: Snow Lion.

Willard, C. (2016). *Growing up mindful: Essential practices to help children and families find balance, calm, and resilience.* Boulder, CO: Sounds True.

Zschucke, E., Gaudlitz, K., & Ströhle, A. (2013). Exercise and physical activity in mental disorders: Clinical and experimental evidence. *Journal of Preventive Medicine and Public Health, 46*(Suppl 1), S12–S21.

CHAPTER 13

SCHOOL-BASED YOGA PROGRAMS: MANUALIZED AND STRUCTURED YOGA PROGRAMS FOR SCHOOLS

Beneath the ups and downs of everyday life
there is a profound state of balance.
By resting for brief periods in that state
we create a resilient and stable mind
even in the face of stress.

Anderson & Sovik (2000, p. 197)

Anderson and Sovik (2000), master yoga teacher trainers at the Himalayan Institute, speak of three of the known outcomes of yoga research in their quote—self-regulation, equanimity, and stress management. Their knowledge comes from practice and the traditional passing down of the practice from teacher to student, generation after generation. As most yoga practitioners know, the research of personal practice is a valid pathway to knowledge. Throughout my years of yoga teacher trainings, when one of us asked how a pose should be taught or what the effects of a particular sequence might be, answers from our teachers did not come easily. We were given the answers in terms of what is known or understood. Then, we were told that these experiences are so different for each of us and that we should try to "live the question," and "be the research." We were told that it is in the practice and the inquiry that we will find our answers.

Looking at things from the long-held yoga perspective that truth and knowledge come from our inner experience, contemporary research methodologies do not necessarily present as a good fit. Right now, researchers are working to standardize and manualize yoga practices, measure outcomes with verbal reports and interviews, track changes using physiological measures such as sleep studies and wrist watches that track heart rate and galvanic skin responses, and look at brain changes using brain imaging. Researchers are doing their best to detect inner transformation, or a different way of being, using respected and validated tools and methods. I have sat in research conference discussions in which we all grappled with the tension between what some saw as the art of yoga teaching and practice and contemporary scientific methods. Collectively we understand that if we are to provide

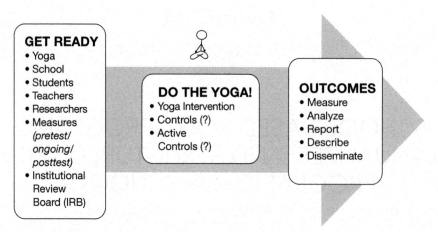

FIGURE 13.1 The process of yoga research in schools.

compelling evidence of the benefits of yoga for children, youth, and adults, we must use contemporary methodologies showing the outcomes based on a scientific method that is respected and valued by academics, administrators, and decision-makers in schools. The body of research is growing. The questions and ways of answering them are becoming increasingly refined and targeted. Each year the methodologies and research designs are more sophisticated and of higher quality.

To school personnel, research sometimes can feel like a daunting and overly complicated process. It is true; it is not easy. There are a lot of moving parts and multiple systems to negotiate (e.g., school systems, university systems, institutional review boards [IRBs]). However, it can be done and done well. Researchers need your help. In order to show the effects of yoga in schools, the research on yoga must be done in schools. Researchers need school personnel willing to see what is possible for students and staff. That means setting aside time and resources for assessment, allowing for control groups and active control groups, committing to the yoga intervention with enthusiasm, and being willing to be active and engaged problem solvers as researchers partner with school personnel to create a high-quality study. The process is illustrated in Figure 13.1. As difficult as it may seem, research can be a fun and rewarding process.

With the research conducted to date on yoga in schools and the growing number of research teams across the country, we are getting closer to being able to explain how yoga works and what the outcomes are. Notably, there is still far more to know than is known. This chapter reviews the current state of yoga research, presenting an overall conceptual model and reviewing outcomes. Next, yoga programs are reviewed and a survey of yoga programs presented. This is followed by what we currently know about contraindications for yoga. Finally, a note on next steps is offered.

THE BODY OF RESEARCH ON YOGA IN SCHOOLS

As detailed in Chapters 9 through 12 of this text, the term *yoga* reflects a set of practices intended to integrate the mind and body, improve self-regulation, and increase capacity for reflective, intentional engagement (Butzer, Bary, Telles, & Khalsa, 2016; Cook-Cottone, 2015;

Forfylow, 2011; Khanna & Greeson, 2013). Nearly universally across programs, school-based practice of yoga entails emphasis on physical postures, breathing exercises, relaxation, and meditation (see Chapter 11; Butzer et al., 2016; Cook-Cottone, 2015; Forfylow, 2011; Khanna & Greeson, 2013). The number of publications in the field of yoga in schools has increased dramatically over the past 20 years (see Figure 13.2).

Although there has been a dramatic increase in the number and quality of yoga-related research publications since 2000 (Butzer et al., 2016), research in the area of yoga lags behind mindfulness research (Cook-Cottone, 2015). Mindfulness research was ignited and then bolstered by the manualization of Mindfulness-Based Stress Reduction (MBSR) and Dialectic Behavioral Therapy (DBT). In the field of yoga practice, there has been some resistance to standardizing and manualizing yoga to conform to empirical methodologies for fear of compromising yoga's authenticity and flexibility, and responsive delivery (Cook-Cottone, 2015). For example, when I teach a yoga class at a studio, I go in with a planned sequence and a theme. However, if the class seems to need something else or I see a need to workshop a pose, I change direction. The ability to see what a class needs and to respond accordingly is part of the *art of teaching yoga*. In a manualized program, this might be seen as a loss of integrity to the intended protocol.

As explained in Chapter 8 in the mindfulness section of this text, there are core scientific requirements for the study of interventions (e.g., feasibility, acceptability, treatment integrity, manualization, use of quality and sensitive outcome measures, active control groups, randomization). Basics such as dosage of yoga (e.g., frequency and duration) have not been adequately addressed in research (Cook-Cottone, 2013; Cook-Cottone, 2015). Currently, researchers believe that yoga is helpful for several reasons including simultaneous relaxation and activation; improved neurological self-regulation; improved sense of well-being and quality of life; as well as an increased awareness and tolerance of bodily sensations, feelings, and physical experience (Butzer et al., 2016; Cook-Cottone, 2015; Simpkins & Simpkins, 2011; van der Kolk et al., 2014; Woodyard, 2011). To help move the field of research forward, Butzer et al. (2016) created a conceptual model for understanding the effects of yoga that was recently updated by Khalsa (personal communication, 2016; see Figure 13.3).

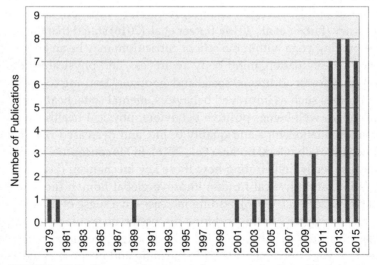

FIGURE 13.2 Quantitative research on yoga in the schools.

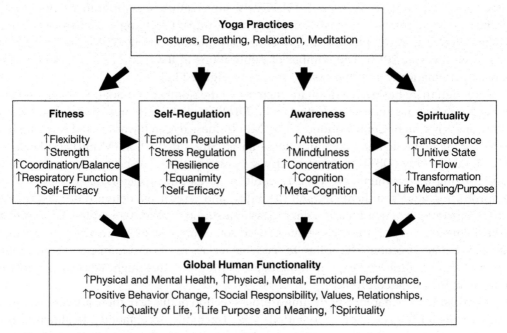

FIGURE 13.3 Conceptualizing school-based yoga effects.
Source: Sat Bir Singh Khalsa, 2016; adapted from Butzer et al., 2016.

Overall, it is theorized that the four core practices of school-based yoga (i.e., posture, breathing, relaxation, and meditation) increase mind-body awareness, self-regulation, and physical fitness (Butzer et al., 2016). Specifically, it is hypothesized that mind-body awareness is increased via improved mindfulness, increased attention, improved concentration and cognitive functioning, and enhanced awareness of the students' individual sense of self as well as their social selves (Butzer et al., 2016). Improvements in self-regulation occur via increases in emotion regulation, stress regulation, resilience over time, increased equanimity, and improved psychological self-efficacy. Third, improved physical fitness occurs via improvements in flexibility, strength, balance, respiratory function, and a strong sense of physical self-efficacy (Butzer et al., 2016). Butzer et al. (2016) stated that the body of research suggests that providing yoga within the school curriculum may be an effective way to help students develop self-regulation, mind-body awareness, and physical fitness. They reason that these effects may foster additional social and emotional learning competencies and positive student outcomes such as improved behaviors, mental state, health, and performance (i.e., improved mood, well-being, positive behaviors, physical health, cognitive and academic performance, relationships and quality of life, and decreased risk for psychological disorders and negative behaviors; Butzer et al., 2016). In his conceptual model Khalsa (2016) takes a broader perspective illustrating how these key mechanism (i.e., mind-body awareness, self-regulation, and physical fitness) improve global human function in each of the ways reported by Butzer et al. (2016), adding increases in a sense of life purpose, meaning, and spirituality (see Chapter 9 of this text for a discussion on secular yoga and spirituality). The new model presented by Khalsa (2016) acknowledges the importance of researchers exploring aspects of yoga outcomes related to meaning and purpose in life as well as spirituality (i.e., a need for purpose and to live our lives in fulfillment of that purpose; Khalsa, 2016; Madden, 2015).

AN OVERVIEW OF OUTCOMES FOR YOGA IN SCHOOLS

As the theoretical model sets the stage for future research, it also provides a framework for understanding the research that has been completed to date. It is important to note that there is a larger body of research on yoga for children and youth with fewer studies based specifically in schools. Research to date presents with a relatively diverse array of interventions using various forms, aspects, and dosages of yoga and few are manualized yoga interventions (e.g., Klein & Cook-Cottone, 2013; Serwacki & Cook-Cottone, 2012). For many years, there were simply too few studies to validly compare outcomes across studies or to meaningfully aggregate outcomes using systematic reviews or meta-analyses. At this point, there have been three major reviews of the research on yoga in schools: Serwacki and Cook-Cottone (2012), Ferreira-Vorkapic et al. (2015), and Khalsa and Butzer (2016).

First, in 2012, my research team published the first review of the extant research on yoga in schools. The objective of our review was to examine the evidence for delivering yoga-based interventions in schools to provide a solid sense of where the research stood. We conducted an electronic literature search to identify peer-reviewed, published studies in which yoga and a meditative component (breathing practices or meditation) were taught to youths in a school setting. Pilot studies, single cohort, quasi-experimental, and randomized clinical trials were considered. We used three independent reviewers to code studies for key components and quality using multiple evaluative criteria (e.g., Did the study describe the method of randomization? Was the sample size justified? Was there a description of withdrawals and drop outs? Was there an intention-to-treat analysis? Did the study report treatment integrity? Was a manual used? Were outcomes well described? Did outcome measures have good reliability? [Serwacki & Cook-Cottone, 2012]).

We identified twelve published studies. Samples for which yoga was implemented as an intervention included youths with autism, intellectual disability, learning disability, and emotional disturbance, as well as youths without special needs (Serwacki & Cook-Cottone, 2012). We found that although the effects of participating in school-based yoga programs appeared to be beneficial for the most part for special needs students, findings included reduced stress, improved cognitive functioning, greater self and social confidence, improved communication and contribution to the classroom, and improved attention and concentration (Serwacki & Cook-Cottone, 2012). For typically developing students, participation in a school-based yoga program was associated with decreased body dissatisfaction, anxiety, negative behaviors, cognitive disturbances (e.g., rumination and intrusive thoughts), impulsivity, emotional and physical arousal as well as increased perceived self-concept and emotional balance (Serwacki & Cook-Cottone, 2012).

The studies reviewed, however, were of predominantly low quality. The methodological limitations included lack of randomization, small samples, limited detail regarding the intervention, and statistical ambiguities, which curtailed the ability to provide definitive conclusions or recommendations. We concluded that the findings spoke to the need for greater methodological rigor and an increased understanding of the mechanisms of success for school-based yoga interventions (Serwacki & Cook-Cottone, 2012).

In 2015, Ferreira-Vorkapic et al. reviewed the literature and conducted a meta-analysis. These authors reported that an extensive search was conducted for studies published between 1980 and October 31, 2014 (PubMed, PsycInfo, Embase, ISI, and the Cochrane Library; Ferreira-Vorkapic et al., 2015). After identifying 48 studies, the authors excluded dissertations, special issues and reviews, unpublished studies, studies with intervention or outcome issues, studies presorting insufficient data, and studies that were not randomized controlled trials. These exclusions from the aggregate analysis highlight the importance of commitment to a high-quality research design—studies with poorer designs simply do not have the impact. Ultimately, the review was based on nine studies, with seven studies depicted in the plot of general effect size in the selected studies (Ferreira-Vorkapic et al., 2015).

Ferreira-Vorkapic et al. (2015) completed an effect size analysis on the remaining studies, through standardized mean difference and Hedges's g, which allowed for the comparison of experimental conditions. Although these studies all evaluated yoga in schools, they were very different in several ways. The studies included either elementary school, middle school, or high school students. The types of yoga utilized included Vinayasa, Ashtanga, Yoga Ed, Kripalu Yoga, Niroga, Mindful Girls Yoga, and Hatha Yoga. The dosage of yoga ranged from 10 to 18 weeks, 15 to 90 minutes per session, and 1 to 5 times a week. Control groups varied as well. Five of the studies used an active control group (i.e., physical education or physical activity) and the other studies used a waitlist or no inventions (Ferreira-Vorkapic et al., 2015).

The general plot of the outcomes shows divided results with half of the studies favoring yoga and the other half favoring controls. In aggregate, the overall effect for yoga was not found to be significant. Appropriately, the authors state, "This is probably due to the heterogeneity of the variables" (Ferreira-Vorkapic et al., 2015, p. 3). To illustrate issues at hand, one of the studies that favored the controls was Haden, Daly, and Hagins (2014). This study compared 15 students in yoga to 15 students in physical education. The yoga group comprised 10 males and five females; the physical education group comprised seven males and eight females. The yoga group engaged in 15 weeks of Ashtanga Yoga (90 minutes a session), three times a week. At the end of the study, there were no significant effects on behavior, aggression, and self-perception but there was an increased negative affect for the yoga group.

There several issues that should be noted to provide context for the Haden et al. (2014) study. First, the sample size was very small, too small to look at gender effects. That leads to the second issue: There is emerging evidence that when middle and high school age male students are assigned to yoga over physical education, they frequently indicate that they feel they are missing out and would prefer the competitive and more vigorous activity in physical education class. We saw this trend in a qualitative study we conducted recently. Once students reached fifth and sixth grades, male students began to voice a preference for physical education over yoga. In discussion on strategies to negotiate this, researchers have argued for research designs that do not make students select yoga or physical education. When putting yoga up against soccer for a 13-year-old male, often soccer wins. That makes sense and it is not what we are trying to study. In this case, we end up with adolescent males filling out the posttest surveys, upset that they had to do yoga and missed soccer, football, track, and weight lifting for 15 weeks. Rather, active control groups should offer noncompetitive activities with similar physical exertion levels. Next, another issue that needs further exploration is the reporting of increased negative affect at posttest among those in the yoga group. Although this might be explained as an expression of the disappointment and frustration resulting from 15 weeks of missing sports, researchers are beginning to look more deeply into this phenomenon. It is hypothesized that the increased awareness of body and feeling states that occurs in yoga practice may make students aware of feelings that they had not noticed prior. More research is needed to better understand this process as well as how to assess more specifically exactly what is occurring.

The issues well illustrated by the Haden et al. (2014) study show what is lost in our understanding of the more nuanced picture of yoga outcomes when studies are aggregated. Notably, when Ferreira-Vorkapic et al. (2015) looked at individual study effects they found positive and a significant effect sizes for mood indicators, tension, and anxiety in the POMS scale, self-esteem, and memory when the yoga groups were compared to control. Ferreira-Vorkapic et al. (2015) noted that future research requires greater standardization and suitability of yoga interventions for children.

In 2016, Khalsa and Butzer published their review of 47 studies with a total sample size of 4,522 participants (one study was not included due to insufficient data). Their review of the research included research conducted in 19 elementary and preschools, six middle schools, seven middle and high schools, and 13 high schools. The sample sizes ranged substantially from a study of 20 participants to a study of 660. The review included 25 randomized controlled trials, seven nonrandomized controlled trials, nine uncontrolled trials, and four qualitative studies (Khalsa & Butzer, 2016). They were conducted primarily in the United States ($n = 30$) and India ($n = 15$). The majority of studies ($n = 41$) were conducted from 2010 onward (Khalsa & Butzer, 2016). Most of the studies (85%) were conducted within the school curriculum. Further, most (62%) were implemented as formal school-based yoga programs (Khalsa & Butzer, 2016). The authors described the field as an infant research field with most of the published research trials preliminary in nature, with numerous study design limitations, including limited sample sizes and relatively weak research designs (Khalsa & Butzer, 2016).

Specific positive *student self-report* outcomes included mood state, self-esteem, self-control, decreased aggression and social problems, self-regulation, emotion regulation, feelings of happiness and relaxation, social and physical well-being, and decreased rumination, emotional arousal, intrusive thoughts, and alcohol use (Khalsa & Butzer, 2016). *Teacher-rated outcomes* included positive findings associated with classroom behaviors, emotion skills, independence, attention skills, transition skills, self-regulation, concentration, mood, ability to function under pressure, attention, adaptive skills, and social skills. Teacher ratings also indicated reductions in performance impairment, hyperactivity, behavioral symptoms, internalizing symptoms, and maladaptive behaviors (Khalsa & Butzer, 2016). *Objective data* collected from school records and academic tests showed positive intervention improvements in student grades and academic performance (Khalsa & Butzer, 2016). Last, *physiological and cognitive outcome measures* showed decreased cortisol concentrations, more stable breathing patterns, improvement in micronutrient absorption, improved strength (i.e., grip and abdominal), improved flexibility, improved heart rate variability, and improved stress reactivity as indicated by skin conductance response (Khalsa & Butzer, 2016). Researchers observed that many positive outcomes were trends ($p < 0.1$) rather than statistically significant ($p < 0.05$). Ultimately, Khalsa and Butzer (2016) concluded that these publications suggest that yoga in the school setting is a viable and potentially efficacious strategy for improving child and adolescent health and therefore worthy of continued research.

When we take all of the research together, we have a good sense of all the work that is yet to be done. Yes, this line of research is in its infancy. It faces the challenge of conducting a rigorous study within the complex system of the school district. As a researcher, I am frequently approached by school personnel to conduct studies. However, once I begin talking about what is required for a solid design, the IRB, pre- and posttests, and informed consent, the enthusiasm quickly wanes. I have also experienced and observed the process of a study slowly falling apart as roadblocks are experienced. Despite these challenges, I know my team and many other teams are committed to making this research happen. It will take teamwork between research and school personnel. Considering the wonderful researchers and school personnel I know, I think we are up to the task (and it's a big one). Here is a list of questions that have yet to be answered.

- Can you really compare Ashtanga, Vinyasa, Kriplau, and Hatha yoga? How are these yoga practices the same? How are they different? What are the yoga ingredients that create change? Do all types of yoga share these ingredients?
- What type of yoga is best for each age? Does it matter? Should we use animal and plant names for kids or is it okay to say Warrior I? Do we need to tell a story, play games, sing songs, or can we just do yoga?
- How much does a research design that uses physical education as the active control group really tell us about the effects of yoga? Are activities conducted in physical education adequately commensurate with yoga?
- What is the best active control group to answer our questions?
- Should all yoga studies be analyzed by gender and age?
- How much does teacher buy-in matter?
- Who teaches better yoga in schools, school-personnel trained as yoga teachers or yoga teachers trained to teach in schools?
- How much does experience with behavioral management matter?
- Does the yoga practice experience of the teacher matter? What if the teacher doesn't practice?
- What is the best way to document the yoga being done in the study? Should we require a manual? Should the manual be somewhat flexible to allow for in-the-moment adaptations?
- Are the programs being implemented with fidelity?
- Should all studies report and control for attendance and participation? Should the level of student engagement in the program be measured (i.e., enthusiastic participation, passive engagement, or active resistance)?
- How are programs adapted for students with special needs? Does this change the integrity measures or manualization? Should this be controlled for?
- Are the samples used in research studies diverse enough?
- What is optimal dosage of yoga? How much does home practice matter? Does it matter if students keep practicing after the intervention or do the effects hold without practice?
- Are all students yoga naïve? Are they mind-body practice naïve? Or do they do other mind-body practices? What if you have four students who are Ti Kwon Do champions in your control group? What about mindful dance?
- Is continued practice necessary for long-term effect?
- How can we compare across studies when studies are not standardized or manualized? Can we standardize and manualize yoga?

YOGA PROGRAM CONTENT

There is a growing number of yoga programs available for your school. To gather the available information, I combined the work of members of my research team with the resources available in published articles and through an independent search of databases and Google. First, Heather Cahill, Killian Cherry, and Rebecca Sivecz of my research team spent an entire semester searching the Internet and research databases to locate yoga programs. This was integrated into the results reported in a 2015 review by Butzer, Ebert, Telles, and Khalsa. Their team completed a survey of school-based yoga programs in the United States. Next, for this overview, an additional search was conducted verifying what my team found, integrating the 2015 survey, and adding further information on the programs.

Using this process, we found a wide variety of programs, ranging in terms of research support, ease of use, and alignment with school standards. I have expanded on a few of the programs as illustrations of unique features. As with mindfulness programs, some programs that self-describe as research-based are referring to a component of their program or a practice that they used in the program (e.g., yoga poses, systematic relaxation, meditation) rather than a study specifically evaluating their program. Some programs say they are research-based, meaning that *yoga* is research-based. Often these programs list general yoga research findings on their web page. Do your research before you bring a program to your school. The following list can give you a good starting point and some things to consider. What follows is a list of school-based yoga program features to consider:

- Be sure the program has clearly defined goals and objectives (Childress & Harper, 2015).
- Review the program for each aspect of school-based yoga (i.e., yoga poses, breathing exercise, relaxation, and meditation; Childress & Harper, 2015).
- Look for a sequence in the lessons plans in which the learning from previous lessons sets the stage for the next lesson (Childress & Harper, 2015).
- Confirm the lesson is age and developmental-level sensitive (Childress & Harper, 2015).
- Look for adaptations for special populations, allowing for variations based on student need and ability (Childress & Harper, 2015).
- Identify resources that will help you keep parents, school personnel, and other teachers informed and empowered to help (Childress & Harper, 2015).
- Look for a match between what is feasible and practical for you to do in your classroom and school and what the program requires (Childress & Harper, 2015).
- Make sure time allotments include time for processing, questions, extra assistance, and breaks (Childress & Harper, 2015).
- Seek out a program with assessment tools or directions so that you can assess understanding in the moment and over time (Childress & Harper, 2015).
- Confirm the program has ways for students to share feedback, reflect, and process activities (Childress & Harper, 2015).
- Look for an integration of closing and reflection activities as well as transitions between lessons (Childress & Harper, 2015).
- Check out program developers. Make sure the program has been developed and reviewed by experienced yoga teachers who know yoga, child development, and how schools work (Childress & Harper, 2015).
- Consider the associated costs of the training and support that is provided after the training.
- Check if there are certifications or continuing education credits offered with the training.
- Look over the research base provided by the authors.

Finally, Childress and Harper (2015) have identified key aspects of a quality yoga curriculum and best practices for yoga in the school in their text, *Best Practices for Yoga in the Schools* (Childress & Harper, 2015; see pp. 24–25 for a quality curriculum). Created by members of the Yoga Service Council and written by contributors across the field of school-based and children's yoga, this is a valuable resource that complements any program or training you choose and will help you choose the right one.

YOGA PROGRAMS FOR SCHOOLS

To provide a general scope of what is available, we can refer to the 2015 survey completed by Butzer et al. Their team looked at school-based yoga programs across the United States. Butzer et al. (2015) queried organizations that offered school-based yoga programs, gathering information on grade level, type of program (e.g., in class, independent class), primary geographical region, number of formally trained instructors, existence of a requirement for basic yoga-teacher certification prior to receipt of training in the program, number of hours of training required, number of schools implementing the program, and number of years that the program has been in service (p. 4). The team identified 36 programs that offered yoga in more than 940 schools. They found that 5,400 instructors had been trained by these programs to offer yoga in educational settings. The training requirements varied substantially across programs. Of the programs, 42% (*n* = 15) of the organizations reported that a basic 200-hour, registered yoga teacher certification by Yoga Alliance is required prior to attending their specialized training (registered yoga teacher [RYT]; Butzer et al., 2015). Some programs offer training for yoga teachers who want to learn how to teach yoga in schools (Butzer et al., 2015). Other programs specifically train classroom teachers, physical education teachers, school mental health professionals, and other school personnel. Trainings range from 200-hour certification to a 1-day in-service for schools. Researchers noted that despite variations across programs in training requirements, locations, services, and grades covered, they shared the common goal of each of the four basic elements of yoga: (a) physical postures, (b) breathing exercises, (c) relaxation, and (d) meditation (Butzer et al., 2015). For the complete review see Butzer et al. (2015) "School-based yoga programs in the United States: A survey."

The take away? The field of school-based yoga is substantial and active across the United States. As with the field of research on school-based yoga, the field of formal programs and trainings also appears to be growing. Just as with research, there is a wide range of quality and complexity across programs. Accordingly, school personnel must be mindful in their choosing. In the following section, I briefly review Yoga 4 Classrooms®, Yoga in Schools, Little Flower Yoga, and Girls Growing in Wellness and Balance: Life Skills, and Yoga to Empower. These programs are detailed to highlight aspects of each program and illustrate various formats. Next, a table of additional programs for which we could retrieve sufficient information is provided (see Table 13.1).

Yoga 4 Classrooms®

Yoga 4 Classrooms is a good example of a high quality, low cost, accessible program for schools. Yoga 4 Classrooms was developed by Lisa Flynn (2013), author of *Yoga for Children: 200+ Yoga Poses, Breathing Exercises, and Meditations for Healthier, Happier, More Resilient Children*; founder and director of Childlight Yoga®; and contributor to *Best Practices for Yoga in Schools* (Childress & Harper, 2015). The program has an extensive informative web page at www.yoga4classrooms.com. This kindergarten through grade 12 program is described as low cost, simple, effective, and sustainable. According to the information provided, the curriculum focuses on physical, social, emotional, and attentional self-regulating strategies and skills. This includes 67 yoga and mindfulness-based activities that are divided into six categories: Let's Breathe, At Your Desk, Stand Strong, Loosen Up, Imagination Vacation, and Be Well (see www.yoga4classrooms.com). Each activity is illustrated and includes discussion points, sub-activities, and ways to tie in the educational curriculum. The program provides a blend of yoga postures, breathing exercises, visualizations, mindfulness activities, creative movement, and community building games. Intentionally, the activities were designed to not overly rely on yoga poses and stretching in order to be more suitable for the classroom space. Many activities can be done standing beside or sitting at desks (www .yoga4classrooms.com). The psycho-educational content is based on wellness, positive psychology, nutrition, and meditation principles.

Trainings include an in-service professional development workshop, which is a 6-hour interactive workshop held on-site for educators/school professionals, a program manual download, a note-taking guide download, and a certificate of completion (www .yoga4classrooms.com). There is also leader training that includes 3-1/2 days of education, support, planning, and teamwork. There is also a residency program that typically follows the in-service professional development workshop for the school staff. According to the web page, the residency training consists of 10 or 18 in-classroom lessons of 30 minutes each (i.e., 5 lessons of 45 minutes for middle school/high school). There is also a parent education component. According to the program information, there are short- and long-term consulting options and multiple trainers throughout the states (www.yoga4classrooms.com). There is also additional training for those who wish to be consultants. Consultants partner with Yoga 4 Classrooms and have a background working in the school setting as well as experience presenting training or consulting. According to the program information, consultants must have attended, at minimum, the Childlight Yoga's basic training (www.childlightyoga .com/basic-level-training), the Yoga 4 Classrooms' 1-day workshop for educators, and the Yoga 4 Classrooms' IMPLEMENT Leader Training, and have extensive experience using, sharing, and growing the Yoga 4 Classrooms program at their school.

The Yoga 4 Classrooms program is comprehensive and well organized. The web page is easy to navigate and provides a base of research support for the rationale, a section on alignment with educational standards, and transparency in the organization sharing information about the of board of directors, trainers, and founder. Fees are clear and accompanying materials are detailed. Yoga 4 Classrooms founder Lisa Flynn (2013) also authored a wonderful set of cards, "Yoga 4 Classrooms Activity Card Deck," filled with activities for the classroom. The deck is very affordable, colorfully illustrated, organized into activity categories, and easy to use. Yoga 4 Schools has collaborated with researchers at University of Massachusetts–Lowell and Brigham and Women's Hospital Medical School to conduct a study of effectiveness. The study found that second graders showed improvement in social interactions with classmates, attention space, ability to concentrate on work, ability to stay on task, academic performance, ability to deal with stress, confidence, self-esteem, and overall mood (Butzer et al., 2015). Third graders showed improvement in creativity, ability to control behaviors, and anger management. Interestingly, the second graders, not the third graders, showed a decrease in salivary cortical concentration, a potential biological marker for stress, from the beginning to end of the Yoga 4 Classrooms intervention (Butzer et al., 2015). Note that the study was small (18 second and 18 third graders) and was not controlled or randomized. Without a control group, it is difficult to determine if results are based solely on the yoga intervention or if they are related to other factors (Butzer et al., 2015).

Yoga in Schools

Yoga in Schools (YIS) is an example of a yoga program created from the perspective of a clinical social worker. YIS was founded in 2004 by Joanne Spence, a clinical social worker, Experienced Registered Yoga Teacher (ERYT), and yoga studio owner (see www.yogainschools.org). She also serves as an advisor to the yoga recreation program at Shuman Juvenile Detention Center and provides yoga therapy to the patients at Western Psychiatric Institute and Clinic. Specifically, YIS is a 501(c) (3) organization that provides yoga programming and teacher training to several school districts in Pittsburgh, Pennsylvania. The program offers mind-body tools for teaching including easy yoga-based exercises to help manage stress; simple and effective classroom management techniques to help with focus, concentration, behavior, and readiness to learn; and brief classroom activities (see www.yogainschools.org). The mind-body tools include yoga breathing, games/activities, yoga-like poses and movements, and time-in (i.e., rest, relaxation, inner listening, and reflection; see www.yogainschools.org).

The program information indicates that, to date, YIS has exposed nearly 20,000 children and 1,000 teachers/staff members to varying levels of yoga programming (see www.yogainschools.org). The program has an extensive web page that details the program's vision, trainings, events, programs, projects, and resources. There is a section that provides research references that support mind-body tools for learning; mindfulness in education research highlights; and evidence for mindfulness programs' effectiveness with school staff.

The program has been evaluated informally as a white paper/program evaluation (see www.yogainschools.org/files/7714/2069/0586/YIS_White_Paper; see also Spence & Hyde, 2013). Using a qualitative design, Andrea Hyde and Joanne Spence queried participants of a YIS professional development program for Health and Physical Education teachers ($n = 74$). They found that program participants experienced both (a) positive personal change and (b) improvement in their professional practice as a result of participating in the yoga training program. Further, participants reported that yoga was a fun way for students to learn about their bodies and the benefits of physical activity and to gain self-control. Teachers saw students gain flexibility, strength, and balance; learn how to relax and calm themselves; and learn how to de-escalate during stress and aggressions. Participants reported that yoga met at least one academic standard, while some teachers reported more. For more about YIS see www.yogainscools.org and Spence and Hyde (2013).

Little Flower Yoga

Little Flower Yoga (LFY) provides a nice illustration of a yoga program that was built from the experiences of a school-based educator drawn to bring yoga into her classroom. Jennifer Cohen Harper, MA, E-RCYT, an educator and yoga teacher, is the founder of LFY. She is also coauthor of *Little Flower Yoga for Kids: A Yoga and Mindfulness Program to Help Your Child Improve Attention and Emotional Balance* (Harper, 2013) and co-author of *Best Practices for Yoga in Schools* (Childress & Harper, 2013). Harper created the LFY program after successful use of yoga in her kindergarten classroom, which ultimately led to requests from other students, teachers, and administrators for their own yoga programs (see www.littlefloweryoga.com).

Affiliated with LFY, the School Yoga Project offers a school-based program delivering yoga and mindfulness practices to students (see www.littlefloweryoga.com/programs/

the-school-yoga-project). According to program information, the School Yoga Project curriculum incorporates learning goals throughout each yoga class as well as teaches instructors how to capitalize on the teachable moments that occur during yoga sessions. The School Yoga Project integrates five elements: connect (i.e., to self, the world around you, and the community), breathe, move, focus, and relax. Yoga classes are 45 minutes in length with 30- to 60-minute options for mat-based classes and a 15-minute option for desk-based classes. The program offers a full 30-week program or a shorter modified curriculum to adapt to school needs and schedules. They also report the ability to modify the curriculum for students with special needs. For more information see their extensive web page for both LFY and the School Yoga Project.

Schools in the New York City area can contract with the School Yoga Project as they are an approved NYC Department of Education vendor. According to program reports, the School Yoga Project currently serves over 3,500 children per week with in-school and after-school yoga classes (see www.littlefloweryoga.com). Additionally, LFY offers a comprehensive, yoga-alliance accredited teacher-training program. The program is a three-level program with each level of training taught as a 2-day intensive or as a 7-day intensive in the summer. Harper also authored a yoga card deck, *Yoga and Mindfulness for Children Card Deck* (www .littlefloweryoga.com/books/yoga-and-mindfulness-for-children-card-deck). The deck corresponds to the five elements of the School Yoga Project (i.e., connect, breathe, move, focus, relax). Although Harper (2013) has cited research to support the use of yoga in schools, there is no published research evaluating her program specifically. In May of 2009, LFY became a founding member of the Yoga Service Council, a nonprofit organization whose mission is to develop a community of professional support in the field of yoga service (see www .littleflower.com).

Girls Growing in Wellness and Balance: Yoga and Life Skills to Empower

The *Girls Growing in Wellness and Balance: Yoga and Life Skills to Empower* (Cook-Cottone, Kane, Keddie, & Haugli, 2013) program is the first eating disorder prevention program to use yoga as the central feature of the intervention (Cook-Cottone, 2015). It is a good example of a disorder-specific, yoga-based prevention program for schools. The protocol is experiential and didactic in nature and includes constructivistic activities in which the participants create their own understanding of concepts such as assertiveness, cultural and media pressures to be thin, and intrapersonal self-regulation. Based on the Attuned Representational Model of Self (ARMS; Cook-Cottone, 2006), the program teaches self-regulations skills such as breath work and yoga asana, integration of thoughts and feelings to make choices, and self-care. Each session begins with an asana practice, includes journaling, and transitions into group sessions that explore key conceptual issues. The 14-session program concludes with the participants creating their own magazine that reflects their personal values of self-development. Each session runs 90 to 120 minutes and ends with guided relaxation or meditation (Cook-Cottone et al., 2013). The program follows body positive guidelines (see Childress & Harper, 2015, pp. 26–27).

Studies of this program show reduction in eating disorder risk and eating disorder symptoms (Scime & Cook-Cottone, 2008; Scime, Cook-Cottone, Kane, & Watson, 2006). Matched controlled analysis shows that the program was equally effective for girls identified as minorities and those who were not (Cook-Cottone, Jones, & Haugli, 2010). Further, a recent study found that the group format may be most effective with girls who are more externally oriented (Norman, Sodano, & Cook-Cottone, 2014). This program was designed for middle school females, but the manual provides adaptation and extension for high school females and adults. Methodical issues include lack of randomization and lower dosage of yoga (i.e., once per week, 45-minute session, for 12 to 14 weeks; Cook-Cottone, 2015).

AN OVERVIEW OF SCHOOL-BASED YOGA PROGRAMS

Based on the search conducted by my team and Butzer and colleagues' (2015) survey, Table 13.1 provides a brief overview of additional school-based yoga programs. Note that if a program's web page or available materials did not provide adequate descriptive data clarifying the program or its services, it was not included. Program names, web pages, and brief descriptions are provided. This is not intended to be a ranking or evaluative survey; the programs are listed in alphabetical order. The purpose is to give you a broad view of the wide variety of programs available. Please go to the program's web page and research the programs in which you are interested. Note that some of the web pages are extensive, providing information on research, administration, training programs, and services offered in a very clear and user-friendly manner. Other web pages are difficult to navigate and lack information and details. The quality of the web page may not reflect the quality of the program. Use the guidance given previously (i.e., yoga program features to consider) and your own research to select your program and training.

TABLE 13.1 Additional Yoga Programs for Schools and Youth

PROGRAM	WEBPAGE	BRIEF DESCRIPTION
Bent on Learning	bentonlearning.org	Bent on Learning is a non-profit organization committed to teaching yoga to New York City public school students. The program was created by yoga teachers who began volunteering to offer classes in schools. They have now taught 18,000 youth. The program collaborates with physical education teachers, school mental health professionals, and administrators to offer yoga to grades K–12 as a gym class, elective, or after-school activity. The program provides yoga, offers training to school teachers, provides age-appropriate guidance to students for home practice, and raises funds for programs. The program cites yoga research and describes the benefits of yoga in schools. Their slogan is, "Where inner city kids find inner peace."
Calming Kids Yoga	calmingkidsyoga .org	Calming Kids Yoga: Creating a Non-Violent World is a non-profit organization committed to reducing bullying and violence in schools, helping students develop coping mechanisms, and increasing students' concentration via provision of yoga education. Yoga is offered in class and as a full yoga session for students in pre-K to grade 12. It offers e-books, online trainings, and a multi-part teacher certification program with curriculum addressing different age groups.

(continued)

TABLE 13.1 Additional Yoga Programs for Schools and Youth (*continued*)

PROGRAM	WEBPAGE	BRIEF DESCRIPTION
Circus Yoga	circusyoga.com	Circus Yoga is designed to connect and empower communities through creative expression, embodied play, and what they call co-authored culture. Although their training is broader, they offer a school residence (i.e., Circus Yoga In-School Residency) for grades K–12, for 2 weeks in which the teacher teaches 6 classes per day and ends with a co-authored show that students provide for their classmates and the community. Circus Yoga also offers programs for therapeutic environments.
Get Ready to Learn	getreadytolearn .net	The Get Ready to Learn program provides pre-K to grade 12 classroom yoga curricula designed to prepare students of all abilities for learning. Developed by occupational therapist Anne Buckley-Reen, OTR-L, RYT, the curriculum uses a series of traditional yoga sequences that incorporate developmental and sensory-motor features. The program is aligned with Response to Intervention (RtI), Positive Behavioral Interventions and Supports (PBIS), and therapeutic classroom goals. Workshops, teacher trainings, and staff trainings are offered. The program also sells *The Kid's Yoga Deck: 50 Poses and Games* by Anne Buckley. Research on the program includes Koenig, Buckley-Reen, and Garg (2012) and Garg et al. (2013).
Go Grounded	gogrounded.com	Go Grounded kids yoga teaches students pre-K to grade 12 grade how to manage their bodies through the alignment of actions and observation of reactions and tendencies without judgment. The teacher-training program begins with coursework to ground the instructor, and offers choices to focus on preschool age children, children with social needs, or yoga in schools. They also offer schools in-service and training programs as well as consultation, online mentoring, and yoga classes provided by Go Grounded's teachers.
Headstand	heasdstand.org	Headstand is a non-profit organization that works to combat stress among disadvantaged K–12 students through mindfulness, yoga, and character education. The curriculum is an in-classroom program that runs for 40 weeks. It is standards-based and classes are integrated into the school curriculum. The program was founded by a public school teacher, Katherine Proire. School programing, teacher training, and consultation are offered.

(continued)

TABLE 13.1 Additional Yoga Programs for Schools and Youth (*continued*)

Program	Webpage	Brief Description
Holistic Life Foundation	hlfinc.org	The Holistic Life Foundation is a non-profit organization committed to nurturing the wellness of children and adults in underserved communities. Founded by Ali and Atman Smith and Andres Gonzalez, the program offers an after-school program called Holistic Me, which teaches students yoga, mindfulness, meditation, centering, and breath work. They offer a Mindful Moment program of 15-minute breath work and meditation recordings at the high school level. They offer a youth and yoga mindfulness training through the Omega Institute. Other programs include a workforce program, mentoring, stress reduction and mindfulness program, environmental programs, and programs that address mental illness and drug treatment. There are opportunities for interns and volunteers. Research on the program includes Ancona and Mendelson (2014); Mendelson et al. (2013); and Mendelson et al. (2010).
Integral Yoga Institute: Yoga at School	iyiny.org	The Integral Yoga Institute: Yoga at School program offers grades K to12 yoga classes that range from 45 to 60 minutes and include yoga poses, breathing, relaxation, and meditation. They offer classes for students as well as teachers, staff, and parents. Integral Yoga will customize a program for your school and help schools look for funding and sponsorships.
Karma Kids Yoga	karmakidsyoga .com	Karma Kids Yoga offers children's yoga teacher training for educators. The course is designed for early childhood educators as well as elementary and secondary school teachers who are looking to integrate yoga techniques in their classes. They offer professional development, an educator's manual, certificate of course completion, and opportunities to Skype the course.
Kripalu Yoga in Schools	kripalu.org/ kyis-teacher -training	Kripalu Yoga in Schools is a yoga teacher training program. According to the web page, this training provides a scientifically validated yoga curriculum appropriate for high school physical education and health classes, or extracurricular settings. Further, the program offers practical guidance on how to effectively partner with high schools, non-profits, and after-school programs serving teens. Teacher trainees are given tips and resources to create professional development workshops for educators. The program is delivered with developmentally appropriate lesson plans, outlining the introduction of postures; centering, breathing, and relaxation techniques; and key yoga concepts. Specifics are offered for working with teens, appropriate verbal communication methods for schools and youth, and opportunities for practice teaching. There have been several studies of this program including: Conboy, Noggle, Frey, Kudesia, and Khalsa (2013); Felver, Butzer, Olson, Smith, and Khalsa (2015); Haden et al. (2014); Noggle, Steiner, Minami, and Khalsa (2012).

(continued)

TABLE 13.1 Additional Yoga Programs for Schools and Youth (*continued*)

PROGRAM	WEBPAGE	BRIEF DESCRIPTION
Lineage Project	lineageproject.org	The Lineage Project offers mindfulness practices for youth at risk (grades 6 to 12). Founded by Soren Gordhamer, the program utilizes yoga and meditation techniques with disenfranchised youth in New York City to help break the cycle of poverty, violence, and incarceration. They offer programs in detention centers, alternative-to-incarceration programs, alternative schools, subsidized housing, and other community sites. Workshops and trainings are offered. The teacher training is a 20-hour program that prepares teachers to use mindfulness and yoga techniques in their communities and schools.
Mindful Practices Yoga	mindful practicesyoga.com	Mindful Practices offers mindfulness and yoga programming for school districts. The program includes professional development workshops as well as toolkits for teachers. The programs can be modified for special education. The founder, Carla Tantillo Philibert, has a background in education, presents nationally and internationally, and has written three books, *Cooling Down Your Classroom*, *Everyday SEL in Elementary School*, and *Everyday SEL for Middle School* (Philibert, 2016a; Philibert, 2016b; Tantillo, 2012). There are also large, laminated pose cards for sale to assist with classroom yoga activities.
Move-into-Learning Program	m.youtube .com/watch?v= aukqfWGYeoA	Provides eight, weekly, 45-minute sessions of yoga, meditation, and breathing exercises set to music along with opportunities for self-expression through writing and visual arts. Focus is on children's hyperactive behavior, with a reported resultant decrease in symptoms of attention-deficit/hyperactivity disorder (ADHD) and inattentiveness according to teacher observations.
Movement and Mindfulness	move-with-me .com/shop/ movement -mindfulness -curriculum/	The program integrates stories, exercise, and self-regulation to build fitness, focus, and learning readiness. The curriculum includes lesson plans for 30 weeks with over 200 movement and mindfulness building activities (stories, cooperative games, mindfulness activities, and music). It also includes nine yoga/movement video classes, 16 skill flash cards, a poster, and three CDs. The program is for kindergarten and first grade.

(*continued*)

TABLE 13.1 Additional Yoga Programs for Schools and Youth (*continued*)

PROGRAM	WEBPAGE	BRIEF DESCRIPTION
Next Generation Yoga	nextgenerationyoga .com	Next Generation Yoga encourages children to use their whole bodies, minds, and intuitive senses as they learn through embodied practice. Founded by Jodi Komitor, MA, E-RYT 500, RCYT, a special educator with a master's degree in learning disabilities from Teachers College, Columbia University, the program uses an interdisciplinary approach that integrates ideals of traditional yoga with creativity and fun. This includes playful yoga poses, animated breathing exercises, and relaxation techniques along with the use of books, props, and sensory elements. The program offers free lesson plans, for-purchase lesson plan books, props, music, and more in its shop. The teacher training for school-based educators is an RCYS through Yoga Alliance program.
Niroga	www.niroga.org/ education/school/	The Niroga Institute is a non-profit organization that offers mindful yoga to individuals, families, and communities. Founder and Executive Director Bidyut Bose received the Jefferson Award for Public Service. Programs serve up to 2,000 students per week in public schools, alternative schools, juvenile court placements, and drug and alcohol rehab placements. The program offers 15-minute transformative life skills in-class sessions, 30–70 minute dynamic mindfulness classes, after school enrichment classes, and transformative peer leadership class during academic school time. The program is designed for underserved schools. Programs are described as trauma-informed and integrate mindful yoga, breathing techniques, and meditation. For more on the program see Bose (2013) and Frank (2012).
Om Schooled	om-schooled.com	Om Schooled trains yoga teachers, classroom educators, and others to teach age-appropriate yoga to grades K to 5 with classes that align with state and physical education standards. Om Schooled teacher trainings were developed by Sarah Herrington after years of developing, managing, and teaching yoga classes in New York City public, private, and charter schools. Training can be completed in person or online. Herrington wrote the book, *Om Schooled: A Guide to Teaching Kids Yoga in Real-World Schools* (2012).
School, Inc.	school-yoga.org	School, Inc. is an acronym for Smiling Calm Hearts Open Our Learning, Inc. It brings social and emotional learning programs rooted in heart-centered mindful movement to underserved public schools by providing professional development for public school teachers and classes for children. Founded by Kelly Wood, E-EYT200, RCYT, RPYT, it offers training for school personnel in mindfulness techniques of storytelling, simple coordinated movement, and calm breathing. The program meets Common Core and California Health and PE Standards.

(*continued*)

TABLE 13.1 Additional Yoga Programs for Schools and Youth (*continued*)

PROGRAM	WEBPAGE	BRIEF DESCRIPTION
The Connection Coalition	theconnection coaltion.org	The Connection Coalition (CoCo) is a non-profit organization, formerly known as Yoga Gangsters, that works in collaboration with youth organizations to provide access to tools that help calm the nervous system and aid in better decision making (i.e., yoga, mindfulness, and meditation). Founded by Terri Cooper, CoCo offers programs in schools, shelters, jails, foster homes, rehabilitation centers, and more (grades K–12). The program offers a weekend certification yoga teacher training in trauma-informed outreach that covers trauma, speaking authentically, sequencing, lesson plans, and practice teaching, as well as issues of privilege and access.
The Newark Yoga Movement	www.newarkyoga movement.org	The Newark Yoga Movement is a non-profit, founded by Debby Kaminsky, committed to bringing life skills to students through the practice of yoga, breathing, and centering at their schools. Servicing grades pre-K to 12, yoga is offered to students at least two times per month. The program integrates into the school schedule with certified yoga teachers and volunteers using yoga to enhance required curriculum. The program also provides continued education, professional development, and teacher support, and utilizes community outreach.
The Sean O'Shea Foundation	seanoshea foundation.org	The Sean O'Shea Foundation supports San Diego and Los Angeles youth (ages 8 to 18) to develop skills that support them to take responsibility for their lives, develop respect for themselves and others, and have confidence in their own potential. They offer CALM (i.e., chair-based activities for learning mindfulness) kids training for school teachers and professionals working with children, yoga for athletes, and a yoga and nutrition program for schools with at-risk students, programs for pregnant teens and teen parents, and yoga and meditation for kids with cancer and their families.
The Sonima Foundation	sonimafoundation .org	The Sonima Foundation, now called Pure Edge: Success Through Focus, trains local educators to teach the Sonima Health and Wellness Curriculum in public schools. It works in partnership with school districts, academic research institutions, and government entities to help develop policies that make health and wellness an essential component of the educational system. They actively support research in the assessment, measurement, and documentation of the benefits of their program. The program includes yoga-based exercises, mindfulness practice, and nutrition education. Research includes Hagins and Rundle (2016) and Wang and Hagins (2016).

(continued)

TABLE 13.1 Additional Yoga Programs for Schools and Youth (*continued*)

PROGRAM	WEBPAGE	BRIEF DESCRIPTION
Yoga Calm	yogacalm.org	Yoga Calm provides yoga teacher training for grades pre-K to 12 through a youth instructor certification program, adult certification program, and yoga for seniors instructor certificate. Founded by Lynea Gillen, MS, RYT, it also offers therapeutic workshops. Yoga Calm has partnered with institutions to provide graduate credits, clock hours, and CEUs. Some courses and certifications are offered online. The program sells Mindful Moments Cards to encourage self-reflection as well as other resources. The founders authored *Yoga Calm for Children: Educating Heart, Mind, and Body* (Gillen & Gillen, 2007). Research specific to the program includes Thomas (2014).
Yoga Child	yogachild.net	Yoga Child is a grades pre-K to 12 yoga teacher training program and yoga provider. Developed by Gail Silver, RCYT, E-RYT, JD (a former Child Advocate attorney), the program offers training in both mindfulness and yoga. Yoga Child provides in-school classes for students and on-site trainings for staff. The founder is author of the children's books, *Anh's Anger* (Silver, 2009), *Steps and Stones* (Silver, 2007), and *Peace, Bugs, and Understanding* (Silver, 2014).
YOGA ed.	yogaed.com	YOGA ed. offers trainings for teaching yoga to grades pre-K to high school (and universities). Their extensive web page links to training programs, resources (for professionals, parents, homeschools, non-profits), videos, a link to a research white paper on the benefits of yoga, and more. There are professional development workshops, specialized trainings (e.g., trauma-sensitive training), and online courses. The program was studied by Khalsa, Hickey-Schultz, Cohen, Steiner, and Cope (2012). Researchers randomly assigned adolescents to YOGA ed. or physical education over 11 weeks. Students showed improvements in anger control and fatigue/ inertia.
Yoga Foster	www.yogafoster .org	Founded by Nicole Cardoza, Yoga Foster is a nonprofit organization that empowers school teachers with yoga and mindfulness techniques for the classroom. Training is provided free of charge to teachers at underserved schools. Yoga Foster provides online training, curriculum, and resources.
Yoga Enriching Schools	yogainschool.org	Yoga Enriching Schools teaches the techniques and tools of yoga in the public school system (grades K to 12). The program is based on Kundalini Yoga and offers yoga as an elective, physical education, and/or after-school program.

(*continued*)

TABLE 13.1 Additional Yoga Programs for Schools and Youth (*continued*)

PROGRAM	WEBPAGE	BRIEF DESCRIPTION
YOGA for Youth	yogaforyouth.org	The YOGA for Youth mission is to provide urban youth (grades 1 to 12) with tools of self-discovery in order to foster hope, discipline, and respect for self, others, and community. The program trains instructors and matches them with facilities, trains teachers to work with youth to apply yoga techniques, funds research studies on yoga, and provides teaching tools for YOGA for Youth teachers and students.
Yoga in My School	yogainmyschool .com	Yoga in My School offers teacher trainings (and a certification), books, classes, and programs for all ages; provides manuals; offers webinars and training videos; and sells lessons plans and provides resources for teachers. It offers training for working with children with special needs, young children, and teens. Founder Donna Freeman (2009) authored a book, *Once Upon a Pose: Doing Yoga With Your Kids Has Never Been Easier.*
YoKid	yokid.org	YoKid teaches yoga and mindfulness to children and youth to support enhanced outcomes for life, health, school, and leadership. Founded by Ellie Burke, MEd, E-RYT 500, and Michelle Kelsey Mitchell, MS, RYT 500, YoKid offers yoga classes for students grades pre-K to 12, as well as the YoKid 20-hour basic kids yoga training, YoKid workshops (e.g., teaching mindfulness to kids and teaching yoga to at-risk kids, pre-K kids, and kids who have experienced trauma), and a 95-hour kid and teen yoga training certification. The YoKid web page offers an extensive set of resources and tools. YoKid hosts the National Kids Yoga Conference (conference.yokids.org).
YogaKids International	yogakids.com/ classroom-yoga/	YogaKids International, Inc., was founded in 1991 by Marsha Wenig. The organization's mission is promotion of peace, health, empowerment, and education. It sells products, offers training, and has a non-profit arm called Go Give Yoga. The organization supports yoga in schools via its Tools for Schools Program. The Tools for Schools Program is designed for ages 5 to 12 and focuses on the whole child by integrating yoga into the classroom. It sells a YogaKids Toolbox that highlights poses, activities, games, breathing, and visualization techniques. A 3-hour teacher training shows school staff how to use the toolbox tools.
Yogis in Service	www .yogisinservice .org	Yogis in Service (YIS®) is a not-for-profit with a mission to provide access to yoga and yoga's tools for stress management YIS provides training for school personnel in trauma-informed yoga provision in schools organized around the 10 principles for growth (see web page). The trauma-informed program is currently being implemented in the city of Buffalo, New York, and is studied in Somalia and Kenya.
108 Monkeys	108monkeys.org	108 Monkeys is a non-profit that offers yoga as an act of social justice as well as a 100-hour yoga service teacher training. It partners with schools, after-school programs, child care centers, mental health clinics, and more.

CEU, continuing education unit; RCYS, registered children's yoga school.

CAUTIONS AND CONTRAINDICATIONS

School administrators, teachers, and parents want to be sure that anything that students do in school is safe. Is yoga safe? The short answer is, "Yes." Overall, researchers say that yoga is safe. In research, we refer to "safe" as being "no more than minimal risk." What does that mean? It means that the probability of physical or psychological harm is no greater than the ordinary encounters a student experiences in daily life. Concerns about yoga and safety peaked in 2012 in response to a *New York Times* piece by William Board, "How yoga can wreck your body." Researchers decided to look into this.

To explore the question, "Is yoga safe?," Cramer et al. (2015) systematically assessed and meta-analyzed the frequency of adverse events in randomized controlled trials of yoga. The researchers identified 301 randomized controlled trials of yoga (1975–2014; a total of 8,430 participants). Of those, 94 reported adverse events (Cramer et al., 2015). Adverse events were coded as serious if they were life-threatening, disabling, or requiring intensive treatment (Cramer et al., 2015). All other adverse events were coded as non-serious. The researchers determined that no differences in the frequency of intervention-related non-serious or serious adverse events and of dropouts due to adverse events were found when comparing yoga with usual care or exercise (Cramer et al., 2015). That is, yoga is no more dangerous than typical exercise. However, when compared with psychological or educational interventions (e.g., health education), more intervention-related adverse events and more non-serious adverse events occurred in the yoga group; serious adverse events and dropouts due to adverse events were comparable between groups. That is, their results indicate that yoga is more risky than deskwork, but not exercise. Overall, the researchers concluded that the findings from their review indicated that yoga appears as safe as usual-care and exercise (Cramer et al., 2015). The authors added that the adequate reporting of safety data in future randomized trials of yoga is crucial to conclusively judge its safety (Cramer et al., 2015). Here are a few tips to considered in regard to safety.

- Be sure the students are physically ready. Cohen and Schouten (2007) recommend requiring a full physical exam prior to the practice of any mind-body practice. School practice should suffice as students are required to have a medical exam on file each year, which clears them for physical education.
- Childress and Harper (2015) note the importance of developmental appropriateness of instruction including physical status and psycho-social functioning. Be sure to engage in developmentally appropriate activities. If you are not sure, check with your school physical therapist, occupational therapist, school nurse, or school mental health professional.
- Teach students about the difference between pain from working hard and pain that indicates injury.
- *Do not do headstands, shoulder stands, or other poses that pose a risk to the developing body.* For safety, Childress and Harper (2015) ask that you avoid poses that require extensive strength and body awareness.
- Teach poses that help students develop balance and strength without risk of injury (Childress & Harper, 2015).
- Instruct only basic breath work. Advanced breathing exercises may not be safe for younger nervous systems and should be avoided (Childress & Harper, 2015). This includes exercises that require holding the breath (Childress & Harper, 2015). Avoid anything that might lead to lightheadedness, discomfort, or difficulty breathing (Childress & Harper, 2015).

- Childress and Harper (2015) implore that school-based yoga teachers stay up to date on the research so that they are aware of any risks that are identified for particular stages of development for children and youth.
- School-based yoga teachers should only instruct poses they feel very confident teaching (Childress & Harper, 2015).
- School-based yoga teachers should get additional training to work with students with disabilities (Childress & Harper, 2015). Further, partner with school-based professionals such as the physical therapist, occupational therapist, and school mental health professionals in order to deliver a safe yoga program.
- Provide students with alternatives and modifications for poses. Always offer choices.

CONCLUSIONS AND FUTURE DIRECTIONS

Overall, the current state of research in area of yoga in schools is in its early stages. Much more research is needed and continued funding and initiatives from the National Center for Complementary and Alternative Medicine (NCCAM; nccam.nih.gov) are necessary for the field to continue to move forward. Overall, yoga in schools can be informed, and is supported by, the current body of research. As the rate of publications in this area is rapidly increasing, school personnel are encouraged to stay informed. As a field we remain committed to more rigorous research (i.e., randomized controlled trials; Forfylow, 2011; Khalsa & Butzer, 2016; Serwacki & Cook-Cottone, 2012). We acknowledge that other standard quality-of-research issues are not yet addressed including: follow-up assessments; over-reliance on use of self-report measures, with less frequent use of performance measures; a need to expand across ethnicity, age, sex, levels of experience, and ranges of disorder-specific issues in order to provide a sufficient body of evidence that can be generalized to particular groups of individuals; as well as a need for studies with larger sample sizes (Forfylow, 2011; Hallgren et al., 2014; Khalsa & Butzer, 2016; McIver et al., 2009; Serwacki & Cook-Cottone, 2012).

Dosage is a key variable that has not been effectively addressed in mindfulness or yoga research (e.g., Cook-Cottone, 2013, 2015). Strongly considered in other fields (e.g., pharmacology), standardized dosages are essentially missing from mindfulness and yogic research. Specifically, frequency, duration, session length, and content of sessions should be detailed and accounted for (Cook-Cottone, 2013; Cook-Cottone, 2015). Relatedly, few studies measure whether or not the treatment or control group members practice meditation, yoga, or breath work at home or outside of the scope of the study intervention (Cook-Cottone, 2013; Cook-Cottone, 2015). Few studies report a content-specific treatment integrity percentage (e.g., were all the breath-work activities completed during the session? Were all of the prescribed yoga-postures implemented; Cook-Cottone, 2013; Cook-Cottone, 2015). Further, few studies assess engagement in other confounding physical activities as an important potentially confounding variable (Cook-Cottone, 2013; Cook-Cottone, 2015). For example, did the treatment or control participants engage in mindful walking or attend a Tai Kwon Do class? Finally, content of interventions must be better detailed. This is especially salient within the context of yoga interventions. Specifically, the type of yoga, aspect of yoga, and amount of each type and aspect of yoga should be detailed and evaluated for efficacy (Cook-Cottone, 2013; Cook-Cottone, 2015; Forfylow, 2011). There is some evidence that the type of yoga utilized may matter (Delaney & Anthis, 2010). Outside of standardized protocols and manualized methods, how are mindful and yogic approaches being integrated?

As our popular culture embraces alternative approaches such as yoga and mindfulness, many schools across the country are implementing yoga in schools and in the classroom. It is critical for the scientific community to continue to carefully evaluate effectiveness honoring both the scientific method as well as the roots and authenticity of these ancient practices (Cook-Cottone, 2015). There are at least two truths at play. Using tools such as the scientific method is necessary within the current cultural zeitgeist (Cook-Cottone, 2015). However, use of qualitative methods and other tools that allow for practices such as mindfulness and yoga to be explored exactly as they are occurring naturalistically is also critical (Cook-Cottone, 2015). It is a dialectic. Perhaps it is in the simultaneous embracing of tradition and change that we will find the effectiveness we seek (Cook-Cottone, 2015).

There are several resources school personnel are encouraged to use. First, get yourself a copy of *Best Practices for Yoga in Schools* (Childress & Harper, 2015). Next, check out www .garrisoninstitute.org/insights-tools/resources/. This is the Garrison Institute's online resource page designed to provide organizations with the necessary tools, information, and guidance in the implementation of mindful practices. These resources can be sorted by topic and type using the web page search tools.

Next, got to K-12YOGA.org/listings/. This is the K-12YOGA.org website designed to bring the yoga and educational communities together by providing resources for finding a yoga instructor to teach in your school, ways to connect to school personnel who have implemented a yoga program, getting trained to be a yoga teacher, updates on the body of research, and ways to disseminate what you have learned. The K-12YOGA.org web page is committed to being a brand-neutral voice in the promotion of the school yoga-mindfulness movement. The creators and maintainers of the web page contend that their goal is to provide an open platform for communities of interest to connect. Ways to search include a zip code locator, fund raising initiatives, provision of a school-based yoga tool kit, a calendar of events, and job listings.

Last, you are encouraged to attend the YoKid International Yoga Conference (conference .yokid.org), Yoga Service Conference (eomega.org/workshops/yoga-service-conference), and Yoga in the Schools Symposium (kriplau.org) to meet with researchers, yoga providers, yoga teacher trainers, and other school personnel. There are opportunities for continuing education, professional growth, trainings, and connecting with professionals who can help you grow in your effectiveness with students. You will also meet people with whom you can collaborate to make research happen at your school, something that will be of huge service to the field of yoga in the schools. I look forward to meeting you!

REFERENCES

Ancona, M. R., & Mendelson, T. (2014). Feasibility and preliminary outcomes of a yoga and mindfulness intervention for school teachers. *Advances in School Mental Health Promotion, 7*, 156–170.

Anderson, S., & Sovik, R. (2000). *Yoga: Mastering the basics.* Honesdale, PA: Himalayan Institute Press.

Bose, B. K. (2013). A necessary catalyst: Dismantling the school-to-prison pipeline with yoga. *Journal of Yoga Service, 1*, 23–28.

Broad, W. (2012). How yoga can wreck your body. *New York Times Magazine.* Published January 5, 2012.

Butzer, B., Bury, D., Telles, S., & Khalsa, S. B. S. (2016). Implementing yoga within the school curriculum: A scientific rationale for improving social-emotional learning and positive student outcomes. *Journal of Children's Services, 11*, 3–24.

Butzer, B., Day, D., Potts, A., Ryan, C., Coulombe, S., Davies, B., … Khalsa, S. B. S. (2015). Effects of a classroom-based yoga intervention on cortisol and behavior in second- and third-grade students: A pilot study. *Journal of Evidence-Based Complementary & Alternative Medicine, 20*, 41–49.

Butzer, B., Ebert, M., Telles, S., & Khalsa, S. B. S. (2015). School-based yoga programs in the United States: A survey. *Advances in Mind-Body Medicine, 29,* 18.

Cohen, M. H., & Schouten, R. (2007). Legal, regulatory, and ethic issues. In J. Lake & D. Spiegel (Eds.), *Complementary and alternative treatments in mental health care* (pp. 21–33). Arlington, VA: American Psychiatric.

Conboy, L. A., Noggle, J. J., Frey, J. L., Kudesia, R. S., & Khalsa, S. B. S. (2013). Qualitative evaluation of a high school yoga program: Feasibility and perceived benefits. *Explore: The Journal of Science and Healing, 9,* 171–180.

Cook-Cottone, C. (2006). The attuned representation model for the primary prevention of eating disorders: An overview for school psychologists. *Psychology in the Schools, 43,* 223–230.

Cook-Cottone, C. (2013). Dosage as a critical variable in yoga therapy research. *International Journal of Yoga Therapy, 2,* 11–12.

Cook-Cottone, C. P. (2015). *Yoga and mindfulness for self-regulation: A primer for mental health professionals.* New York, NY: Springer Publishing.

Cook-Cottone, C., Jones, L. A., & Haugli, S. (2010). Prevention of eating disorders amongminority youth: A matched-sample repeated measures study. *Eating Disorders, 18,* 361376.

Cook-Cottone, C. P., Kane, L., Keddie, E., & Haugli, S. (2013). *Girls growing in wellness and balance: Yoga and life skills to empower.* Stoddard, WI: Schoolhouse Educational Services, LLC.

Childress, T., & Harper, J. C. (2015). *Best practices for yoga in the schools.* Best Practices Guide Vol. 1. Atlanta, GA: YEC-Omega Publications.

Cramer, H., Ward, L., Saper, R., Fishbein, D., Dobos, G., & Lauche, R. (2015). The safety of yoga: A systematic review and meta-analysis of randomized controlled trials. *American Journal of Epidemiology, 182,* 281–293.

Felver, J. C., Butzer, B., Olson, K. J., Smith, I. M., & Khalsa, S. B. S. (2015). Yoga in public school improves adolescent mood and affect. *Contemporary School Psychology, 19,* 184–192.

Ferreira-Vorkapic, C., Feitoza, J. M., Marchioro, M., Simões, J., Kozasa, E., & Telles, S. (2015). Are there benefits from teaching yoga at schools? A systematic review of randomized control trials of yoga-based interventions. *Evidence-Based Complementary and Alternative Medicine.* doi:10.1155/2015/345835

Flynn, L. (2013). *Yoga for children: 200+ yoga poses, breathing exercises, and meditations for healthier, happier, more resilient children.* Avon, MA: Adams Media.

Forfylow, A. L. (2011). Integrating yoga with psychotherapy: A complementary treatment for anxiety and depression. *Canadian Journal of Counseling and Psychotherapy, 45,* 132–150.

Frank, J. (2012). *Results of TLS evaluation* (Research Report, October 2012). Retrieved from http://www.niroga.org/research/papers.php

Freeman, D. (2009). *Once upon a pose: Doing yoga with your kids has never been easier.* Bloomington, IN: Trafford Publishing.

Garg, S., Buckley-Reen, A., Alexander, L., Chintakrindi, R., Ocampo Tan, L. V. C., & Patten Koenig, K. (2013). The effectiveness of a manualized yoga intervention on classroombehaviors in elementary school children with disabilities: A pilot study. *Journal of Occupational Therapy, Schools, & Early Intervention, 6,* 158–164.

Gillen, L., & Gillen, J. (2007). *Yoga calm for children: Educating heart, mind, and body.* Portland, OR: Three Pebble Press.

Haden, S. C., Daly, L., & Hagins, M. (2014). A randomised controlled trial comparing the impact of yoga and physical education on the emotional and behavioural functioning of middle school children. *Focus on Alternative and Complementary Therapies, 19,* 148–155.

Hagins, M., & Rundle, A. (2016). Yoga improves academic performance in urban high school students compared to physical education: A randomized controlled trial. *Mind, Brain, and Education.* doi:10.1111/mbe.12107

Harper, J. C. (2013). *Little flower yoga for kids: A yoga and mindfulness programs to help your children improve attention and emotional balance.* Oakland, CA: New Harbinger Publications.

Herrington, S. (2012). *Om schooled: a guide to teaching kids yoga in real-world schools.* San Marcos, CA: Addriya.

Khalsa, S. B. S., & Butzer, B. (2016). Yoga in school settings: A research review. *Annals of the New York Academy of Sciences, 1373,* 1–12.

Khanna, S., & Greeson, J. M. (2013). A narrative review of yoga and mindfulness as complimentary therapies. *Complimentary Therapies in Medicine, 21,* 244–252.

Khalsa, S. B. S., Hickey-Schultz, L., Cohen, D., Steiner, N., & Cope, S. (2012). Evaluation of the mental health benefits of yoga in a secondary school: A preliminary randomized controlled trial. *The Journal of Behavioral Health Services & Research, 39,* 80–90.

Klein, J., & Cook-Cottone, C. (2013). The effects of yoga on eating disorder symptoms and correlates: A review. *International Journal of Yoga Therapy, 2,* 41–50.

Koenig, K. P., Buckley-Reen, A., & Garg, S. (2012). Efficacy of the get ready to learn yoga program among children with autism spectrum disorders: A pretest–posttest control group design. *American Journal of Occupational Therapy, 66,* 538–546.

Madden, T. (2015). Journeys of purpose: A review of literature about work and spirituality. *International Journal of Religion & Spirituality in Society, 5,* 69–76.

Mendelson, T., Dariotis, J. K., Feagans Gould, L., Smith, A. S. R., Smith, A. A., Gonzalez, A. A., & Greenberg, M. T. (2013). Implementing mindfulness and yoga in urban schools: A community-academic partnership. *Journal of Children's Services, 8,* 276–291.

Mendelson, T., Greenberg, M. T., Dariotis, J. K., Feagans Gould, L., Rhoades, B. L., & Leaf, P. J. (2010). Feasibility and preliminary outcomes of a school-based mindfulness intervention for urban youth. *Journal of Abnormal Child Psychology, 38,* 985–994.

Noggle, J. J., Steiner, N. J., Minami, T., & Khalsa, S. B. S. (2012). Benefits of yoga for psychosocial well-being in a US high school curriculum: A preliminary randomized controlled trial. *Journal of Developmental & Behavioral Pediatrics, 33,* 193–201.

Norman, K., Sodano, S. M., & Cook-Cottone, C. (2014). An exploratory analysis of the role of interpersonal styles in eating disorder prevention outcomes. *The Journal for Specialists in Group Work, 39,* 301–315.

Philibert, C. T. (2016a). *Everyday SEL in elementary school: Integrating social-emotional learning and mindfulness into your classroom.* New York, NY: Routledge.

Philibert, C. T. (2016b). *Everyday SEL in middle school: Integrating social-emotional learning and mindfulness into your classroom.* New York, NY: Routledge.

Scime, M., & Cook-Cottone, C. (2008). Primary prevention of eating disorders: A constructivist integration of mind and body strategies. *International Journal of Eating Disorders, 41,* 134–142.

Scime, M., Cook-Cottone, C., Kane, L., & Watson, T. (2006). Group prevention of eating disorders with fifth-grade females: Impact on body dissatisfaction, drive for thinness, and media influence. *Eating Disorders, 14,* 143–155.

Serwacki, M., & Cook-Cottone, C. (2012). Yoga in the schools: a systematic review of the literature. *International Journal of Yoga Therapy, 22,* 101–110.

Silver, G. (2007). *Steps and stones.* Berkeley, CA: Plum Blossom Books.

Silver, G. (2009). *Anh's anger.* Berkeley, CA: Plum Blossom Books.

Silver, G. (2014). *Peace, bugs, and understanding.* Berkeley, CA: Plum Blossom Books.

Simpkins, A. M., & Simpkins, C. A. (2011). *Meditation and yoga in psychotherapy: Techniques for clinical practice.* New York, NY: Wiley.

Spence, J., & Hyde, A. (2013). Yoga in schools: Delivering district-wide yoga education. *Journal of Yoga Service, 1,* 53–59.

Tantillo, C. (2012). *Cooling down your classroom: Using yoga, relaxation, and breathing strategies to help students learn to keep their cool.* Chicago, IL: Mindful Practices.

Thomas, E.M. (2014). *Yoga and breathing and relaxation techniques used during the school day and their effects on school-aged children* (Wayne State University Thesis Paper 357). Retrieved from http://digitalcommons.wayne.edu/oa_theses/357

van der Kolk, B. A., Stone, L., West, J., Rhodes. A., Emerson, D., Suvak, M., Spinazzola, J. (2014). Yoga as an adjunctive treatment for posttraumatic stress disorder: A randomized controlled trial. *Journal of Clinical Psychiatry, 75,* e1–e7.

Wang, D., & Hagins, M. (2016). Perceived benefits of yoga among urban school students: A qualitative analysis. *Evidence-Based Complementary and Alternative Medicine, 7.* doi:10.1155/2016/8725654

Woodyard, C. (2011). Exploring the therapeutic effects of yoga and its ability to increase quality of life. *International Journal of Yoga, 4,* 49–54.

PART IV

MINDFUL SELF-CARE FOR STUDENTS AND TEACHERS

CHAPTER 14

MINDFUL SELF-CARE

Because no matter the challenges we confront . . .
There is no escaping this reality,
no matter what others, or we, try to say about it.
If we don't care for ourselves,
we'll be limited in how we can care for others.
It is that simple.
And it is that important—
for you, for others, and for our planet.

Daniel Siegel (*The Mindful Therapist*, 2010, p. 3)

MINDFUL SELF-CARE AND SELF-REGULATION

At their core, mindfulness and yogic approaches are pathways to self-care (Cook-Cottone, 2015; Herrington, 2012; Hyde, 2012; Jennings, 2015). Self-care, as a contemporary practice is defined as the daily process of being aware of and attending to one's basic physiological and emotional needs, including the shaping of one's daily routine, relationships, and environment as needed to promote self-care (Cook-Cottone, 2015; Norcross & Guy, 2007). As well said by Rechtschaffen (2014), "Caring for yourself is always a good idea" (p. 20). Essentially, self-care is the foundation of physical and emotional well-being (Cook-Cottone, 2015). Without self-care, we can become susceptible to exhaustion, emotionally and physically burned out, fatigued, and depleted and unable to give of ourselves (Herrington, 2012; Jennings, 2015; Sutterfield, 2013). Jennings (2015) explains how she knows when she is in need of self-care. It is when her thoughts turn negative, she feels unappreciated, and she notices that she is slipping into guilt trips or blame (Jennings, 2015). The key is to see this for what it is—*you need self-care*—and not believe the burnout stories you are telling yourself. Self-care is associated with positive physical health, emotional well-being, and mental health. Steady and intentional practice of self-care is seen as protective by preventing the onset of mental health symptoms, job/school burnout, and improving work and school productivity (Cook-Cottone, 2015; Figure 14.1).

It is just as important for school personnel and caretakers to engage in self-care as it is for the students (Cook-Cottone, 2015; Harper, 2013; Norcross & Guy, 2007; Sayrs, 2012; Shapiro & Carlson, 2009; Siegel, 2010). Those specializing in the neurobiology of the brain

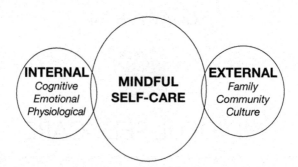

FIGURE 14.1 Mindful self-care.
Source: Cook-Cottone, 2015; used with permission.

and behavior agree. For example, Siegel (2010) emphasizes the significance of attending to the development of your own inner life in order to do your job well. Self-care allows you to bring a healthy and positive presence to your work, in addition to bringing resilience to your life (Cook-Cottone, 2015; Siegel, 2010). I like to think of it this way: Consider that you cannot give what you do not have (Cook-Cottone, 2015). A teacher who presents as overworked, exhausted, depleted, and overly self-sacrificing, even if not articulated, does not inspire. Siegel (2010) says it this way: "Caring for yourself, bringing support and healing to your own efforts to help others and the larger world in which we live, is an essential daily practice—not a luxury, not some form of self-indulgence" (p. 3).

I first developed the self-care scale for use with a yoga-based eating disorder prevention program (Cook-Cottone, Kane, Keddie, & Haugli, 2013a). The initial version of the scale addressed nutrition, hydration, exercise, soothing, rest, and medicines/vitamins. Appropriate for use with children of middle school age and above, the scale assesses self-care behaviors including eating healthy foods in moderation, drinking enough water, exercising at least 1 hour a day and not to excess, engaging in relaxation and rest behaviors throughout the day, and taking medicines prescribed and not taking those that are not (e.g., alcohol). Like the Mindful Self-Care Scale (MSCS), the children's self-care scale allows for an assessment of self-care behaviors across domains.

Self-care practice is self-regulating (see Figure 14.2; Cook-Cottone, Tribole, & Tylka, 2013; Herrington, 2012). Self-care, mindful, and yogic practices can provide a foundation for self-regulation. Self-care is the thing to do now in order to feel better later. Ironically, many people say that they will take better care of themselves and do healthy things such as yoga and mindfulness once they feel better emotionally. Conversely, school personnel and students should engage in self-care, yoga, and mindfulness practices as a foundation for feeling better (Cook-Cottone, 2015; Cook-Cottone et al., 2013b). Emotional regulation is inextricably linked to physiological stability and homeostasis (Cook-Cottone, 2015; Cook-Cottone et al., 2013). Daily self-care practices can enhance physiological stability and support emotional regulation (Cook-Cottone, 2015; Linehan, 1993). You are happier and feel better because you do the self-care work.

To be a self-regulated teacher means you know that you are offering the students the very best version of yourself. Childress and Harper (2015) remind us that being of service in the field of mindfulness and yoga is the intentional sharing of our own practices. This should be done within the context of conscious relationships with others that are supported by ongoing personal reflection and inquiry (Childress & Harper, 2015). Mindful self-care goes

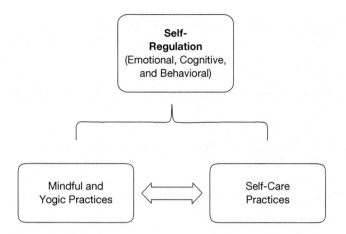

FIGURE 14.2 Self-care and self-regulation
Source: Cook-Cottone, 2015; used with permission.

beyond a basic assessment of and engagement in self-care behaviors. It is the integration of the practice of mindful awareness and self-care. Mindful self-care is the closing aspect of embodied self-regulation designed to help both students and school personnel negotiate personal needs and challenges and external demands (see Figure 14.1 and Chapter 3, Principle of Embodied Growth and Learning 1, Worth: I am worth the effort). Mindful self-care begins with self-awareness and self-monitoring (Cook-Cottone, 2015; Norcross & Guy, 2007).

The Mindful Self-Care Scale–Long (MSCS–L) is an 84-item scale that measures the self-reported frequency of self-care behaviors (Cook-Cottone, 2015). This scale is intended to help individuals identify areas of strength and weakness in self-care behavior, as well as assess interventions that serve to improve self-care. The scale addresses 10 domains of self-care: nutrition/hydration, exercise, soothing strategies, self-awareness/mindfulness, rest, relationships, physical and medical practices, environmental factors, self-compassion, and spiritual practices (see Figure 14.3). There are also three general items assessing the individual's general or more global practices of self-care. Research is currently being conducted on this specific self-care scale to evaluate psychometric properties and association of the scale with self-regulation. See gse.buffalo.edu/about/directory/faculty/cookcottone for a full version of the scale with formatting instructions and updates of research outcomes.

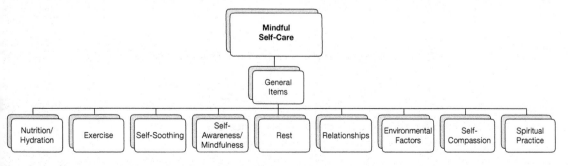

FIGURE 14.3 Domains of mindful self-care.

MINDFUL SELF-CARE: HOW TO USE THIS CHAPTER

The Mindful Self-Care process involves four steps: (a) mindful awareness of self-care as essential to well-being, (b) assessment of self-care domains, (c) assessment-driven self-care goal setting, and (d) engagement in self-care behaviors (see Figure 14.4; Cook-Cottone, 2015). The four steps are discrete phases of an ongoing process, a continuous mindful awareness of one's own self-care behaviors, continual assessment, and goal setting (Cook-Cottone, 2015). Mindful self-care is a process of constant remembering (Cook-Cottone, 2015). It is easy for school personnel, parents, and students to get pulled away from their own self-care by external contingencies and the needs of others (see Figure 14.1; Cook-Cottone, 2015). Accordingly, mindful self-care involves a remembering of the self (Cook-Cottone, 2015).

This chapter is presented domain-by-domain in order to facilitate a mindful and intentional review of personal self-care. Each domain is defined and domain-specific questions follow. Whether you are working with students or exploring your own self-care, work through the chapter one domain at a time. Read the definition and then carefully answer the questions. The directions for scoring accompany each set of questions. Please note that some questions are reversed scored. Once the domain is scored, average the scores across the domain. Note, averages of 0 to 2 in a domain suggest that that area of self-care can be targeted for improvement (Cook-Cottone, 2015). The specific items are prescriptive in nature. For example, if you or your students are not hydrating adequately, the item, "I drank 6 to 8 glasses of water" can be easily translated to a goal, "I will drink 6 to 8 glasses of water each day." Take the test, set the goals, and get your self-care going.

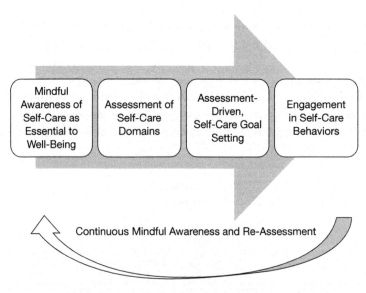

FIGURE 14.4 The mindful self-care process.
Source: Cook-Cottone, 2015; used with permission.

General (G)

The general self-care items were designed to provide a broad sense of variety of self-care strategies utilized, planning of self-care, and creativity and exploration of self-care. Norcross and Guy (2007) warn that there is no single self-care strategy that alone can help you or your students manifest well-being. Further, for some individuals, one beloved hobby or leisure pursuit can be more effective than working to engage in a variety of self-care strategies (Cook-Cottone, 2015; Norcross & Guy, 2007). For my daughter Chloe, a long run, and for my daughter Maya, sitting at the piano and singing, make all the difference. You want to look for a few things that really work, a lot of things that help keep you steady.

TABLE 14.1 Self-Care General Items

Ask yourself, "This past week how many days did I do the following?" You can give yourself the following scores: 0 = *never* (0 days), 1 = *rarely* (1 day), 2 = *sometimes* (2–3 days), 3 = *often* (4–5 days), and 4 = *regularly* (6–7 days). Your score for this section can range from 0 to 15.

- I engaged in a variety of self-care strategies (e.g., mindfulness, support, exercise, nutrition, spiritual practice).
- I planned my self-care.
- I explored new ways to bring self-care into my life.

Nutrition and Hydration

Norcross and Guy (2007) identify nutrition and hydration as critical aspects of self-care. A healthy body responds to the unavoidable stress in life better than an unhealthy body (Davis, Eshelman, & McKay, 2008; Harper, 2013). First, addressing basic nutritional needs can deeply affect self-regulation (Cook-Cottone, 2015). Addressing nutritional needs includes both eating a healthy amount of healthy foods, as well as engaging in the planning needed to make that happen (Cook-Cottone, 2015). Drops in sugar levels, insufficient or excessive energy intake, nutrient deficits (i.e., low iron intake, low vitamin D and B12 levels) have all been identified in variations in mood and sense of well-being and can be dysregulating (Cook-Cottone, 2015). See the *American Dietetic Association Complete Food and Nutrition Guide* (Duyff, 2011) and *The Relaxation and Stress Reduction Workbook*, Sixth Edition (Davis et al., 2008) for nutritional guidelines and tools for enhancing nutrition.

Second, it is well accepted that water is essential for life, and maintaining recommended levels of hydration is critical to healthy functioning (i.e., 1.2 liters per day or about 6–8 glasses; Benelam & Wyness, 2010; Cook-Cottone, 2015). If water losses are not replaced, dehydration occurs (Benelam & Wyness, 2010). At extreme levels, dehydration is very serious and can be fatal. Mild dehydration (i.e., 2% loss of body weight) can result in headaches, fatigue, and reduced physical and mental performance and too much water can result in hyponatremia (low levels of sodium in the blood; Benelam & Wyness, 2010). The items following can give you and your students a sense of basic nutrition and hydration self-care practices.

TABLE 14.2 Self-Care Nutrition/Hydration Items

Ask yourself, "This past week how many days did I do the following?" You can give yourself the following scores: 0 = *never* (0 days), 1 = *rarely* (1 day), 2 = *sometimes* (2–3 days), 3 = *often* (4–5 days), and 4 = *regularly* (6–7 days). For the items that state "reverse score" score as: 4 = *never* (0 days), 3 = *rarely* (1 day), 2 = *sometimes* (2–3 days), 1 = *often* (4–5 days), and 0 = *regularly* (6–7 days). Your score for this section can range from 0 to 28.

- I drank at least six to eight cups of water.
- Even though my stomach felt full enough, I kept eating (reverse score).
- I adjusted my water intake when I needed to (e.g., for exercise, hot weather).
- I skipped a meal (reverse score).
- I ate breakfast, lunch, dinner, and, when needed, snacks.
- I ate a variety of nutritious foods (e.g., vegetables, protein, fruits, and grains).
- I planned my meals and snacks.

Exercise

A review of the literature indicates that the association between exercise and well-being has been well-documented (Cook-Cottone, 2015; Norcross & Guy, 2007). Exercise reduces stress by releasing endorphins into the blood stream, decreasing muscle tension, increasing alpha wave activity, improving strength and flexibility, lessening fatigue, increasing resting metabolism, ridding your body of toxins, improving blood flow to the brain, and reducing risk for those with stress-related medical conditions (Cook-Cottone, 2015; Davis et al., 2008). Further, you learn lessons on your mat, in your running shoes, and at the gym that you can apply to your life (e.g., persistence pays off, my breath is powerful, I can handle this; Cook-Cottone, 2015; Davis et al., 2008). The beneficial effects of regular exercise include improvements on measures of cognition and psychological well-being in healthy individuals (Cook-Cottone, 2015; Hopkins, Davis, VanTieghem, Whalen, & Bucci, 2012). The items following address planning, duration, frequency, and quality of exercise, as well as the amount of sedentary activity present. Assessment can aid in the development of specific physical activity goals.

TABLE 14.3 Self-Care Exercise Items

Ask yourself, "This past week how many days did I do the following?" You can give yourself the following scores: 0 = *never* (0 days), 1 = *rarely* (1 day), 2 = *sometimes* (2–3 days), 3 = *often* (4–5 days), and 4 = *regularly* (6–7 days). For the items that state "reverse score" score as: 4 = *never* (0 days), 3 = *rarely* (1 day), 2 = *sometimes* (2–3 days), 1 = *often* (4–5 days), and 0 = *regularly* (6–7 days). Your score for this section can range from 0 to 28.

- I exercised at least 30 to 60 minutes.
- I took part in sports, dance, or other scheduled physical activities (e.g., sports teams, dance classes).
- I did sedentary activities instead of exercising (e.g., watched TV, worked on the computer) (reverse score).
- I sat for periods of longer than 60 minutes at a time (reverse score).
- I did fun physical activities (e.g., danced, played active games, jumped in leaves).
- I exercised in excess (e.g., when I was tired, sleep deprived, or risking stress/injury) (reverse score).
- I planned/scheduled my exercise for the day.

Self-Soothing

Self-soothing is an effective tool in emotional regulation (Cook-Cottone, 2015; Linehan, 1993). Self-soothing is a positive, healthy response to feeling stressed, distressed, or an intense emotional reaction (Cook-Cottone, 2015). Self-soothing includes relaxation techniques, deep breathing, pursuit of stimuli or activities that are calming and relaxing (Cook-Cottone, 2015). There are many other ways to self-soothe. For example, reading, writing, and cultivating sensory awareness are all effective forms of self-soothing (Cook-Cottone, 2015; Davis et al., 2008; Norcross & Guy, 2007). Students can learn to use self-soothing in response to a trigger and planned as a preventive tool (Cook-Cottone, 2015; Davis et al., 2008; Norcross & Guy, 2007). The items that follow assess a wide range of self-soothing behaviors.

TABLE 14.4 Self-Care Self-Soothing Items

Ask yourself, "This past week how many days did I do the following?" You can give yourself the following scores: 0 = *never* (0 days), 1 = *rarely* (1 day), 2 = *sometimes* (2–3 days), 3 = *often* (4–5 days), and 4 = *regularly* (6–7 days). For the items that state "reverse score" score as: 4 = *never* (0 days), 3 = *rarely* (1 day), 2 = *sometimes* (2–3 days), 1 = *often* (4–5 days), and 0 = *regularly* (6–7 days). Your score for this section can range from 0 to 52.

- I used deep breathing to relax.
- I did *not* know how to relax (reverse score).
- I thought about calming things (e.g., nature, happy memories).
- When I got stressed, I stayed stressed for hours (i.e., I couldn't calm down) (reverse score).
- I did something physical to help me relax (e.g., taking a bath, yoga, going for a walk).
- I did something intellectual (using my mind) to help me relax (e.g., read a book, wrote).
- I did something interpersonal to relax (e.g., connected with friends).
- I did something creative to relax (e.g., drew, played an instrument, wrote creatively, sang, organized).
- I listened to relax (e.g., to music, a podcast, radio show, rainforest sounds).
- I sought out images to relax (e.g., art, film, window shopping, nature).
- I sought out smells to relax (lotions, nature, candles/incense, smells of baking).
- I sought out tactile or touch-based experiences to relax (e.g., petting an animal, cuddling a soft blanket, floated in a pool, put on comfy clothes).
- I prioritized activities that help me relax.

Self-Awareness/Mindfulness

Self-awareness and mindfulness are fundamental and unique features of mindful self-care (Cook-Cottone, 2015). These self-care practices include formal and informal mindful and yogic practices (e.g., mindful awareness, yoga practice, and meditation; Cook-Cottone, 2015). Well reviewed and detailed throughout this text as well as in Cook-Cottone (2015), self-awareness, one-mindedness, and active practices, such as meditation and yoga, are emphasized as they are increasingly acknowledged for their effectiveness as self-care practices (Cook-Cottone, 2015; Linehan, 1993; Norcross & Guy, 2007; Sayrs, 2012; Shapiro & Carlson, 2009).

TABLE 14.5 Self-Care Self-Awareness/Mindfulness Items

Ask yourself, "This past week how many days did I do the following?" You can give yourself the following scores: 0 = *never* (0 days), 1 = *rarely* (1 day), 2 = *sometimes* (2–3 days), 3 = *often* (4–5 days), and 4 = *regularly* (6–7 days). For the items that state "reverse score" score as: 4 = *never* (0 days), 3 = *rarely* (1 day), 2 = *sometimes* (2–3 days), 1 = *often* (4–5 days), and 0 = *regularly* (6–7 days). Your score for this section can range from 0 to 40.

- I had a calm awareness of my thoughts.
- I had a calm awareness of my feelings.
- I had a calm awareness of my body.
- I carefully selected which of my thoughts and feelings I used to guide my actions.
- I meditated in some form (e.g., sitting meditation, walking meditation, prayer).
- I practiced mindful eating (i.e., paid attention to the taste and texture of the food, ate without distraction).
- I practiced yoga or another mind/body practice (e.g., Tae Kwon Do, Tai Chi).
- I tracked/recorded my self-care practices (e.g., journaling, used an app, kept a calendar).
- I planned/scheduled meditation and/or a mindful practice for the day (e.g., yoga, walking meditation, prayer).
- I took time to acknowledge the things for which I am grateful.

Rest

The rest domain of self-care includes getting enough sleep, taking restful breaks, and planning time in your schedule to rest and restore (Cook-Cottone, 2015; Harper, 2013). First, sleep is a critical aspect of self-care for both students and teachers. The National Sleep Foundation recommends 7 to 9 hours of sleep for adults per day (sleepfoundation .org). The National Sleep Foundation's recommendations for children and youth are as follows: preschoolers, between 10 and 13 hours of sleep; school-age children, between 9 and 11 hours; and teenagers, between 8 and 10 hours (Hirshkowitz et al., 2015). Lack of sleep and too much sleep are associated with negative outcomes. Both short and long duration of sleep are predictors, or markers, of cardiovascular outcomes (Cappuccio, Cooper, D'Elia, Strazzullo, & Miller, 2011; Cook-Cottone, 2015). Researchers have noted cognitive effects of sleep deprivation (i.e., speed and accuracy; Lim & Dinges, 2010). Further, review of the literature suggests that insomnia impacts in diverse areas of health-related quality of life (Kyle, Morgan, & Espie, 2010). See the National Sleep Foundation for tips on addressing problems with sleep and ways to induce and maintain sleep (sleepfoundation.org).

Next, rest involves taking breaks from the current activity (Cook-Cottone, 2015; Harper, 2013; Norcross & Guy, 2007). This can look very different depending on what you or your students are doing. For example, if your students have been sitting all day or engaged in testing, rest might be a brief walk (Cook-Cottone, 2015). Rest for someone who is teaching yoga all day might be taking time to sit and have some green tea. Taking a break from electronics is relevant to nearly everyone. Planned breaks and relaxation are vital (Cook-Cottone, 2015; Norcross & Guy, 2007). Seemingly counterproductive, breaks can actually create more time and energy (Cook-Cottone, 2-15; Norcross & Guy, 2007). Breaks and relaxation can be days off, lengthier vacations, as well as short 5- to 10-minute breaks away from work, the computer, or interpersonal interactions (Cook-Cottone, 2015; Norcross & Guy, 2007). Taking breaks is consistent with the Principle of Embodied Growth and Learning: Sustainability, 9: I find balance between effort and rest (see Chapter 3). Sleep, rest, and taking breaks are all addressed in the items following.

TABLE 14.6 Self-Care Rest Items

Ask yourself, "This past week how many days did I do the following?" You can give yourself the following scores: 0 = *never* (0 days), 1 = *rarely* (1 day), 2 = *sometimes* (2–3 days), 3 = *often* (4–5 days), and 4 = *regularly* (6–7 days). For the items that state "reverse score" score as: 4 = *never* (0 days), 3 = *rarely* (1 day), 2 = *sometimes* (2–3 days), 1 = *often* (4–5 days), and 0 = *regularly* (6–7 days). Your score for this section can range from 0 to 28.

- I got enough sleep to feel rested and restored when I woke up.
- I planned restful/rejuvenating breaks throughout the day.
- I rested when I needed to (e.g., when not feeling well, after a long work out or effort).
- I took planned breaks from school or work.
- I planned/scheduled pleasant activities that were not work or school related.
- I took time away from electronics (e.g., turned off phone and other devices).
- I made time in my schedule for enough sleep.

Relationships

Supportive relationships enhance well-being (Cook-Cottone, 2015; Norcross & Guy, 2007; Shin et al., 2014). Being mindful of the nature of the relationships that you are in is a critical aspect of mindful self-care (Cook-Cottone, 2015). Norcross and Guy (2007) identify a range of potentially nurturing relationships: colleagues, staff, supervisors, peer support groups, clinical teams, community professionals, friends, spouse/partner, family, employee assistance professionals, and consultants. The supportive aspects of relational self-care are operationalized in the items: "I felt supported by people in my life," "I made time for people who sustain and support me," and "I feel like I had someone who would listen to me if I became upset." For school personnel, this can include undergoing your own personal therapy and/or securing a mentor, supervisor, or team support (Cook-Cottone, 2015; Norcross & Guy, 2007). In a meta-analysis of studies on burnout, Shin et al (2014) found that seeking social support was negatively associated with burnout. That is, seeking support may be protective.

An important aspect of healthy relationships is appropriate boundaries (Cook-Cottone, 2015; Norcross & Guy, 2007; Sayrs, 2012). In relationships, a boundary "denotes maintenance of a distinction between self and other—what is within bounds and what is out of bounds" (Norcross & Guy, 2007, p. 93). Norcross and Guy (2007) recommend that relationship boundaries (e.g., student to teacher, spouse to spouse, partner to partner) be clear and flexible. The self-care process of setting boundaries is operationalized in the following items: "I felt confident that people in my life would respect my choice if I said 'no'" and "I knew that, if I needed to, I could stand up for myself in my relationships."

TABLE 14.7 Self-Care Relationship Items

Ask yourself, "This past week how many days did I do the following?" You can give yourself the following scores: 0 = *never* (0 days), 1 = *rarely* (1 day), 2 = *sometimes* (2–3 days), 3 = *often* (4–5 days), and 4 = *regularly* (6–7 days). For the items that state "reverse score" score as: 4 = *never* (0 days), 3 = *rarely* (1 day), 2 = *sometimes* (2–3 days), 1 = *often* (4–5 days), and 0 = *regularly* (6–7 days). Your score for this section can range from 0 to 28.

- I spent time with people who are good to me (e.g., support, encourage, and believe in me).
- I scheduled/planned time to be with people who are special to me.
- I felt supported by people in my life.
- I felt confident that people in my life would respect my choice if I said "no."
- I knew that, if I needed to, I could stand up for myself in my relationships.
- I made time for people who sustain and support me.
- I felt that I had someone who would listen to me if I became upset (e.g., friend, counselor, group).

Physical and Medical

The physical and medical domain of self-care addresses the medical care and keeping of the body (Cook-Cottone, 2015). The items speak to maintenance of medical and dental care, practicing daily hygiene, adherence to medical advice (e.g., taking prescribed medicines or vitamins and brushing teeth); and avoiding substance abuse (Cook-Cottone, 2015). Despite cultural messages to the contrary, substance use should not be confused with self-care. Norcross and Guy (2007) refer to substance abuse as a form of unhealthy escape. For students under 18, engaging in medical or physical self-care is not completely under their control. However, this section can reinforce value of good physical and medical care.

TABLE 14.8 Self-Care Physical and Medical Items

Ask yourself, "This past week how many days did I do the following?" You can give yourself the following scores: 0 = *never* (0 days), 1 = *rarely* (1 day), 2 = *sometimes* (2–3 days), 3 = *often* (4–5 days), and 4 = *regularly* (6–7 days). For the items that state "reverse score" score as: 4 = *never* (0 days), 3 = *rarely* (1 day), 2 = *sometimes* (2–3 days), 1 = *often* (4–5 days), and 0 = *regularly* (6–7 days). Your score for this section can range from 0 to 32.

- I engaged in medical care to prevent/treat illness and disease (e.g., attended doctor visits, took prescribed medications/vitamins, was up to date on screenings/immunizations, followed doctor recommendations).
- I engaged in dental care to prevent/treat illness and disease (e.g., dental visits, tooth brushing, flossing).
- I took/did recreational drugs (reverse score).
- I did *not* drink alcohol.
- I practiced overall cleanliness and hygiene.
- I accessed the medical/dental care I needed.
- I did not smoke.
- Answer only if over 21 years of age: I did not drink alcohol in excess (i.e., more than one or two drinks [*one drink = 12 ounces beer, 5 ounces wine, or 1.5 ounces liquor*]).

Environmental Factors

In their review of the literature, Norcross and Guy (2007) note that most approaches to self-care focus on changing the behaviors of the individual without adequately addressing environmental factors. The physical environment can affect well-being (Cook-Cottone, 2015; Norcross & Guy, 2007). The comfort and appeal of lighting, furniture, decorations, flooring, and windows can make a difference in the overall tone of a space (Cook-Cottone, 2015; Norcross & Guy, 2007). Barriers to daily functioning can play a large role in stress. Similar to the concept of micro-aggressions that can add up over time, *micro-stressors* can aggregate, chipping away at resiliency and the ability to cope. Is there a door knob that needs fixing? Would it help to take some time and clean your study or work area? Organize your classroom? It is easy to underestimate the power of unaddressed micro-stressors. Self-care involves noticing and addressing these types of environmental issues (Cook-Cottone, 2015). As mentioned, the environmental factors domain also addresses maintaining an organized work space, balancing work for others and addressing your own initiatives, wearing suitable clothes, and doing small things to make each day a little bit better.

TABLE 14.9 Self-Care Environmental Factors Items

Ask yourself, "This past week how many days did I do the following?" You can give yourself the following scores: 0 = *never* (0 days), 1 = *rarely* (1 day), 2 = *sometimes* (2–3 days), 3 = *often* (4–5 days), and 4 = *regularly* (6–7 days). For the items that state "reverse score" score as: 4 = *never* (0 days), 3 = *rarely* (1 day), 2 = *sometimes* (2–3 days), 1 = *often* (4–5 days), and 0 = *regularly* (6–7 days). Your score for this section can range from 0 to 36.

- I maintained a manageable schedule.
- I avoided taking on too many requests or demands.
- I maintained a comforting and pleasing living environment.
- I kept my work/schoolwork area organized to support my work/school tasks.
- I maintained balance between the demands of others and what is important to me.
- Physical barriers to daily functioning were addressed (e.g., needed supplies for home and work were secured, light bulbs were replaced and functioning).
- I made sure I wore suitable clothing for the weather (e.g., umbrella in the rain, boots in the snow, warm coat in winter).
- I did things to make my everyday environment more pleasant (e.g., put a support on my chair, placed a meaningful photo on my desk).
- I did things to make my work setting more enjoyable (e.g., planned fun Fridays, partnered with a co-worker on an assignment).

Self-Compassion

Self-compassion entails "treating oneself with kindness, recognizing one's shared humanity, and being mindful when considering negative aspects of oneself" (Neff, 2011, p. 1). Compassion decreases the effects of stress, increases social connectedness, and elicits kindness toward ourselves and others (Sutterfield, 2013). Norcross and Guy (2007) address self-compassion throughout their text. However, it is most saliently addressed in their chapter on cognitive restructuring. In this chapter the authors cite several rigid, overarching beliefs that care providers hold that can lead to burnout. These include thoughts such as: the belief that a teacher must be successful with all students, that the teacher must be one of the most outstanding teachers, and that the teacher be liked by all students. Students can have rigid beliefs as well (i.e., "I must get all As," "My teachers must never be disappointed in me," "Everyone at school must like me," "I must look effortlessly perfect at all times"). Although I have seen it across the array of self-regulation difficulties, rigid beliefs such as these share perfectionism, a quality incompatible with self-compassion. In some pockets of our culture, perfectionism is held as achievable and honorable. In practice, I actively discourage perfectionism by defining it as *romanticized rigidity* (Cook-Cottone, 2015). Students typically laugh and then get it. By dropping perfectionism and labeling it as just another way to be rigid, students can more easily move toward more compassionate ways of thinking about behaviors, goals, and the self (Cook-Cottone, 2015). Self-compassion is the focus of a very recent and growing body of research and appears to play a role in self-regulation (Cook-Cottone, 2015). For example, self-compassion has been found to be negatively correlated with emotional regulation difficulties (Vettese, Dyer, Li, & Wekerle, 2011) and self-compassion can help students reach achievement goals and cope with academic failure (Neff, Hsieh, & Dejitterat, 2005).

TABLE 14.10 Self-Care Self-Compassion Items

Ask yourself, "This past week how many days did I do the following?" You can give yourself the following scores: 0 = *never* (0 days), 1 = *rarely* (1 day), 2 = *sometimes* (2–3 days), 3 = *often* (4–5 days), and 4 = *regularly* (6–7 days). For the items that state "reverse score" score as: 4 = *never* (0 days), 3 = *rarely* (1 day), 2 = *sometimes* (2–3 days), 1 = *often* (4–5 days), and 0 = *regularly* (6–7 days). Your score for this section can range from 0 to 28.

- I noticed, *without judgment*, when I was struggling (e.g., feeling resistance, falling short of my goals, not completing as much as I'd like).
- I punitively/harshly judged my progress and effort (reverse score).
- I kindly acknowledged my own challenges and difficulties.
- I engaged in critical or harsh self-talk (reverse score).
- I engaged in supportive and comforting self-talk (e.g., "My effort is valuable and meaningful").
- I reminded myself that failure and challenge are part of the human experience.
- I gave myself permission to feel my feelings (e.g., allowed myself to cry).

Spiritual Practice

Spirituality involves inspiration from something greater than yourself (Cook-Cottone, 2015; Harper, 2013; Norcross & Guy, 2007). Specifically, spirituality can be sourced from a sense of mission, purpose, and value as well as from religion (Cook-Cottone, 2015; Harper, 2013; Norcross & Guy, 2007; Sayrs, 2012). Spirituality is a seeking. Spirituality can be a source of strength and meaning (Harper, 2013; Norcross & Guy, 2007). The spirituality items address bringing meaning or purpose into work or school life as well as your personal life (Cook-Cottone, 2015). Cultivating spiritual moments, connections, and experiences are also addressed.

TABLE 14.11 Self-Care Spiritual Practice Items

Ask yourself, "This past week how many days did I do the following?" You can give yourself the following scores: 0 = *never* (0 days), 1 = *rarely* (1 day), 2 = *sometimes* (2–3 days), 3 = *often* (4–5 days), and 4 = *regularly* (6–7 days). For the items that state "reverse score" score as: 4 = *never* (0 days), 3 = *rarely* (1 day), 2 = *sometimes* (2–days), 1 = *often* (4–5 days), and 0 = *regularly* (6–7 days). Your score for this section can range from 0 to 24.

- I experienced meaning and/or a larger purpose in my *work/school* life (e.g., for a cause).
- I experienced meaning and/or larger purpose in my *private/personal* life (e.g., for a cause).
- I spent time in a spiritual place (e.g., church, meditation room, nature).
- I read, watched, or listened to something inspirational (e.g., watched a video that gives me hope, read inspirational material, listened to spiritual music).
- I spent time with others who share my spiritual worldview (e.g., church community, volunteer group).
- I spent time doing something that I hope will make a positive difference in the world (e.g., volunteered at a soup kitchen, took time out for someone else).

MINDFUL SELF-CARE SCALE–SHORT

The 84-item MSCS–L is a good way to look at your broader self-care practices within the context of self-regulation or having students carefully assess their own self-care behaviors as part of a reflective exercise. I do this for my Self-Care and Service course at the University at Buffalo. In this course, students create a service learning project and simultaneously engage in active self-care. Their self-care practice receives a grade equal in weight to their service project. Use of the long version of this scale is perfect for that level of self-refection. However, we wanted to create a psychometrically sound scale that was shorter and easier to use for researchers and those in the helping professions that can be completed in several minutes. Dr. Wendy Guyker and I set out to create the Mindful Self-Care Scale–Short (MSCS–S; see gse.buffalo.edu/about/directory/faculty/cook-cottone for full details of the analysis and the psychometric properties of the scale).

After receiving institutional review board approval from our university, participants were recruited. Data were screened for duplicate, erroneous, or missing information. The 448 participants' data were analyzed. A factor analysis resulted in a 33-item scale with six subscales (see Figure 14.5): First, internal self-practices: Self-Compassion and Purpose and Physical Care: second, external practices: Supportive Structure and Supportive Relationships; last, practices that help create embodied attunement by integrating features of the internal self and the external self: Mindful Awareness and Mindful Relaxation (see the appendix to this chapter, "The MSCS–S" for a list of questions and scoring directions; Cook-Cottone & Guyker, 2016).

Specifically for the internal self-practices, the Physical Care scale includes items addressing hydration, nutrition, and exercise. These items detail ways in which you can take care of your body. Next, the Self-Compassion and Purpose scale items include the things we do to mentally cope when times get tough. We considered calling it the mindful grit scale. These things include acknowledging your challenges and difficulties, engaging in positive self-talk, feeling your feelings, and finding a larger sense of purpose in your life and work.

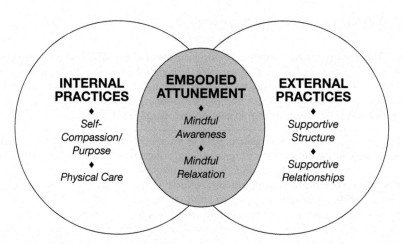

FIGURE 14.5 Embodied self-care practices–short form.

It is exactly these practices that can keep us going when we experience failure and setbacks. They help organize our emotional and cognitive selves so we can stay in the bigger game of being present and engaged in our lives.

The scales that address the needs of the external self are Supportive Structure and Supportive Relationships. First, Supportive Structure included keeping your work area organized, maintaining a manageable schedule, balancing the demands of others and what is important to you, and maintaining a comfortable living environment. Second, the Supportive Relationships scale includes items that help you evaluate your relationships in terms of support, encouragement, and reliability. Also, items evaluate your relationships for good boundaries (i.e., "I felt confident people in my life would respect my choice if I said, 'no.'" These two scales help you look carefully at your immediate environment and relationships as a source of support and comfort for your own self-care.

Last, Mindful Awareness and Mindful Relaxation scales support attunement between the inner and outer selves. They are embodied as you engage in your world in a way that helps you stay internally attuned. The Mindful Awareness scale includes four items that get to the essence of mindful awareness. They ask you if you had a calm awareness of your thoughts, feelings, and body and if you carefully selected which thoughts and feelings you used to guide your actions in your world and with others. The Mindful Relaxation subscale assesses the ways you engaged in the world and with your self to relax. For example, did you read a book, connect with friends, listen to soothing text or music, or find nature (Harper, 2013)? Each of the items requires an interface between your awareness and the outside world in a calm and engaged manner.

CONCLUSION

Mindful self-care is a foundational self-regulating practice (Cook-Cottone, 2015). It is a constant practice of bringing awareness to self-care, assessing self-care practices, setting self-care goals, and actively engaging in self-care practices (Cook-Cottone, 2015). This chapter reviewed self-care and mindful self-care and provided a domain-by-domain review, each with a set of questions to facilitate self-assessment. As with the long form, you can use the short form to assess, and re-assess your own self-care or that of your students. The purpose of the MSCS–S is to give you an embodied, actionable way to connect and attune your mind, body, and actions in a manner that shows an appreciation for your body and mind as it is right now and the circumstances and people in your world. Rechtschaffen (2014) recommends turning to organizations that take a self-care and personal renewal approach to teacher development: Inner Resilience Program (www.innerresilience-tidescenter.org), CARE for Teachers (www.garrisoninstitute.org/signature-programs/care-for-teachers), SMART in Education (passageworks.org/courses/smart-in-education), and Parker Palmer's Courage and Renewal Programs (www.couragerenewal.org/parker). See also Jennings's (2015) Chapter 5, "The Heart of Teaching." Jennings reviews her perspective on self-care and provides step-by-step guidance for developing a nurturing self-care practice.

It is in the turning inward with curiosity, care, respect and loving-kindness that we are empowered as we endeavor outward. As I close the book, I add one of my mother's quotes. Recall that as an English teacher, she began each class with a quote and journal writing. As I commenced writing this book, my father sent me all of the quotes he could find. Some are from magazines, pages pulled from the binding. Others are written in her handwriting on scraps of paper, or a dog-eared page (mom would never write in a book). Today, I found this one, on a scrap of paper in mom's writing. I looked for the source and no one is sure who wrote it. It has been attributed to many authors such as Thoreau, Emerson, and Morrow. What we do know, is that it is a gift from those who have come and gone and perhaps know best how to guide us.

What lies behind us and what lies before us
is nothing compared to what lies within us.

Notes from my Mom,
Elizabeth G. Cook
(1940–2015)

REFERENCES

Benelam, B., & Wyness, L. (2010). Hydration and health: A review. *Nutrition Bulletin, 35*, 3–25.

Cappuccio, F. P., Cooper, D., D'Elia, L., Strazzullo, P., & Miller, M. A. (2011). Sleep duration predicts cardiovascular outcomes: A systematic review and meta-analysis of prospective studies. *European Heart Journal, 32*, 1484–1492.

Childress, T., & Harper, J. C. (Eds.) (2015). Best practices for yoga in the schools. *Best Practices Guide* (Vol. 1). Atlanta, GA: YEC- Omega Publications.

Cook-Cottone, C. P. (2015a). *Mindfulness and yoga for embodied self-regulation: A primer for mental health professionals*, New York, NY: Springer Publishing.

Cook-Cottone, C. P., & Guyker, W. (2016, manuscript in preparation). The mindful self-care scale: Mindful self-care as a tool to promote physical, emotional, and cognitive well-being.

Cook-Cottone, C. P., Kane, L. S., Keddie, E., & Haugli, S. (2013a). *Girls growing in wellness and balance: Yoga and life skills to empower*, Stoddard, WI: Schoolhouse Educational Services, LLC.

Cook-Cottone, C. P., Tribole, E., & Tylka, T. (2013b). *Healthy eating in schools: Evidenced-based interventions to help kids thrive*. Washington, DC: American Psychological Association.

Davis, M., Eshelman, E. R., & McKay, M. (2008). *The relaxation and stress reduction workbook* (6th ed.). Oakland, CA: New Harbinger Publications.

Duyff, R. L. (2011). *American dietetic association complete food and nutrition guide*, New York, NY: Houghton Mifflin Harcourt.

Harper, J. C. (2013). *Little flower yoga for kids: A yoga and mindfulness programs to help your children improve attention and emotional balance.* Oakland, CA: New Harbinger Publications.

Herrington, S. (2012). Om schooled: a guide to teaching kids yoga in real-world schools. San Marcos, CA: Addriya.

Hirshkowitz, M., Whiton, K., Albert, S. M., Alessi, C., Bruni, O., DonCarlos, L., … Hillard, P. J., (2015). National Sleep Foundation's sleep time duration recommendations: Methodology and results summary. *Sleep Health, 1*, 40–43.

Hopkins, M. E., Davis, F. C., VanTieghem, M. R., Whalen, P. J., & Bucci, D. J. (2012). Differential effects of acute and regular physical exercise on cognition and affect. *Neuroscience, 215*, 59–68.

Hyde, A. (2012). The yoga in schools movement: Using standards for educating the whole child and making space for teacher self-care. *Counterpoints, 425*, 109–126.

Jennings, P. A. (2015). *Mindfulness for teachers: Simple skills for peace and productivity in the classroom,* New York, NY: W. W. Norton.

Kyle, S. D., Morgan, K., & Espie, C. A. (2010). Insomnia and health-related quality of life. *Sleep Medicine Reviews, 14*, 69–82.

Lim, J., & Dinges, D. F. (2010). A meta-analysis of the impact of short-term sleep deprivation on cognitive variables. *Psychological Bulletin, 136*, 375.

Linehan, M. M. (1993). *Skills training manual for treating borderline personality disorder,* New York, NY: The Guilford Press.

Neff, K. D. (2011). Self-compassion, self-esteem, and well-being. *Social and Personality Psychology Compass, 5*, 1–12.

Neff, K. D., Hsieh, Y. P., & Dejitterat, K. (2005). Self-compassion, achievement goals, and coping with academic failure. *Self and Identity, 4*, 263–287.

Norcross, J. C., & Guy, J. D. (2007). *Leaving it at the office: A guide to psychotherapist self-care.* New York, NY: The Guilford Press.

Rechtschaffen, D. (2014). *The way of mindful education: Cultivating well-being in teachers and students,* New York, NY: W. W. Norton.

Sayrs, J. H. (2012). Mindfulness, acceptance, and values-based interventions for addiction counselors: The benefits of practicing what we preach. In Steven C. Hayes & Michael E. Levin (Eds.), *Mindfulness and acceptance for addictive behaviors: Applying contextual CBT to substance abuse and behavioral addictions* (pp. 187–215). Oakland, CA: New Harbinger.

Shapiro, S. L., & Carlson, L. E. (2009). *The art and science of mindfulness: Integrating mindfulness into psychology and the helping professions,* Washington, DC: American Psychological Association.

Shin, H., Park, Y. M., Ying, J. Y., Kim, B., Noh, H., & Lee, S. M. (2014). Relationships between coping strategies and burnout symptoms: A meta-analytic approach. *Professional Psychology: Research and Practice, 45*, 44–56.

Siegel, D. J. (2010). *The mindful therapist: A clinician's guide to mindsight and neural integration,* New York, NY: W. W. Norton.

Sutterfield, J. (2013). Self-care as a foundation for social action: How to thrive and sustain personal well-being in the field of yoga service. *Journal of Yoga Service, 1*, 33–37.

Vettese, L. C., Dyer, C. E., Li, W. L., & Wekerle, C. (2011). Does self-compassion mitigate the association between childhood maltreatment and later emotion regulation difficulties? A preliminary investigation. *International Journal of Mental Health and Addiction, 9*, 480–491.

APPENDIX

THE MINDFUL SELF-CARE SCALE–SHORT (MSCS–S)

The Mindful Self-Care Scale–Short (MSCS–S, 2016) is a 33-item scale that measures the self-reported frequency of behaviors that measure self-care behavior. These scales are the result of an Exploratory Factor Analysis (EFA) of a large community sample. The subscales are positively correlated with body esteem and negatively correlated with substance use and eating disordered behavior. (Please check the text for the published citation.) Note that there are an additional six clinical questions and two general questions for a total of 42 items. (The long-form has 84 questions and 10 subscales. It can be found on Dr. Catherine Cook-Cottone's faculty web page.)

    Self-care is defined as the daily process of being aware of and attending to one's basic physiological and emotional needs including the shaping of one's daily routine, relationships, and environment as needed to promote self-care. Mindful self-care addresses self-care and adds the component of mindful awareness.

    Mindful self-care is seen as the foundational work required for physical and emotional well-being. Self-care is associated with positive physical health, emotional well-being, and mental health. Steady and intentional practice of mindful self-care is seen as protective by preventing the onset of mental health symptoms, job/school burnout, and improving work and school productivity.

    This scale is intended to help individuals identify areas of strength and weakness in mindful self-care behavior as well as assess interventions that serve to improve self-care. The scale addresses six domains of self-care: physical care, supportive relationships, mindful awareness, self-compassion and purpose, mindful relaxation, and supportive structure. There are also six clinical items and three general items assessing the individual's general or more global practices of self-care.

Check the box that reflects the frequency of your behavior (how much or how often) within past week (7 days):

THIS PAST WEEK, HOW MANY *DAYS* DID YOU DO THE FOLLOWING?	NEVER 0 DAYS	RARELY 1 DAY	SOMETIMES 2 TO 3 DAYS	OFTEN 4 TO 5 DAYS	REGULARLY 6 TO 7 DAYS
Example: I drank at least 6–8 cups of water	1 Never	2 Rarely	3 Sometimes	4 Often	5 Regularly
Scoring:	5	4	3	2	1
If reverse-scored:	Never	Rarely	Sometimes	Often	Regularly

The questions on the scale follow.

Physical Care (Eight Items)

Score	Item
1 2 3 4 5	I drank at least 6–8 cups of water.
1 2 3 4 5	I ate a variety of nutritious foods (e.g., vegetables, protein, fruits, and grains).
1 2 3 4 5	I planned my meals and snacks.
1 2 3 4 5	I exercised at least 30 to 60 minutes.
1 2 3 4 5	I took part in sports, dance, or other scheduled physical activities.
5 4 3 2 1	I did sedentary activities instead of exercising (e.g., watched TV, worked on the computer) (*reverse score*).
1 2 3 4 5	I planned/scheduled my exercise for the day.
1 2 3 4 5	I practiced yoga or another mind/body practice (e.g., Tae Kwon Do, Tai Chi).
	Total
	Average for subscale = Total/Number of items

Supportive Relationships (Five Items)

Score	Item
1 2 3 4 5	I spent time with people who are good to me (e.g., support, encourage, and believe in me).
1 2 3 4 5	I felt supported by people in my life.
1 2 3 4 5	I felt that I had someone who would listen to me if I became upset (e.g., friend, counselor, group).
1 2 3 4 5	I felt confident that people in my life would respect my choice if I said "no."
1 2 3 4 5	I scheduled/planned time to be with people who are special to me.
	Total
	Average for subscale = Total/Number of items

Mindful Awareness (Four Items)

Score	Item
1 2 3 4 5	I had a calm awareness of my thoughts.
1 2 3 4 5	I had a calm awareness of my feelings.
1 2 3 4 5	I had a calm awareness of my body.
1 2 3 4 5	I carefully selected which of my thoughts and feelings I used to guide my actions.
	Total
	Average for subscale = Total/Number of items

Self-Compassion and Purpose (Six Items)

SCORE	ITEM
1 2 3 4 5	I kindly acknowledged my own challenges and difficulties.
1 2 3 4 5	I engaged in supportive and comforting self-talk (e.g., "My effort is valuable and meaningful").
1 2 3 4 5	I reminded myself that failure and challenge are part of the human experience.
1 2 3 4 5	I gave myself permission to feel my feelings (e.g., allowed myself to cry).
1 2 3 4 5	I experienced meaning and/or a larger purpose in my _work/school_ life (e.g., for a cause).
1 2 3 4 5	I experienced meaning and/or larger purpose in my _private/personal_ life (e.g., for a cause).
	Total
	Average for subscale = Total/Number of items

Mindful Relaxation (Six Items)

SCORE	ITEM
1 2 3 4 5	I did something intellectual (using my mind) to help me relax (e.g., read a book, wrote).
1 2 3 4 5	I did something interpersonal to relax (e.g., connected with friends).
1 2 3 4 5	I did something creative to relax (e.g., drew, played an instrument, wrote creatively, sang, organized).
1 2 3 4 5	I listened to relax (e.g., to music, a podcast, radio show, rainforest sounds).
1 2 3 4 5	I sought out images to relax (e.g., art, film, window shopping, nature).
1 2 3 4 5	I sought out smells to relax (lotions, nature, candles/incense, smells of baking).
	Total
	Average for subscale = Total/Number of items

Supportive Structure (Four Items)

SCORE	ITEM
1 2 3 4 5	I kept my work/schoolwork area organized to support my work/school tasks.
1 2 3 4 5	I maintained a manageable schedule.
1 2 3 4 5	I maintained balance between the demands of others and what is important to me.
1 2 3 4 5	I maintained a comforting and pleasing living environment.
	Total
	Average for subscale = Total/Number of items

Clinical (Six Items; Not to Be Averaged)

SCORE	ITEM
1 2 3 4 5	I took time to acknowledge the things for which I am grateful.
1 2 3 4 5	I planned/scheduled pleasant activities that were not work or school related.
1 2 3 4 5	I used deep breathing to relax.
1 2 3 4 5	I meditated in some form (e.g., sitting meditation, walking meditation, prayer).
1 2 3 4 5	I rested when I needed to (e.g., when not feeling well, after a long workout or effort).
1 2 3 4 5	I got enough sleep to feel rested and restored when I woke up.

General (Three Items; Not to Be Averaged)

SCORE	ITEM
1 2 3 4 5	I engaged in a variety of self-care strategies.
1 2 3 4 5	I planned my self-care.
1 2 3 4 5	I explored new ways to bring self-care into my life.

Total Score Summary
(Be sure you have correctly scored your reverse-scored items.)

AVERAGED SCORE	SCALE
_____	Physical Care
_____	Self-Compassion and Purpose
_____	Supportive Structure
_____	Supportive Relationships
_____	Mindful Awareness
_____	Mindful Relaxation

Shade in Your Average Score for Each Scale in the Following

5						
4						
3						
2						
1						
Scale	Physical Care	Self-Compassion and Purpose	Supportive Structure	Supportive Relation	Mindful Awareness	Mindful Relaxation

INDEX